Midwifery: Best Practice 2

EDUCATION CENTRE LIBRARY
WITHDRAWN BLACKBURN

D0550421

BLACKBURN EDUCATION CENTRE
LIBRARY

TB07825

For Books for Midwives:

Senior Commissioning Editor: Mary Seager
Development Editor: Kim Benson
Project Manager: Mandy Galloway
Cover Design: Temple Design

Midwifery: Best Practice 2

Edited by

Sara Wickham RM MA BA(Hons) PGCE(A)
Senior Lecturer in Midwifery, Anglia Polytechnic University

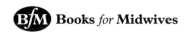 **Books** *for* **Midwives**

An Imprint of Elsevier

EDINBURGH LONDON NEW YORK OXFORD PHILADELPHIA ST LOUIS SYDNEY TORONTO 2004

Books for Midwives
An imprint of Elsevier Limited

© 2004, Elsevier Limited. All rights reserved.

No part of this publication may be reproduced, stored in a retrieval
system, or transmitted in any form or by any means, electronic,
mechanical, photocopying, recording or otherwise, without either the
prior permission of the publishers or a licence permitting restricted
copying in the United Kingdom issued by the Copyright Licensing
Agency, 90 Tottenham Court Road, London W1T 4LP. Permissions
may be sought directly from Elsevier's Health Sciences Rights
Department in Philadelphia, USA: (+1) 215 238 7869, fax: (+1) 215 238
2239, e-mail: healthpermissions@elsevier.com. You may also complete
your request on-line via the Elsevier homepage
(http://www.elsevier.com), by selecting 'Customer Support' and
then 'Obtaining Permissions'.

EDUCATION CENTRE
LIBRARY
ACC. No. TB07825
CLASS No. 618.2 MID.

ISBN 0 7506 8805X

British Library Cataloguing in Publication Data
A catalogue record for this book is available from the British Library

Library of Congress Cataloguing in Publication Data
A catalog record for this book is available from the Library of
Congress

Note
Medical knowledge is constantly changing. As new information
becomes available, changes in treatment, procedures, equipment and
the use of drugs become necessary. The editor and the publishers
have taken care to ensure that the information given in this text is
accurate and up to date. However, readers are strongly advised to
confirm that the information, especially with regard to drug usage,
complies with the latest legislation and standards of practice.

Note
The publisher has made every effort to obtain permission to
reproduce all borrowed material.

Printed in China

The
publisher's
policy is to use
**paper manufactured
from sustainable forests**

Contents

EDUCATION CENTRE LIBRARY
ROYAL INFIRMARY, BLACKBURN

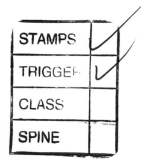

STAMPS ✓
TRIGGER ✓
CLASS
SPINE

Introduction

I think it is fair to say that just about everybody involved in the writing and production of the first volume of *Midwifery: Best Practice* was pleasantly stunned by just how well the book was received in its first few months of publication. Clearly, midwives enjoyed the compilation of articles, stories and 'added extras' that the book provided. Delighted by this success, we have been spurred on to produce this next volume, which not only includes articles from *The Practising Midwife*, but some from *Midwifery* and a few longer pieces which have been written especially for this book.

Each of the main sections begins with an introduction to the topic area and material within, and concludes with a few questions for reflection, which can be used for personal reflection, group discussion, workshops or towards PREP requirements. We have stayed with the division of articles into the main areas of 'Pregnancy', 'Being With Women', 'Labour and Birth' and 'The Postnatal Experience' in an attempt to organise the material in a logical way. Of course, in doing this there is a need to acknowledge that these are artificially imposed dividing lines that reflect our tendency as an industrialised society to compartmentalise aspects of childbearing rather than being the way in which women view their own journey. There are also four 'Focus on...'

sections which include a smaller selection of material on themes relevant to current practice. The final section, 'Stories and Reflection' is a collection of the kind of short pieces for which *The Practising Midwife* has become known and treasured by midwives.

This is a book that has benefited from a team of midwives, and I am very grateful to them all for their help and support. Thanks to all of the authors who gave permission for their previously published work to be included in the book, and to Tricia Anderson, Gemma Purrett, Shona Hamilton, Lorna Davies and Nessa McHugh for writing original pieces for the book against what turned out to be a fairly tight deadline. I am certain that the editing and production of a book like this would be far less pleasant without the support of women like Mary Seager, Kim Benson and Catharine Steers at Elsevier, who make the process so straightforward. Thanks also to Jilly Rosser, Tricia Anderson, Julia Magill-Cuerden, Jenny Hall and Ann Thomson for their work in editing *The Practising Midwife* and *Midwifery*. And, by no means least, I would like to thank Ishvar, who supports me in more ways than I can express.

Sara Wickham

Acknowledgements

We would like to thank all those who have contributed to this edition of *Midwifery: Best Practice*.

Jo Alexander, Tricia Anderson, Kathleen Baird, Maria Barrell, Susan Battersby, Nicky Bean, Beverley Beech, Cecily M Begley, Joanna Berry, Alison Blenkinsop, Jane Bowler, Marion Borkent-Polet, Mario-Paul Cassar, Jenny Chambers, Sue Cripps, Leslie L Davidson, Lorna Davies, Ruth Deery, Susan Downe, Anna Fielder, Jenny Fraser, Jo Garcia, A Rashid Gatrad, Sheila Glenn, Jacqueline K Gibson, Kerry M Grimes, Christine Grabowska, Shona Hamilton, Marion HB Heres, Virginia Howes, Hannah Hulme Hunter, Carol Hughes, Johanne Jakeway, Sandy Kirkman, Sally Marchant, David Marshall, Linda Mason, Majid Mirmiran, Mary Newburn, Mary Nolan, Nessa McHugh, Jacqueline E Parsons, Maria Pel, Sally Price, Gemma Purrett, Andrea Robertson, Isobel Ryder, Aziz Sheikh, Debbie Singh, Susan M Stratigos, Pieter E Treffers, Helen Wallace, Irene Walton, Lois Wattis, Joan Webster, Frances Wedgwood, Rosalind Weston, Sandra L Wheatley.

Focus on:
Normal birth

SECTION CONTENTS

Is there a future for normal birth?

Soo Downe

We have very little evidence in the accepted sense of the word about the physiology of normal birth. Most of the studies which have attempted to examine this topic have done so from the perspective of births which have been medicalised. As Friedman comments at the outset of his seminal 1956 paper:

'The continuity of patient selection was intermittently disturbed by the not infrequent multipara whose delivery was imminent upon arrival the hospital, and whose labour curve, therefore, was valueless.'[1]

This suggests that women labouring at home, and anyone arriving in advanced spontaneous labour, were not included in the analysis. A more recent investigation of the progress of labour has been carried out in a hospital setting, but where there were very few external pressures to curtail a labour if all was going well.[2] This work has suggested that the chronological parameters of physiological labour extend at least twice as far as Friedman proposed. However, Friedman's curves remain the standard for many labour wards and intrapartum research studies.

There have been a number of reports on the subject of normal birth from official bodies over the last few years.[3-6] The nature of normality expressed in these reports varies considerably.

The only prospective study undertaken in this area seems to be that of Williams and colleagues.[7] This was a large, well-designed prevalence study, covering Scotland and England, and involving 3160 low risk primigravid women giving birth between February 1993 and January 1994. The authors noted the unexpectedly high rates of intervention found in the study (Box 1).

More recently, Mother And Baby magazine, in collaboration with BUPA, reported a survey of 2000 unselected women, both multigravid and primigravid, who responded to an internet survey.[8] For some of the intervention rates in this study see Box 2.

Box 1 Labour intervention rates[7]
Artificial rupture membranes 53%
Augmentation 38%
Episiotomy 46%

Box 2 Intervention rates[8]
Induced labours 27%
Episiotomy 29%
Caesarean section 26%

Of the respondents, 23% were reported to be 'down and shocked by the whole experience'. The authors of the survey comment:

'forget bean bags and water music, only 7% of women in the UK today are lucky enough to have a completely natural birth.'

The method of recruitment to this survey carried a high risk of bias. However, it continues the theme of very high levels of intervention across the board. Both these studies looked at the nature of interventions regardless of type of birth. In a currently unpublished prevalence study, the author of this paper and her colleagues looked at the nature of interventions which preceded births which were termed 'normal' or 'spontaneous'.[9] The study took place in five consultant units in one regional health authority over a randomly selected series of five weeks in 2000. Five interventions were chosen using the criteria proposed by the Association for Improvements in the Maternity Services. These were induction and acceleration of labour, epidural analgesia, episiotomy, and artificial rupture of membranes. Of the total of 1464 births, 956 were recorded as being normal or spontaneous. During the five weeks of the study, physiological birth according to this definition was experienced by 16.9% of primigravid women (103/609), 30.1% of multigravid women (257/855), and 24.6% of all women (360/1464).

According to his speech at the Royal College of Midwives Congress in Torquay (May 2001), Alan Milburn, Secretary of State for Health, wants to increase choice for women, and specifically their access to out of hospital birth. The long-standing arguments about safety (and, more latterly, cost), seem to have been swept aside. There are to be better buildings, more continuity of care, a guarantee of access to a dedicated midwife 100% of the time during labour and crucially, more midwives to do all this.

This is indeed good news. More, if the evidence on the provision of support in labour is to be believed, it should even lead to more physiological births, less postnatal morbidity for mother and baby, and, consequently, an increase in public health. But will it?

Professional debates about the nature of physiological birth have been on-going since the time when the majority of women were attended by midwives, and when home birthing was the norm. In the middle of the last century, Thaddeus Montgomery, an obstetrician, was driven to state:

I have stated on numerous occasions that there is no more need to interfere with the course of normally progressing labor than there is to tamper with good digestion, normal respiration, and adequate circulation.[10]

It appears that his words were, and still are, largely unheeded. This suggests that the mere provision of more midwives and increasing access to out of hospital births may not be the answer to the problem of high intervention rates in labour. There are fundamental questions to be asked about the processes which have brought us to this point. Numerous historical analyses have been undertaken of the changing nature of maternity and obstetric care.[11-14] The majority of these note the shifting of power from lay to professional midwives, and the parallel rise in control of the barber surgeons as they evolved the profession of obstetrics. Other authors also note the apparently counter-intuitive fact that as scientific medicine began to predominate, the wellbeing of many women in labour deteriorated.[15] The notion that midwives and obstetricians espouse opposing philosophical approaches to birth is widespread. Birth as on the one hand a prospectively normal event, and on the other hand only normal in retrospect is widely acknowledged to be the standard dichotomy. However, the belief that midwives are universally aligned to the former ideal, and obstetricians to the latter one does not seem to be borne out by the evidence given in the studies above. Many of the interventions found to be prevalent in the processes of normal birth are carried out by or brokered by midwives.

While some midwives employ subtle tactics to circumvent these rules, such as delaying an internal examination to allow the women to get a bit further in

the hope that intervention can be avoided, others seem to have adopted the rites and mores of the establishment wholeheartedly. One of the most common indicators of this state of affairs is the frequency with which the following scenario occurs in some labour wards:

A woman is progressing well in her first labour, and coping. It has been established within the last hour that her cervix is 5 centimetres dilated (or 6 or 7, depending on the woman and the day). Suddenly, she loses control, she is intensely uncomfortable, she insists she can't cope, and she wants an epidural. The anaesthetist is called, the epidural is sited, the woman has a heavy show, or feels a bit strange, the midwives check the situation – the cervix is full dilated. Some hours later, failure to progress is diagnosed, and the baby is born by forceps, or a ventouse.

Are midwives still the guardians of the normal? Recently, a supervisor of midwives is reported to have told a local lay representative that continuous fetal monitoring was widely used in her unit because the midwives were not competent to undertake intermittent monitoring with a pinard stethoscope. More usually, continuous fetal monitoring is utilised because there are not enough midwives to care for women on a one-to-one basis. Since there is good research evidence that both the use of continuous electronic fetal monitoring and of epidural analgesia are strongly linked to interventions in labour, we midwives are at the very front line of the kind of decision making which supports or interrupts the normal labour process. When we do hold the belief that labour is a normal process, we seem to be in an apparently irreconcilable position of wanting to defend the normality of labour while finding it almost impossible to continuously challenge the culture and constraints of the organisations within which we work. This is partly because there is very little research and reflection on the complexity of the normal birth process. Official definitions tend to take a purely clinical approach. The World Health Organization for example, produced a clear and balanced publication addressing many aspects of normal birth. Despite this, the authors offer the following definition:

We define normal birth as: spontaneous in onset, low-risk at the start of labour and remaining so throughout labour and delivery. The infant is born spontaneously in the vertex position between 37 and 42 completed weeks of pregnancy. After birth mother and infant are in good condition...[4]

In one of the few published descriptive papers in this area, Deborah Gould constructed a synthesis of the key aspects of normal birth, based on observations of labouring women.[16] She constructs four defining attributes of labour from her data. While the second criterion is common to many definitions in emphasising, for example, painful uterine contractions and progressive effacement, dilation, and descent, the other three offer a different perception on the nature of the normality of labour:

1 Physiologically normal labour naturally follows a sequential pattern
2 ...(usual criterion for a low risk labour and birth) ...
3 It is strenuous work
4 Movement has a crucial role

However, although these attributes bring more depth to an understanding of natural processes of normal birth, they are still apparently focused on physical processes. In contrast, women writing about their experiences of labour often focus on the acute psychological transition which takes place. Anais Niin expressed this psychic tension in the following quote:

He wants to interfere with his instruments while I struggle with nature, with myself, with my child, and with the meaning I put into it all, with my desire to give and to hold, to keep and to lose, to live and to die... [17]

This sense of the awe-full nature of the process of normal birth, of the profound effects of the shock of confronting life and death and its consequences for the whole of the future for the woman, her baby and her family is very rarely found in official definitions of normal birth. One of the few attempts to capture this is given in the 1993 Myles Textbook for Midwives:

Normal labour is... the physiological transition from pregnancy to motherhood (which) heralds an enormous change in each woman physically and psychologically... every system in the body is affected and the experience represents a major rite de passage in the woman's life... [18]

This experience could be either positive or negative for women. If the data above are generalisable across this and other countries, it may be assumed that the impact is negative for a significant minority of women. Leonie van der Hulst postulates that this is because of the adoption of 'obstetrical dooming', which she defines as

the belief that a woman who is pregnant or in labour inevitably is submitted to some fate, or that she is bound to find herself in an undesirable situation while giving birth. [19]

This lack of faith in the normal birth process seems to be pervading both professions and societies at large, and it may seem to be inexorable. [20] It is ironic that this is also a unique time in human history when in many parts of the world women and babies are very unlikely to die during the process of birth. This strongly suggests that survival is not the only or even the most important determinant of faith in the process of birth.

It seems that it is time to examine some of the more subtle benefits of the normal birth process, as a first step in restoring faith in the benefits of physiological process.

Some work is beginning to emerge on this subject. It appears that both mothers and babies who experience normal labours and births may benefit physiologically from the process when compared to either emergency or elective caesarean sections. [21-24] Anecdotally, there are women's birth stories which suggest that, even in the midst of intense adversity, such as a profoundly disabled baby or a stillbirth, a physiologically and psychologically uninterrupted labour and birth can be literally life-saving for both the mother and her family. In contrast, the birth of an apparently normal baby after a disempowering distressing 'normal' birth can leave psychic scars, which engender both physical and psychological morbidity, and even a risk of suicide for many years after the event. These stories have been shared by word of mouth or in internet groups. More recently, their importance has been formally acknowledged. [25] They now need to be encouraged and collected more formally, so that a body of knowledge can be built which reflects the fundamental importance of the normal physiological process of birth to individual women, their babies and their families, and to the public and social health of society as a whole.

It may be that this work would be easier within a new philosophical approach to midwifery research and practice. The concept of salutogenesis has been developed over the last thirty years by Aaron Antonovsky, a researcher and philosopher. [26] This term is the opposite of pathogenesis. It is about the generation of and study of wellbeing, as opposed to the examination of illness. The concept is perfectly suited to maternity care, and, specifically, to midwifery, if midwives are indeed the guardians of normality. There are a number of movements which provide hope for an expansion of normal birth, and for an opportunity to explore a salutogenic approach. As free-standing birthing units and home births expand, there is an opportunity to observe the physiological processes of birth in action. If these developments can happen within the context of a belief in the public health benefits of the normal processes of birth itself, then we not only have a paradigm for birth which can grow rapidly, but we also have an opportunity to undertake research about the physiology of the birthing process which is almost impossible to undertake in current large consultant units. Perhaps, then, we can finally fulfill the current Royal College of Midwives Vision, which states that:

Maternity services should demonstrate, in their policies and practice, an underpinning philosophy of pregnancy and birth as normal physiological processes, with a commitment to positive reduction in unnecessary medicalisation of normal pregnancy and birth. [27]

REFERENCES

1. Friedman EL. Labor in multiparas: A graphicostatistical analysis. Obstet Gynaecol 1956; 8(6): 691-703.
2. Albers L. The duration of labour in healthy women. J Perinatology 1999; 19(2): 114-9.
3. Clinical Standards Advisory Group. Women in normal labour. London: HMSO, 1995.
4. World Health Organization Department of Reproductive Health and Research. Care in normal birth: A practical guide. Geneva: WHO, 1997.
5. Royal College of Midwives. Debating midwifery: Normality in midwifery. London: RCM 1997.
6. Troop P, Goldacre M, Mason A et al (Eds). Health outcome indicators: Normal pregnancy and childbirth. Report of a working group to the Department of Health. Oxford: National Centre for Outcomes Development, 1999.
7. Williams FL, Florey CV, Ogston SA et al. UK study of intrapartum care for low risk primigravida: A survey of interventions. J Epid Comm Health 1998; 52(8): 494-500.
8. Mother and Baby magazine and BUPA 2001. The Birth and Motherhood Survey 2000. www.bupa.co.uk/healthy-living/baby-centre/survey/survey5.html
9. Downe S, McCormick C, Beech B 2001. Labour interventions associated with normal birth. Unpublished paper, available from SM Downe. email sdowne@uclan.ac.uk
10. Montgomery T. Physiologic considerations in labor and the puerperium. Am J Obstet Gynaecol Oct 1958.
11. Ehrenreich B, English D. Witches, midwives and nurses: A history of women healers. London: Writers and readers publishing cooperative, 1976.
12. Oakley A. Women confined: Towards a sociology of childbirth. Oxford: Martin Robertson, 1980.
13. Arney WR. Power and the provision of obstetrics. London: University of Chicago Press, 1982.
14. Towler J, Bramhall J. Midwives in history and society. London: Croom Helm Press, 1998.
15. Loudon I. Death in childbirth: An international study of maternal care and maternal mortality, 1800-1950. Oxford: Clarendon Press, 1992.
16. Gould D. Normal labour: A concept analysis. J Adv Nurse 2000; 31(2): 418-27.
17. Niin A, reproduced in: The Body Shop. Mamatoto. London: Virago Press, 1991.
18. Bennett VR, Brown LK (Eds). Myles Textbook for Midwives (12th ed). Edinburgh: Churchill Livingstone, 1993.
19. Van der Hulst L. Protector of the normal birth process. Midwifery Today 1994; 32: 14-5.
20. Machin D, Scamell M. The experience of labour: Using ethnography to explore the irresistible nature of the bio-medical metaphor during labour. Midwifery 1997; 13(2): 78-84.
21. Hemminki E. Impact of caesarean section on future pregnancy: A review of cohort studies. Paediatric and Perinatal Epidemiology 1996; 10(4): 366-79.
22. Lowe NK, Reiss R. Parturition and fetal adaptation. JOGNN 1996; 25(4): 339-49.
23. Gronlund MM, Nuutila J, Pelto L et al. Mode of delivery directs the phagocyte function of infants for the first six months of life. Clinical and Experimental Immunology 1999; 116(3): 521-6.
24. Creedy DK, Shochet IM, Horstall J. Childbirth and the development of acute trauma symptoms: Incidence and contributing factors. Birth 2000; 27(2): 104-11.
25. Kirkham MJ. Stories and childbirth. In: Kirkham MJ and Perkins ER (Eds). Reflections on Midwifery. London: Bailliere Tindall, 1997.
26. Antonovsky A. The implications of salutogenesis: An outsider's view. In: Turnbull et al (Eds). Cognitive coping families and disability. Baltimore: Paul Brookes, 1993.
27. Royal College of Midwives. Vision 2000, executive summary. London: RCM, 2000.

What is normal childbirth?

The midwife practitioner's view

Rosalind Weston

Within the last week I have had the privilege of being the midwife for four birthing women. All laboured in upright positions, freely walking, standing, kneeling, leaning forward or rocking, moaning and groaning through their contractions but breathing rhythmically. One actually fell asleep in her husband's arms – the endorphins had cut in! She awoke rejuvenated and alert, and able to give birth with confidence. Jowett[1] and Odent[2] both recognise the influence of stress hormones and endorphins which can either impede or facilitate the progress of normal labour. These endorphins are most likely to be released when a woman can be assured of privacy, warmth, security and when her 'rational' neo-cortex brain is not being stimulated by such things as bright lights and unnecessary questions.

Davis[3] challenges the midwifery community to define what makes for normal childbirth. I would suggest that it is a labour and birth in which a woman is free to 'tap into her inner resources' of strength, and her innate abilities to give birth without interventions such as syntocinon or an epidural. This means keeping intrusive vaginal examinations to a minimum,[4] and midwives being able to recognise progress of labour without them. Arbitrary time limits have no place in a spontaneous physiological birth.

Throughout the world, women in labour, surrounded by their closest friends and family, spontaneously change their position, naturally adopting upright stances, often until the fierce contractions of later labour are so intense that they feel the need to 'be grounded' by being close to the floor, or a strong person. Lefeber[5] and Priya[6] show how normal childbirth in developing countries is culturally situated in the family, according to the traditions of the society in which the woman lives. If she is surrounded by women who believe that their bodies are designed for giving birth, she is more likely to trust her ability to give birth with confidence, and without medicalised intervention. We in the sophisticated West have much to learn from our sister midwives and birthing women in these countries.

In the later half of the twentieth century the 'medical model' has propelled women towards an alien hospital environment. According to O'Connor[7] for most women 'comfort' means freedom from anxiety rather than soft sofas and pretty curtains.

The 'medical model' encourages women to expect choices that appear to offer a high degree of perceived comfort and safety. Women are also choosing to have elective caesareans and booking their epidurals in advance. Will this in ten years time become normal practice for childbirth? Do Brazilians really need a 75% rate of caesarean section? Could it happen here? Surely there is a need to highlight the morbidity rates of what is, after all, a major operation? I eagerly await the full results of the National Sentinel Caesarean Section Audit.

Marsden Wagner,[8] of the World Health Organization, has written a penetrating study entitled 'Pursuing the Birth Machine – The Search for Appropriate Birth Technology'. It is a brilliant extended resume of international conferences on the virtues and otherwise of insufficiently tested technologies.

The 'official story,' as Mavis Kirkham[9] describes the midwife's record of a labour, may have very little in common with the experienced described by the woman. These records risk reducing the wonder of a woman's childbirth to a purely clinical event. Students and others who read these notes learn only one side of the story. The integration into family life is barely touched upon. How much more beautiful and powerful if women can be encouraged to write (or draw) their recollections of their birth, and for these to be included in the official records. This would go a long way to redressing the balance of power, and give a greater understanding for a midwife of a woman's perception of her labour.

How can our daughters learn about natural childbirth if 98% of births occur under secluded hospital conditions where whole families attending a woman in labour can be an unwelcome intrusion on the smooth running of the labour ward? How can the students I meet learn the art of birth if they have never seen a 'natural' childbirth in which women are not continuously monitored or labouring immobile in bed with an epidural?

Some women and midwives might contend that an epidural is 'normal' simply because it is so common. Should we not be following Sutton's[10] advice to implement more effective ways of improving optimal fetal positioning into our antenatal teaching? This would undoubtedly reduce occipito-posterior positions and the pain which is so often associated with these labours. Leap[11] is another who advocates 'working with women in the pain of labour', thus helping to keep childbirth normal.

As I reflect on the four women and their babies, Ruby, Jade, Lauren and Robert, I wonder whether, as a result of their normal physiological births, they will be able to pass on their knowledge of (and confidence in) an unimpeded birth to their children's children? I hope and pray they will!

REFERENCES

1 Jowett M. Childbirth Unmasked. Peter Wooller, 1993.
2 Odent M. The Nature of Birth and Breastfeeding. London: Bergin & Garvey, 1992.
3 Davis L. Keeping Birth Normal. MIDIRS Midwifery Digest 2000; 10(1): 57-8.
4 Hobbs L. Assessing Cervical Dilatation without VEs: Watching the Purple Line. The Practising Midwife 1998; 1(11): 34-5.
5 Lefeber Y. Midwives without Training. Van Gorcum, 1994.
6 Vincent PJ. Birth Without Doctors. London: Earthscan Publications, 1991.
7 O'Connor M. Birth Tides. London: Pandora, 1995.
8 Wagner M. Pursuing the Birth Machine – The Search for Appropriate Birth Technology. Camperdown, Australia: Ace Graphics, 1994.
9 Kirkham M, Perkins E. Reflections on Midwifery. Baillière Tindall, 1997.
10 Sutton J. Occipito-posterior positioning and some ideas about how to change it. The Practising Midwife 2000; 3(6): 20-2.
11 Leap N. Pain in Labour: Towards a Midwifery Perspective. MIDIRS Midwifery Digest 2000; 10(1): 49-53.

What is normal childbirth?

The educational perspective

Sandy Kirkman

Normal can mean natural, physiological or unenhanced, or it can mean that which is most commonly seen.[1] A difficulty that midwife teachers face in the developed world today is that they teach the first, but students commonly see labour which is interfered with in some way. It is the epitome of the theory-practice gap and causes new students much grief. The dilemma, from an educational point of view, is that the physiological and the research-based information must be imparted to students, but we know they may often see something very different in practice.

In other mammals, gestation lasts for more precise periods. Shepherds leave the ram in the field of ewes on successive days so that the lambing will be spread over a corresponding period of days some weeks later. Rats and cats too have very precise gestation periods.[2] Not so humans – the period is around 280 days plus or minus ten so there is no precise date on which the baby is due. Similarly, no one is exactly sure what precise mechanism makes labour start but it would seem that it is much more efficient when it starts spontaneously, than when it is induced by prostaglandins or by artificial rupture of the membranes. In the recent past there was a belief that the placenta was a deciduous organ and it began to fail serially from 37 weeks onwards, thus inductions were carried out to escape this evil. It has now been shown that the placenta does not lose much function until well after 44 weeks.[3] So, it could be expected that students would see labours which started spontaneously at or after term, where no drugs or stimulants were given to make it start, and where the membranes were left intact until they ruptured spontaneously. I wonder.

Mammals walk about in labour, only settling into one position for expulsion of the offspring. Studies in women have shown that both upright position and ambulation reduce the timespan of labour and the need for pain relief.[4] The very worst position in which to labour is the 'stranded beetle' where the woman is on her back, or is semi-recumbent.[5] If the woman labours at home and can choose her position, she rarely adopts the recumbent, but, in hospital, she may be asked to adopt that position to enable the staff to site an intravenous infusion in her arm, or to access her abdomen. This might be for palpation of descent/contractions, for the attachment of CTG electrodes, or when an epidural has been sited. As it seems to be the position which helps the staff the most, she may well opt to stay in it for a quiet life.

Vets monitor the progress of labour in farm animals behaviourally. My old district midwife used to use that method too. If the woman was cleaning the house she would speed to the labour call. If the woman paused to catch her breath in the middle of a sentence, my midwife would motion me upstairs with a lift of her eyebrows. Despite all the work in the late sixties by O'Driscoll et al,[6] the cervix may not dilate at exactly one centimetre per hour, and it might not need Syntocinon to make it begin to do so. In normal labour the uterine contractions increase in length, strength and frequency and the upper and lower poles of the uterus enjoy a co-ordinated and rhythmic action. If this does not progress smoothly, the problem could be a poor maternal position, poor cervical stimulation, lack of calories and/or fluid. Jean Sutton's outstanding work on optimum fetal positioning[7] bears some examination in the context of normal labour.

Laboring mammals eat when they are hungry and drink when they are thirsty; the uterus needs calories and fluids to carry out its work. Spurious arguments about Mendelson's disease[8] have kept eating and drinking in labour in humans in hospital labour wards to a bare minimum. Women may not want to eat in labour, but if they are hungry they are listening to their bodies. Denying food and fluid on the grounds that they might vomit is not logical when the outcome is an IV infusion of sugar and water. The drugs most commonly used for pain relief in labour have been shown consistently to be poor analgesics and to have adverse effects on the length of labour, gastric emptying times and suckling,[9-11] so you might expect them to be used less often.

In mammals labour might seem to have begun and then stop again. In humans the use of the partogram feeds an expectation that all labours will be completed within 12 hours, and the second stage within one hour. The second stage is usually defined as from the full dilatation of the cervix to the complete expulsion of the baby, but how do we know the cervix is fully dilated unless a vaginal examination is carried out? If the second stage is defined from the onset of an urge to bear down it is quite often very short. This modern uncertainty of what is normal is why Wagner[12] suggests that we no longer know what we don't know.

Assisted delivery is rare in animals. In humans the HOOP trial[13] has cast doubt on the management of the perineum and attendants might not touch either the head or the perineum until the face appears. However, in examining the term 'normal labour' the forceps and ventouse delivery rates, the episiotomy rate and the caesarean section rate should all be assessed. Normal might include instrumental delivery if the woman has accepted it and is happy with the outcome.[1] Students are still taught the positions of the occiput in the second stage of labour, about OP position and the possible outcomes. Malrotations of the occiput will need operative delivery but current rates indicate that simpler measures are not being tried first.

Without oxytocic drugs the placenta is delivered in about twenty minutes. Blood loss has been shown to be greater in physiological third stages.[14] Students see a few physiological third stages but if these are after managed first and second stages the physiology might be a little altered.

REFERENCES

1 Gould D. Normal labour: A concept analysis. Journal of Advanced Nursing 2000; 31(2): 418-27.

2 Johnson M, Everitt B. Essential Reproduction. Edinburgh: Blackwell, 1980.

3 Reynolds LP, Redmer DA (1995) Utero-placental vascular development and placental function. Journal of Animal Science 1995; 73(6): 1839-51.

4 Read JA, Miller FC, Paul RH. Randomised trial of ambulation versus oxytocin for labour enhancement. American Journal of Obstetrics & Gynaecology 1981; 139: 669-72.

5 MIDIRS and the NHS Centre for reviews and dissemination. Positions in labour and delivery. Bristol: MIDIRS, 1996.

6 O'Driscoll K, Jackson RG, Gallagher JT. Prevention of prolonged labour. British Medical Journal 1969; 2: 177-80.

7 Sutton J. A midwife's observation of how the birth is influenced by the relationship of the maternal pelvis and the fetal head. Journal of the Association of Chartered Physiotherapists in Women's Health 1996; (79): 31-3.

8 Crawford JS. Maternal mortality from Mendelson's syndrome. Lancet 1986; 1: 920-1.

9 Thomson AM, Hillier VF. A re-evaluation of the effect of pethidine on the length of labour. Journal of Advanced Nursing 1994; 19(3): 448-56.

10 Oloffson CH, Ekblom A, Ekman-Orderberg G. Lack of analgesic effect of systemically administered morphine or pethidine on labour pain. British Journal of Obstetrics and Gynaecology 1996; 103(10): 968-72.

11 Reynolds F. Opioids in labour – no analgesic effect. Lancet 1997; 349 (9044): 4-5.

12 Wagner M. Pursuing the Birth Machine: the search for appropriate birth technologies. Camperdown, Australia: ACE Graphics, 1994.

13 McCandlish R, Bowler U, van Asten H et al. A randomised controlled trial of care of the perineum during second stage of normal labour. British Journal of Obstetrics and Gynaecology 1998; 105(12): 1262-72.

14 Rogers J et al. Active versus expectant management of third stage of labour: the Hinchinbrooke randomised controlled trial. Lancet 1998; 351: 693-9.

What is normal childbirth?

A consumer perspective

Mary L Nolan

When I had my first daughter seventeen years ago, I was quite sure what a 'normal birth' was. At this point in my life, I had no particular axe to grind in the realms of maternity care. I had trained as a general nurse and done the 13 weeks midwifery course during which I had seen a variety of births, from the easy to the difficult. I attended NCT classes with a teacher who had given birth to all three of her children by caesarean section, and who was therefore, not a tub-thumper for spontaneous vaginal delivery at all costs. My concept of normal birth preceded my nurse training and my antenatal classes, and wasn't particularly influenced by either. I was much more influenced by my mother's experiences which she had told me about briefly. Her two births were a normal cephalic presentation (me) and a face presentation (my brother) and she delivered us both flat on her back with no pain relief or assistance from forceps. She advised me to 'do as I was told' (by the hospital staff) and 'get on with it'.

I have never been especially inclined to 'do as I am told', but I certainly felt that women should 'get on' with giving birth and I was absolutely confident that I could deliver my baby unaided. For me, a normal birth meant that I would do my own thing in labour, have no drugs for pain relief, and push my baby out myself. Any variation on this theme would be 'abnormal'. I had no flexibility built into my plans – and, as luck (if it was luck) would have it, I had two births which were normal by my own inflexible definition.

This was back in the mid 1980s. For the last 14 years, I have been teaching antenatal classes for the NHS and the NCT, and writing, lecturing and broadcasting on pregnancy, birth and parenting. My definition of normal birth has not changed, although I would consider that having gas and air or using a TENS machine would not make labour 'abnormal'. However, I am increasingly and uneasily aware that for many, if not most, of the mothers and fathers with whom I come into contact, normal birth now accommodates a variety of experiences that I would certainly not consider normal. The NCT is busily engaged at present in drawing up a Birth Policy to complement its Baby Feeding Policy published in May 1999. At every meeting of the Advisory Group, of which I am a member, the issue to which all discussions eventually return is that of what constitutes a 'normal' or 'straightforward' vaginal birth. Endless talk moves us little closer to a definition with which we are all happy. We have consulted NCT mothers, whose comments on what 'straightforward vaginal birth' means have been fascinating:

Straightforward vaginal birth is not the same as birth without pain relief, or 'active birth'.

At the time, I certainly considered the birth of my first baby to have been a normal birth. I didn't have a caesarean. However, I did have gas and air, meptid, syntocinon and syntometrine. I think 'normal' is more to do with a state of mind than with what happens to you clinically.

I wouldn't say that pethidine was part of a normal birth.

To me, straightforward vaginal birth means a birth which is uncomplicated i.e. the baby isn't 'helped' into the world with any kind of intervention – ventouse or forceps.
A prostaglandin induction can be part of a normal labour if the labour progresses normally from there. A syntocinon induction wouldn't be part of a normal labour.

I don't think having an epidural is 'normal'; that's definitely a medical intervention and alters the course of the labour. I'm not sure about episiotomy – if it's just to help the baby out and you would have torn anyway...

A normal birth is one that the mother is satisfied with i.e. she participated, felt empowered, was in control and is content with the outcome.

'Straightforward vaginal birth' starts spontaneously, and continues at its own pace without drugs to speed it up. The mother pushes her baby out into the world herself. Pethidine, TENS and gas and air could be part of a normal vaginal birth.

What is quite clear from this fascinating exercise is that the concept of normal birth is, as an editorial in this journal not so long ago suggested, 'Going, Going, Gone!' Consumers define normal birth in medical terms and rarely in midwifery terms. None of the women we consulted defined normal birth in social terms. The women who favoured a midwifery model of birth could still only define 'normal' as not being 'medical'. It is as if, to paraphrase Denis Walsh's acute comment, 'normal birth is what is left after obstetrics has defined risk'.

Needless to say, the implications for midwives and women are huge if normal birth is now perceived as incorporating a whole barrage of drugs and interventions. Our back is against the wall if we believe that women are made strong and launched into motherhood with their self-esteem sky-high when they achieve a non-medicated, spontaneous birth with no interventions.

Like the woman whose comments on normal birth I cited above, I sometimes wonder whether I am 'out of touch with reality' in defining normal birth the way I do. The funny thing is that, whether I teach classes for the NCT or the NHS, the vast majority of women (and their men) tell me that 'if they can manage it' they would love to be able to give birth themselves. On closer questioning, this turns out to mean that they would like:

- not to have any drugs
- not to have their labour interfered with, and
- to push their baby out unaided (triumphantly).

What is troubling is that this image of themselves giving birth is sadly acknowledged by most women to be 'a dream', unlikely to be realised.

A curriculum for normality

Tricia Anderson

As the normal birth rate continues to fall steadily and now less than half the women in the UK can be expected to give birth naturally, it is becoming imperative that we re-look at midwifery knowledge, education and skills for normal birth if we are to reverse this downward trend.

With the renewed interest in midwife-led care, out-of-hospital birth centres and homebirth as key strands in the government's strategy to try to achieve this, midwives are needed who can take the vision forward – strong, articulate midwives who can work autonomously using their initiative, taking responsibility and using their diagnostic and decision-making skills to the full. The trouble is that there is now a generation of midwives who have spent their whole working lives inside consultant obstetric units where they have been unable to exercise these skills. Clinical decisions have been made either by the clock, the protocol, the labour ward sister or the registrar, with the ordinary midwife simply following the rulebook. In one large consultant unit, a senior labour ward midwife last year told a student who was worrying about her inability to do vaginal examinations, 'Oh, I wouldn't worry about learning to do VEs – the doctors end up doing them all and making all the decisions anyway.' Another senior labour ward midwife told a new student on her first day, 'Now then, let me get one thing straight: I don't believe in all that research-based nonsense they teach you at university – here we just follow the policies.'[1] Like an unused muscle, the decision-making capacity of the brain slowly atrophies and eventually dies. Mavis Kirkham calls midwives today 'the lost generation' of midwifery.[2]

But these 'lost generation' midwives are currently mentoring the next generation of students, and as we all know, the resulting fracas can be uncomfortable and stressful. The eager new student midwife, armed with her research, her internet information, her new knowledge gained from a Jean Sutton or Andrea Robertson study day, her ideology of woman-centred care, her mantras of evidence-based practice and informed choice and her never-ending questions can be quite a nightmare for a midwife who has spent ten or fifteen years following a medicalised, active management approach to maternity care, and who was never taught to question or challenge in her own education.

In this approach to maternity care, normal birth is something that happens almost by accident or default when a woman comes into the labour ward and pushes out her baby herself. Multigravid woman are quite good at it, as they can usually manage it within the limited time frame they are allowed: first timers less so. Give or take a bit, midwifery care consists of writing notes, doing routine observations, assessing the need for pain relief and administering it, and being the one to catch the baby should it manage to be born within a certain time frame. If it doesn't, the doctor must be called. Key midwifery skills for this lost generation focus on being able to run an intravenous drip through, process paperwork, manage epidural infusions, suture and so on. 'Lost generation' midwives tell students there is no need to understand the mechanism of labour or the different diameters and types of pelvis. Why bother? The normal birth 'bit' comes when the vertex is in the birth canal and gloves are put on ready to 'deliver'. If it doesn't come, call a doctor. Normal birth – where the midwife's expertise used to reign supreme – is becoming more and more narrowly defined. It used to include breeches and twins, anterior and posterior babies, face presentations – now it seems to include only full-term singleton, vertex, left occipito anterior babies. Is it any wonder that the normal birth rate is now less than 50%?

One problem is that normal birth is considered 'easy'. It's something that first year student midwives think they have all wrapped up, as they eagerly progress onto more challenging, complicated births. They make hugely worrying, complacent remarks such as, 'I'm OK with the normal now...' Every midwife thinks she can 'do' normal birth – even high dependency specialists think they can attend a normal birth without effort. Updating in more 'complex' skills such as epidural top-ups, CTG interpretation, suturing and so on require annual updating: normal birth itself is considered so simple that no refreshing is necessary and it can be happily left to the first year students.

But normal birth is far from easy. In fact, it's so complex, tantalising and immense that I am quite sure I shall never understand it! Tiny timid women who look as though they wouldn't say boo to a goose give birth to enormous babies like shelling peas; athletic, strong women labour for days and days and finally push out a small baby in total exhaustion; women who wait for their husbands to arrive (or go away!) before they will push their babies out, compound presentations, asynclitisms, posterior babies, steep pelvic inclines, narrow pelvic outlets... the variations of women and babies are infinite, and the midwife's task is to help each and every one give birth normally. A competent midwife needs to be able to use her midwifery skills and knowledge to help the vast majority of women who have no underlying medical complications give birth safely without medical assistance. That's what being a midwife means. The World Health Organization concluded this should be in the region of 90% of all women. This will not be achieved by just rubbing backs, mopping brows, being nice and waiting until the baby comes out.

A wise midwife once said to me that you only really grow up as a midwife when you first use your midwifery knowledge to get a baby out and safely born that was not going to come easily.

So a knowledge and understanding of midwifery for normal birth needs to reach back over the lost generation and go back to the earlier midwives in the 1950s and 1960s who cared for most women at home with good outcomes, when transfer was a rare event.[3] But it is not simply going back: the exciting new challenge is to synthesise their old-fashioned skills with contemporary knowledge gained from new research and technology. Midwifery tricks to assist slow labours, to diagnose compound presentations or get out stubborn placentas without syntometrine need to be on the curriculum for our next generation. Lost skills such as manually turning posterior babies, flicking out nuchal arms or 'chinning' large babies need to be rediscovered. And physiology, physiology, physiology!!! Revisiting the different types of pelvis and its impact on the mechanism of labour and solutions for each one, learning how to maximise maternal pelvic diameters to assist an asynclitic posterior baby to rotate, learning midwifery tricks to help a baby stuck on the ischial spines... now that's what I call a curriculum for normal birth.

Education for normal birth needs to include how to assess maternal and fetal well-being with confidence without using electronic fetal monitoring or fetal blood sampling, how to get a slow labour moving without rupturing membranes or putting up syntocinon, tricks to get a slow second stage going without using harmful coached pushing, and psychological techniques for dealing with pain and panic. It needs to cover alternative ways to assess that a woman's labour is going well without resorting to internal examinations, means of differentiating between a slow meandering labour that will be fine and the rare obstructed labour that won't be, and decision-making skills to judge when intervention is necessary without resorting to simple artificial time limits. It needs to include the physiology of the myometrium and how it links with the limbic system of the emotions, an understanding of oxytocin receptors and cervical cells, and the psychology of relationships, trust and pain and fear.

What I am describing goes far beyond the scope of a first year student and is not found in one or two convenient textbooks; it is something that takes decades to even begin to master. But the knowledge is there if you search hard enough. It can be found in the experiences and minds of some of our most venerated elder midwives, being rediscovered by some of our younger ones, being shared at midwifery conferences and workshops around the world, being researched and developed by some of our brightest midwifery brains.

There is no place for a lack of humility when faced with the vast complexities of 'normal birth'. It's not something to be left for the first year students; it is a constant, fascinating, perplexing challenge – a life's work at the very least! So don't consign the 'easy' normal births to the students, and don't write off anxious primigravidas with OP positions to the ventouse or the operating theatre... On the contrary, send in your most experienced midwives to these more complex situations and throw down the gauntlet, saying to them, 'I want you to use every ounce of your midwifery knowledge and skill to help this woman give birth normally.'

Now *that's* normal birth.

REFERENCES

1   Personal communication, 2002
2   Personal communication, 2003

3   Allison J (1996). Delivered at Home, Chapman and Hall, London

Pregnancy

If there is one thing I try to remember when visiting women during their pregnancy, it is that their contact with midwives (and the maternity services in general) is but a small part of their journey of pregnancy. Yet some of the things we do in the time we spend with pregnant women, such as calculating their expected date of birth, offering information about tests and responding to a woman's need for advice about issues which are relevant for her, can have effects which last way beyond the few minutes we spend together.

Following on from some of the work which was published in the early days of *The Practising Midwife*, Gemma Purrett has written an original article which summarizes her work on how we can improve our calculations of women's estimated dates of birth by taking into account individual variations on this. It seems incredible to me that we are still using standardised measurements of length of pregnancy, despite living in a society where we are generally encouraged to embrace difference! Other ways in which we can increase choices and options for women are outlined in the article by Andrea Robertson, who offers tips on using antenatal groups to enable parents to make informed choices about antenatal tests.

Midwives are sympathetic to the fact that, although some 'symptoms' of pregnancy may be common, they can have a significant impact on women's experiences. Rachel Allen offers a useful overview of the possible causes and potential treatments of nausea and vomiting in pregnancy and Johanne Jakeway draws on her personal experience of hyperemesis gravidarum as well as her midwifery knowledge in this area. Her article not only crushes some of the common myths about this condition but also discusses an Internet support group (still going strong at the time of writing) to which women who are facing this situation can turn.

Another complication of pregnancy that can be both traumatic for women and potentially fatal for babies is obstetric cholestasis. Emily McDermott's article provides an overview of the diagnosis and management of this condition, while Jenny Chambers shares her own experience of this condition, highlighting the very real heartbreak that can be caused when professionals fail to provide the appropriate diagnosis and treatment.

All too often the kind of research studies whose results make headlines are speedily turned into recommendations which are given to all women without real consideration of their validity. The issue of folic acid supplementation is one example of this, and Judith Ockenden's article provides a very useful insight into this area. In this time of growing consumer awareness about food, this may be another area which, as consumers, we need to watch – to ensure that we are making our own choices about what we put into our bodies, rather than having these choices dictated to us by governments and/or the food industry.

In considering some of the problems and dilemmas which can be associated with pregnancy, it's also nice to remember that this is a joyful, happy time for most women; an experience which our knowledge and skills (such as in massage) can positively enhance. Mario-Paul Cassar offers some useful techniques – and illustrations of these – which can help women not only in pregnancy, but throughout the childbearing years and beyond.

How long?

Calculating individualised due dates

Gemma Purrett

Although seemingly trivial, the issue of calculating a woman's estimated date of birth (EDB) is something which is done all over the world, every day, with a potentially huge impact on a woman and her pregnancy. For many women this date represents the exact point when they expect to have their babies, but unfortunately the reality is often a major disappointment, because this is rarely the case. Current practice in relation to the calculation of an EDB usually involves an obstetric calculator, which utilises Naegele's rule, and in most cases, although not all, an early dating ultrasound. The result of these practices can often be more than one due date and this can cause significant confusion for a woman and her family. The resulting EDB is often that calculated by the ultrasound scan, particularly if there is a discrepancy between the two dates.

It is a sad fact that these kind of practices within today's maternity services lead women to believe they cannot trust their bodies and should accept intervention as a necessary part of pregnancy and childbirth. In many ways it reinforces their belief that women should comply with a 'health professional' *who knows best*, perhaps not knowing that the methods currently employed are not always particularly effective. The current basis for obstetric calculators, Naegele's rule, does utilise some of the valuable information that pregnant women have relating specifically to themselves, making their EDB somewhat more individualised, but this is often disregarded when an ultrasound scan reveals different findings. This practice can disempower women, and place them in a position where they question their knowledge and perhaps, on a greater level, their ability to be pregnant and give birth without medical intervention.

It is interesting to consider that, whilst intervention like ultrasound is frequently used in today's maternity services to improve the accuracy of pregnancy dating, there is still a national rate of labour induction of more

than 21%.[1] This statistic includes induction for reasons other than 'post-dates', but approximately one third of this number are women whose pregnancy is medically defined as 'prolonged'.[1] Apart from the question of whether this induction rate is acceptable, the point that neither Naegele's rule nor ultrasound appear to be particularly effective should be considered.

The key question that seems to underpin this important issue is how long does pregnancy really last? This is a surprisingly difficult question to answer. The calculation of the EDB predominantly utilises Naegele's rule, which assumes pregnancy length is forty weeks (280 days). There is, of course, a degree of error accepted around this, extending from approximately thirty-seven weeks to forty-one or forty-two weeks, subject to local opinion. So where has this specific period of time evolved from?

The practice of dating pregnancy goes back to the time of Aristotle, who developed the principle that pregnancy lasted two hundred and eighty days or ten calendar months.[2] This was then further reinforced by the New Testament account of the birth of Christ and the nine month 'gestation' from the Feast of the Annunciation in March until Christmas day.[3] It was then from Hermann Boerhaave's observations that Franz Carl Naegele's rule evolved.[3] This rule is now commonplace in everyday midwifery and obstetrics, providing women with a non-invasive method of calculating their EDB. However, this has never been substantiated by any large scale research study.[2]

The vast majority of research relating to this subject considers the accuracy of ultrasound in comparison with Naegele's rule. Which, given that Naegele's rule is an unproved theorum, means that ultrasound is almost bound to come out on top. Researchers sometimes consider how long the average pregnancy lasts, but this is rarely the main focus of a study. The fact that this is rarely the principal research question constitutes a significant problem, but understandably a study of this nature would be very difficult to carry out, primarily because so many women are now induced at some point – particularly when they are considered 'overdue'.

There are many other factors that can influence research findings, such as augmentation of a woman's labour, instrumental delivery or caesarean section. Most significantly, there are ethical issues surrounding the continuation of pregnancy past a certain number of weeks, based on research regarding the increased possibility of stillbirth at this point.[4] Overall it must be said that there is only a very limited amount of research on the true length of pregnancy, which is frustrating, particularly when considering the implications it has not only for women, but also financially for the health service.

Naegele's rule can be, and is, calculated in many ways. Most frequently the formula utilised consists of the addition of seven days to the first day of the last menstrual period (LMP), minus three months.[3] The basis for this rule is the assumption that an individual has a twenty-eight day menstrual cycle, and therefore ovulation occurs on day fourteen, resulting in a probable date of conception two weeks later.[3] It is evident, perhaps unsurprisingly, that this is not always the case for every woman, creating a point of possible inaccuracy. Variation in the length of the pre-conceptual follicular phase has been highlighted by Gardosi,[5] who describes it as a major source of error in the calculation of the EDB. In actual fact, ovulation often occurs later than mid-cycle resulting in a pregnancy lasting longer than would be predicted by Naegele's rule.[5]

The considerable variation between the interval of the first day of the LMP and the day of ovulation has been well documented. Saito et al[6] found that more than 20 per cent of their research sample ovulated after twenty-five days and 11 per cent exceeded thirty-five days. Wilcox et al[7] found in their sample of 221 women that only 10 per cent ovulated on day 14; in the 696 cycles studied ovulation took place as early as the eighth day and as late as the sixtieth. Both groups of researchers considered that the assumption that ovulation occurs at 14 days is based on outdated information and should be reconsidered.

These results indicate a significant point of possible error in relation to the calculation of the EDB using Naegele's rule. In essence, if the time of ovulation exceeds the expected fourteen days from the LMP, the point of conception could also be delayed. The result would be a clinically 'prolonged' pregnancy that might fall into the category where induction of labour is indicated, which could possibly lead a woman further into the well-documented 'cascade of intervention'. Essentially what this means is Naegele's rule frequently under-estimates the length of pregnancy, a point which has been well documented.[5,6,8-10]

Whilst the efficacy of Naegele's rule is being questioned, it is important to also consider ultrasound and its effectiveness. The research to date has frequently favoured ultrasound dating as being more accurate at calculating the EDB than Naegele's rule. However, this method is still contributing to a significant labour induction rate. It should be remembered that ultrasound itself is a form of gestational dating; it calculates the point of gestation of the baby, based on certain measurements. The EDB is then calculated using the same basis as Naegele's rule, that pregnancy lasts 280 days. If this is the element of the rule that is inaccurate then both methods could theoretically be improved upon.

The controversy surrounding whether ultrasound should be used independently to date pregnancy continues to this day. Overall, it is accepted and supported as a beneficial intervention in *some* cases,[11] but perhaps skills should be concentrated on improving the other non-invasive procedures that might be just as effective. This point is particularly pertinent when we consider that a full evaluation of ultrasound has not been made yet, and we may still be unaware of the possible *subtle* effects that ultrasound may have on unborn babies.[12] This may become more significant as the power of the ultrasound machinery used, and the amount of time taken to carry out scans increase, especially on women who are considered 'high-risk'.

The view that Naegele's rule could be adjusted and therefore made more accurate is supported by a considerable body of the literature available in this area, which primarily finds pregnancy lasts longer than the currently assumed 280 days. For instance, Olsen and Clausen[13] suggest that the substitution of 283 days for 280 would render the EDB more accurate. This is supported by the largest published cohort study by Bergsjo et al.[14]

Other factors have also been shown to influence the EDB, including a woman's parity, ethnic group and height. In particular, the difference between multiparous and primiparous women seems very significant. It has long been considered by some midwives to be an almost forgone conclusion that many women expecting their first baby will go past their due date.[15] Based on this perhaps it should be questioned why so little has been done to examine this further, and perhaps alter what is considered to be the average length of a first pregnancy.

Mittendorf et al[16] found that pregnancy lasted 288 days for primiparous women and 283 days for multiparous women – both significantly longer periods than stated by Naegele's rule. It should be noted, however, that the sample used was small. Interestingly, and perhaps more importantly, was the way in which this study calculated the EDB, which was from the point of assumed ovulation and not the LMP. Therefore if a woman's cycle lasted twenty-eight days, then ovulation was assumed to occur on day fourteen, but if the cycle length was longer or shorter then the equivalent number of days was added or subtracted. This could in theory have improved the accuracy of the actual EDB calculated, by making it more specific to the individual woman. The findings of this study have also been supported by Berjso[14] and Smith.[17]

Ethnicity may also be a factor. Mittendorf et al[16] found that the duration of pregnancy in black women was approximately eight and a half days less than that in white women. A prospective study of Japanese women found pregnancy length on average was 278 days.[6] These findings make sense if consideration is given to the anatomical differences that can be expected to exist between different ethnic groups. Although this information is minimal, it is reasonable to consider that an adjustment, such as this, might make a substantial difference to the accuracy of Naegele's rule.

The influence of height on the length of pregnancy is another interesting issue. Again the information available is very restricted but one study showed that the proportion of pregnant women undelivered by their EDB was strikingly influenced by maternal height. Women over 1.75m were, in more than 60 per cent of cases, still pregnant by their EDB, compared with less than 40 per cent of women who were less than 1.45m tall.[18] Of course this information is of limited use on its own, but its significance should not be underestimated. The obvious question is: why do these variables influence pregnancy length? Whatever the reason may be, it makes more sense to consider applying them to practice and therefore utilising this information rather than just ignoring it.

Sutton[19] has also suggested that the increased incidence of occipito-posterior (OP) positioning in babies may impact on the duration of pregnancy. Anecdotally, midwives recognise postmaturity as a common feature in babies presenting in an OP position. The fact that these women may be more likely to experience intervention to speed up their labour in conjunction with an inaccurate EDB can have disastrous consequences for a mother and baby.

The impact of all of this on the pregnant woman should not be forgotten. From a very early point in their pregnancy women's knowledge is often questioned and in many cases undermined, immediately putting them in a 'patient' focused setting. This early intervention is essentially the start of a time when the medical model of care, which is often very prominent in hospital-based maternity units, probably becomes most apparent. Ideally, the midwifery model of care, which encompasses shared responsibility and involvement in a woman's care, should be utilised, but this is often not the case.

So, what can be done in everyday practice? Most obviously, a good explanation of the theory behind the

Figure 2.1.1 Factors in time from last menstrual period to estimated date of birth

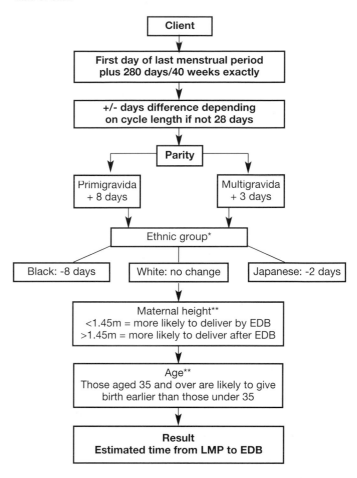

* If women do not fit exactly into one of these ethnic groups, continue without change.
** Maternal height and age are factors for guidance only, and should not be used to alter the predicted date of birth.

length of pregnancy and the calculation of the EDB should be made, thus ensuring that a woman understands the efficacy of the date she is being given, whether based on her LMP or an ultrasound scan. One way of reducing the specificity of the EDB would perhaps be to give an entire week labelled as when someone is due. [20]

By taking many of the above points into consideration, a more accurate method of calculating an EDB may be reached. An example of one such tool is included in Figure 2.1.1. This tool differentiates between primiparous and multiparous women, and also considers the differences identified between ethnic groups. This information is very minimal and therefore can only be used if an individual fits exactly into one group or another, but it is a start. It would seem that the most obvious way of benefiting women would be by using the information that they have about themselves, valuing it rather than disregarding it when another technology isn't in agreement. It should be noted, however, that this tool can only be used when an accurate LMP is available, for obvious reasons. This tool has been formulated using the available research, but has not yet been tested to measure its efficacy. However, it would seem possible that this tool could be utilised in practice alongside current methods in order to assess its validity, but this obviously must be in situations where the point of birth has not been artificially altered.

While there is a clear need to update the way we calculate the EDB, it may not be necessary – or possible – to aim for absolute perfection. Are we really justified in trying to gain some kind of control or supreme knowledge over this fascinating process that we will probably never fully understand? In addition to this we should question whether women actually want an absolute EDB, or whether perhaps the element of the unknown is a positive and exciting thing rather than a negative. For many, the specific nature of the EDB is probably the underlying factor that causes unnecessary anxiety not only for women, but also for those around them, all of whom wait for the day with eager anticipation. In some ways this may be putting undue pressure on a woman to do what has been predicted.

Whatever the outcome of this article, changes need to be made. An improvement in the accuracy of the EDB could have major financial implications for the NHS, allowing more money to go into other areas that would be more beneficial. The ongoing costs of labour induction, and with these the greater likelihood of interventions such as augmentation, additional analgesia and the increased chance of caesarean section should all be counted, in addition to the routine ultrasound scans that are frequently offered to women. Of course the costs can be counted in many ways, psychologically and physically, as well as financially.

Ultimately everyone should be moving towards the same goal, of improving the experiences that women and their families have. With this in mind, the fact that pregnancy and birth are natural processes should not be forgotten. As health professionals it should be our role to move women through these elements as safely as possible, taking care not to disregard information that is right in front of us.

REFERENCES

1 Department of Health. NHS Maternity Statistics, England: 1998-99 to 2000-01. London: HMSO; 2002.

2 Rosser J. Calculating the EDD: which is more accurate, scan or LMP? The Practising Midwife 2000; 3(3): 28-9.

3 Baskett TF, Nagele F. Naegele's rule: A reappraisal. British Journal of Obstetrics and Gynaecology. 2000;107: 1433-5.

4 National Institute for Clinical Excellence Inherited Clinical Guideline D, Induction of Labour. London: NICE; 2001

5 Gardosi J. The menstrual history: Old limitations, new prospects. Ultrasound Obstetrics and Gynaecology 1999;13: 84-5.

6 Saito M, Yazawa K, Hashigushi A, Kumasaka T, Nishi N, Kato K. Time of ovulation and prolonged pregnancy. American Journal of Obstetrics and Gynaecology 1972;112(1):31-8.

7 Wilcox AJ, Dunson D, Day Baird D. The timing of the 'fertile window' in the menstrual cycle: Day specific estimates from a prospective study. British Medical Journal 2000; 321:1259-62.

8 Berg AT (1991) Menstural cycle length and the calculation of gestational age. American Journal of Epidemiology. 133, 585-9.

9 Mongelli M, Wilcox M, Gardosi J. (1996) Estimating the date of confinement: Ultrasonographic biometry versus certain menstrual dates. American Journal of Obstetrics and Gynaecology. 174, 278-81.

10 Nguyen TH, Larsen T, Engholm G, Moller H. (1999) Evaluation of ultrasound estimate date of delivery in 17,450 spontaneous singleton births: Do we need to modify Naegele's rule? Ultrasound Obstetrics and Gynaecology. 14, 23-8.

11 Anderson T. (2000) How to calculate an EDD. The Practising Midwife. 3(3), 12-3.

12 Beech BA, Robinson J. (1996) Ultrasound? Unsound. London, Association for Improvements in the Maternity Services.

13 Olsen O, Clausen JA. (1997) Routine ultrasound dating has not been shown to be more accurate than the calendar method. British Journal of Obstetrics and Gynaecology. 104, 1221-2.

14 Bergsjo P, Denman DW, Hoffman HJ, Meirik O. (1990) Duration of human singleton pregnancy, a population based study. Acta Obstetricia et Gynecologica Scandinavica. 69, 197-207.

15 Kitzinger S. (1982) The experience of childbirth. Middlesex, Penguin Books Ltd.

16 Mittendorf R, Williams MA, Berkey CS, Cotter PF. (1990) The length of uncomplicated human gestation. Obstetrics and Gynaecology. 75, 929-32.

17 Smith GCS. (2001) Use of time to event analysis to estimate the normal duration of human pregnancy. Human Reproduction. 16(7), 1497-500.

18 Saunders N, Paterson C. (1991) Can we abandon Naegele's rule? The Lancet. 337-600-1.

19 Sutton J. (2001) Let birth be born again. Middlesex, Birth Concepts.

20 Stevenson J. (1994) More on EDD. Midwifery Matters. Autumn, 62, 15-7.

Pregnancy tests
A vital topic for prenatal education

Andrea Robertson

At a recent in-service weekend for the faculty involved in our Graduate Diploma of Childbirth Education, we reviewed the information available to parents regarding the pregnancy tests offered as part of normal pregnancy care. Although the care offered by hospital doctors and midwives often varies considerably, there are a number of tests that are regarded as routine. We looked at the evidence available and discussed the implications for informed choice by parents. Our first task was to participate in a role play of a typical prenatal visit where the doctor is explaining the outcomes of various prenatal tests to a couple who are expecting their first baby. Elaine explained that this role play was an exact transcription of an interview that she had taped as part of a research project, so had to be 'real'. What an eye-opener! Those of us playing the parts quickly realised how difficult it would have been for parents to make any sense of what was being discussed and also how hard it would be to ultimately make a decision about whether to have the tests being offered or not.

Reviewing this information and participating in a role play like this makes you reassess the way we present the various issues surrounding prenatal test and diagnosis in our classes. It emphasises again the key role parenthood education programmes play from the very start of pregnancy. Where else will parents find a knowledgeable person, not directly involved in their care and therefore (hopefully) unbiased who will facilitate a discussion of the topic, the emotional and practical issues it raises whilst supporting and enabling informed choice to be made? I doubt that the midwife in the busy prenatal clinic will have time and I think it unlikely that the doctor who may be ordering the tests will take the time required to ensure s/he has obtained informed consent.

We must recognise the enormous dilemmas faced by parents and make sure they have access to the information they need at a time when they are facing the issues, that is, in early pregnancy. We must also recognise

that we must protect our midwifery and medical colleagues from charges of withholding information by ensuring that parents are truly informed about the options they have. If the reality is that these busy colleagues don't have enough time for individual counselling, it must be provided in another forum, and the early pregnancy programme provides an ideal forum.

I firmly believe that every prenatal programme should incorporate at least two sessions for parents who are 12 – 16 weeks pregnant. It is around this time in pregnancy that parents are confronted by a series of often major decisions that may well have a major impact on the physical and emotional health of themselves and their babies. There are often other concerns that would benefit from talking through, such as the enormous changes taking places in their lives, the practical aspects of producing the healthiest baby possible, the options and choices regarding health care for the pregnancy and birth. Indeed, the most influential decision they make will be the choice of caregiver and birth place: the evidence is very clear that it is these two factors, above every other consideration, that will determine the final outcome of the birth. An early pregnancy class provides an opportunity to explore these issues and perhaps learn about alternatives. The steps that can be taken to change the type of care, seek a second opinion and gain further information as a framework to underpin the final choice can also be offered.

It's the prenatal tests, however, that often produce the greatest confusion. The explanation given by the midwife or doctor may have been completely unintelligible to the woman. She may have said she understood the discussion (rather than appear stupid), may have accepted the written information (without a hope of reading what it says) or may have felt flustered or overcome by the sudden announcement that testing is being offered (what is wrong with my baby that I have to have all these tests?). Many caregivers may believe that parents want and need to have as many tests as possible and encourage parents ('it's for the good of your baby' or 'it will set your mind at rest'). They may be unaware of the emotional trauma that may result and the possible deleterious effects a screening test may precipitate. Michel Odent has written about the 'Nocebo' effect and its implications for maternal wellbeing. Before parents are offered any screening or diagnostic tests as part of their pregnancy care, it is useful for them to have learned of and practise the most important questions that need to be asked:

'What is the test you are offering me?'
'What do you expect the test to reveal?'
'How will the test be carried out?'
'What are the advantages and disadvantages of this test? Specifically, are there any risks to the baby?'
'How will the results alter your care or treatment of me?'
'What will happen if I decline the test/procedure?'

Although some women do receive extensive counselling prior to genetic testing, many need follow-up and a chance to talk through the issues in a more relaxed and informal setting. Again, an early pregnancy group can offer a chance to explore concerns with others in a similar situation. Sharing experiences and learning more about the implications of testing before it is done ensures parents have fully considered their options.

You may also need to provide support for those parents who choose not to test. It is unusual for parents to decline (avoid using that judgmental word 'refuse') ultrasounds or other offered tests but not rare and these parents often feel very isolated after taking this decision. Given that we know so little about the overall effects and even advisability of many of these prenatal tests, we must be prepared to support and recognise parent's right to protect their baby through taking other avenues open to them. No one can guarantee that the baby will be healthy or that any particular test is safe, therefore parents must have the right to choose and be supported in their decision. A group of peers, led by a competent educator with good facilitation skills might just counteract the prejudice and pressure often exerted on parents by friends and family (and some unthinking health professionals!).

The way you tackle the presentation of these issues will be important. Small group discussion and a chance to examine various viewpoints will be essential. Centring the discussion on the specific tests being offered also avoids tedious exploration of issues that are not relevant.

This is one topic that is not going to go away, especially with the headlong rush to screen, test, prod, poke, examine and assess in the hope that all this surveillance will reduce the anxiety experienced by mothers and the numbers of damaged babies being born. I certainly am glad I had a chance to talk through these issues with my colleagues at the study day – is this an area you need to bone up on too?

Are we failing women?

Advice for nausea and vomiting in pregnancy

Rachel Allen

About 70% of women experience nausea and vomiting in pregnancy (NVP), beginning in about the 4th week of gestation, and generally resolving by the 12th week. It has been said to be present in the morning and to generally recede during the day.[1,2] It tends to be regarded as a minor disorder of pregnancy, yet research has shown that as many as a third of women with the complaint find it a serious problem which adversely affects the quality of their lives.[3]

It has also been demonstrated that it may be more prevalent than previously thought. In a trial involving 160 women in Canada,[4] 80% reported nausea lasting all day and this had only resolved by week 14 in 50% of cases. By 22 weeks, 90% of cases had resolved. The researchers conclude that 'traditional teachings about nausea and vomiting of pregnancy are contradicted by our findings'. They also found that the nausea experienced was as bad as that experienced by patients undergoing cancer chemotherapy. Although a small study, it mirrors the results found in a previous larger study involving 1000 women.[5]

What is the cause?

For something so common, surprisingly little is known about its aetiology, although oestrogen, progesterone, HCG and altered thyroid function are all thought to play a part. Profet[1] has offered a theory that it is the body's way of protecting the fetus against potential toxins during organogenesis. She supports this argument with the fact that those with NVP are less likely to miscarry, but it has also been suggested that if this were the case, NVP would also be evident in animals. Other theories have also been proposed, and have been summarised[2] as

- physiological changes, such as reduced gastric motility or reflux oesophagitis
- metabolic changes, such as carbohydrate deficiency, vitamin B deficiency

- genetic incompatibility
- position of corpus luteum
- psychological factors.

It is known to be associated with multiple pregnancy and some trials have also found it to be more common in young and primigravid women and in severe pre-eclampsia, although the evidence across trials is not conclusive.

Women who smoke have been found to have fewer symptoms than non-smokers, and the more severe the vomiting in early pregnancy, the longer the symptoms were likely to last.[6]

Does it predict pregnancy outcomes?

There is a theory amongst midwives that NVP is worse in women carrying female babies, but trials have so far been inconclusive.[6] However this may lie with the fact that it is difficult to quantify the severity of NVP, especially from questionnaires which are often collected postnatally.

Trials which have evaluated neonatal outcomes have found no differences in congenital defects between those who had vomited and those who had not.[7] NVP has also been shown to protect against miscarriage, especially in the context of a threatened miscarriage, and it also appears to protect against postnatal depression.[7] There is an association between severe cases of NVP and low birth weight.[6,7]

What can the midwife do about it?

One study showed that midwives were providing fragmented and even contradictory advice to women on the subject.[8] Typical advice was to eat carbohydrates little and often, to eat something before rising, to rest or even to exercise. However, women often found this information insufficient and seldom effective.

As midwives are aware, many of the remedies come from a complementary field in the form of oils, herbs, acupressure, acupuncture, hypnosis or homeopathy. These can sometimes be difficult for a midwife to evaluate, making her wary of handing out advice. However midwives should have some basic information to help women, and this article will highlight some of the more common treatments and what advice midwives can give.

Essential oils and herbs

Tiran[9] provides a comprehensive account of which oils to use for nausea in pregnancy. She recommends mandarin, tangerine, sweet orange, lime, grapefruit and ginger. Women can also eat grapefruit, and make ginger tea from a piece of ginger in boiling water. Contraindicated oils in pregnancy are basil, cedarwood, clary sage, camomiles, fennel, juniper, lavender, marjoram, peppermint, nutmeg, rose and rosemary, although there is controversy over peppermint.

Stapleton[10] also provides advice on herbs for NVP, recommending chamomile, meadowsweet, spearmint, ginger or aniseed. She recommends these be taken as tea or frozen in ice cubes. She also discusses the fact that the effects are often short lived and that the body quickly develops a tolerance, so rotating herbs may be of benefit. For more severe cases a trained herbalist will be able to prescribe something stronger.

It is easy to see from this why the average practising midwife is confused, as camomile as an oil is contraindicated by Tiran but recommended as a tea by Stapleton. This may be because oils are stronger, or due to a difference in professional opinion. Unfortunately I was unable to find any additional information on the subject, but midwives can feel confident in mentioning ginger or the citrus oils.

The use of ginger

Ginger has been evaluated in one trial[11] although it only involved 27 women with hyperemesis gravidarum. These women were given ginger capsules 250mg four times a day and compared with a control group given a placebo of 250mg of lactose four times daily. There was a considerable reduction in both nausea and vomiting in the ginger group, but it is difficult to translate these quantities into ginger found in normal foodstuffs. To complicate the issue further, Davis[1] has questioned the safety of ginger in large doses, and there are no adequate trials to provide analysis of this question.

In light of present evidence, it would seem safe for midwives to suggest the use of ginger as found in food stuffs, such as tea, biscuits, drinks etc. The typical amount found in ginger capsules is about 12gms, in excess of that used in the trials, and should probably not be recommended to women without further evidence as to its safety.

Acupressure

A review of studies for this intervention[11] has demonstrated a benefit in the treatment of postoperative emesis, chemotherapy-associated emesis and motion sickness. The main criticism of trials is that it is difficult to provide an adequate placebo, and the effect may therefore be in part attributable to psychological factors. Some of the trials[12] indeed reflected this, with the greatest effect gained from the Neiguan point, followed by a dummy point, followed by no intervention. Many of the trials[12,14] also had as much as a 30 or 40% drop-out rate, which could potentially bias results, especially as numbers were small to begin with. One of the more recent and larger trials[13] (161 women) actually found no difference in nausea rates between the treatment group, the dummy (placebo) group and the no intervention group. This was a trial which achieved a 92.5% completion rate; this may account for the different results when compared with the other studies, or it may be due to other unrecognised factors.

However, the majority of trials from both a nursing and midwifery perspective have found this intervention to be effective. Even if this is due to a placebo effect, it is a cheap and safe option which could be recommended to clients. Tiran[9] stresses the importance of finding the right spot on the wrist, the Neiguan point. To do this the distance from the wrist crease to the elbow is calculated and divided by 12. This will give the distance of 1 Chinese anatomical inch; the point is 2 anatomical inches from the wrist crease, between the two tendons.

Pyridoxine supplementation (vitamin B6)

The two randomised controlled trials on pyridoxine supplementation for nausea and vomiting involved 59[15] and 342[16] women respectively. In the first study there was a marked improvement in severe nausea and vomiting but no improvement in mild nausea. The second trial used smaller doses of pyridoxine (30mg as opposed to 75mg daily) and found a reduction in nausea but not in vomiting. However overall the trials were effective and this corresponds with the results of the first trials on the subject in the 1940s[11] Unfortunately neither trial reported on neonatal outcomes. However Sahakian et al[15] state that the available evidence suggests no teratogenic risk with supplementation up to 40mg a day.

The exact action of pyridoxine is not known, as levels of serum B6 have not been shown to be related to the severity of NVP.[11] Supplementation may therefore be effective due to some other factor than simply a deficiency. Pyridoxine, except in extremely high doses, is unlikely to be harmful and has even been shown to have a beneficial effect on the placental vascular bed, leading to increased birth weight.[17] As NVP has been associated with severe pre-eclampsia,[2] which also affects the placental bed, there may be an association which we are as yet unaware of. It is also thought to protect against dental caries, although the research dates from the 1960s and has not been repeated.[17]

Interestingly grapefruit, a treatment suggested by herbalists for NVP, contains vitamin B6. Other sources of vitamin B6 include tuna, mackerel, banana, avocado, raisins, sunflower seeds, and hazelnuts.[2] If the midwife is hesitant about recommending supplements, she could suggest these foodstuffs as a safe alternative, as it has been shown that women taking even low doses of pyridoxine in the form of multivitamins have a reduced incidence of nausea.[11] It is thought however that this is due to enhanced nutritional status rather than to such a small dose.

Implications for the midwife

Tiran[9] along with the UKCC[18] stress the importance of not advising or prescribing anything about which the midwife has not been properly trained. However as a result of this it could be that women are not receiving adequate information on a subject which adversely affects them. This leaves midwives with a dilemma. It is easy to suggest ginger, yet there is no suggested dose or evaluation. The same issues apply to vitamin B6 supplementation. Although the available evidence indicates that these are safe options, as yet no large scale studies have been carried out to exclude the possibility of rare teratogenicity. However nothing obvious has emerged either. The use of

sea bands is less controversial as it non-invasive and unlikely to lead to long-term effects.

Maybe all the midwife needs to do is to acknowledge the fact that these therapies may work for individual women, although high doses have not been evaluated. However this still leaves the woman with inadequate information and an unsolved problem. The midwife can continue to suggest small meals and eating before rising, yet in order to fulfil her duty of care to her client, she needs to provide information in keeping with the needs of the woman. If in doubt a midwife could suggest consulting a herbalist or homeopath. In this way she protects her professional accountability yet provides women with an alternative.

The interventions appear to be very individual to women, especially the use of such things as oils and herbs, and the woman may need more support and input than just experimenting by trial and error on her own. Of course in some cases all the woman may need is support and understanding from the midwife. As yet no trials on the positive effect of support have been carried out.

At the moment NVP is something which women are expected to cope with on their own, often because there is no easy answer which suits all women. Yet it should be acknowledged as a problem and possibly Trusts should start taking a more proactive role in its treatment by providing oils or acupressure bands for women to try. More midwives could be trained in alternative therapies and cascade their knowledge to others within their Trust so that midwives are able to answer the needs of women. In this way women will be able to experiment and find something which suits their needs, while the additional support and interest may in itself help to ease the condition.

REFERENCES

1 Stables D. Physiology in childbearing. London: Bailliere Tindall, 1999.
2 Lindsay P. Vomiting. In: Sweet B. Mayes Midwifery. 12th edition. London: Bailliere Tindall, 1997.
3 O'Brien B, Naber S. Nausea and vomiting during pregnancy: effects on the quality of women's life. Birth 1992; 19: 138-143.
4 Lacroix R, Easton E, Melzack R. Nausea and vomiting during pregnancy: a prospective study of its frequency, intensity, and patterns of change. Birth 1992; 182(4): 931-7.
5 Whitehead SA, Andrews PLR, Chamberlain GVP. Characterisation of nausea and vomiting in early pregnancy: a survey of 1000 women. Journal of Obstetrics and Gynaecology 1992; 12: 364-9.
6 Zhou Q, O'Brien B, Relyea J. Severity of nausea and vomiting during pregnancy: what does it predict? Birth 1999; 26(2): 108-14.
7 Deuchar N. Nausea and vomiting in pregnancy: a review of the problem with particular regard to psychological and social aspects. British Journal of Obstetrics and Gynaecology 1995; 102(1): 6-8.
8 Dilorio C. The management of nausea and vomiting in pregnancy. Nurse Practitioner 1988; 13(5): 23-4, 26-8.
9 Tiran D. Complementary therapies for nausea in pregnancy. Modern Midwife 1996; 6(3): 19-21.
10 Stapleton H. Herbal medicines for the disorders of pregnancy. Modern Midwife 1995; 5(4): 18-22.

11 Murphy PA. Alternative therapies for nausea and vomiting of pregnancy. Obstetrics and Gynaecology 1998; 91(1): 149-55.
12 Dundee JW, Sourial FB, Ghaly RG et al. P6 acupressure reduces morning sickness. J R Soc Med 1988; 81: 456-7.
13 O'Brien B, Relyea MJ, Taerum T. Efficacy of P6 acupressure in the treatment of nausea and vomiting during pregnancy. Am J Obstet Gynecol 1996; 174: 708-15.
14 Belloumini J, Litt RC, Lee KA et al. Acupressure for nausea and vomiting of pregnancy: a randomized blinded study. Obstet Gynecol 1994; 84: 245-8.
15 Sahakian V, Rouse D, Sipes S et al. Vitamin B6 is effective therapy for nausea and vomiting of pregnancy: a randomized, double-blind placebo-controlled study. Obstet Gynecol 1991; 78(1): 33-36.
16 Vutyavanich T, Wongtrangan S, Rkuangsri R. Pyridoxine for nausea and vomiting of pregnancy: a randomized, double-blind, placebo-controlled trial. Am J Obstet Gynecol 1995; 173: 881-4.
17 Mahomed K, Gulmezoglu AM. Pyridoxine (vitamin B6) supplementation in pregnancy. In: The Cochrane Library, Issue 4, 2000. Oxford: Update Software.
18 UKCC. Standards for the administration of medicines. London: UKCC, 1992.

Hyperemesis Gravidarum
Not just morning sickness!

Johanne Jakeway

Most of you may not be aware that Charlotte Brontë, who died in 1855, four months into her first pregnancy, did so as a result of severe vomiting. Her sufferings were written in her diaries in detail, describing her nights of vomiting with no reprieve at all. Does this sound familiar? It certainly did in my case.

In past times severe pregnancy sickness or Hyperemesis Gravidarum (HG) was a significant cause of maternal deaths. The only form of treatment available then was a therapeutic abortion.

Nowadays, the outcome is not so bleak. Thankfully, maternal morbidity and mortality are extremely rare and with the advancement of medicine and intravenous therapy, complications such as Wernicke's encephalopathy (owing to thiamine deficiency) can be avoided.

Hyperemesis Gravidarum does however continue to be a tiring and miserable condition that can have profound effects on the woman and her family. Despite this, it remains a complication of pregnancy that is neither understood nor widely acknowledged throughout the medical profession. As a result, many sufferers and their families are not receiving the appropriate emotional support that they desperately require.

About HG

Hyperemesis Gravidarum is a severe and debilitating form of morning sickness. A HG sufferer will prefer to use the term 'any time of the day sickness' as being a more accurate description. It has been described as intractable vomiting before the twentieth week of pregnancy resulting in disturbed nutritional status (Long & Russell, 1993).

Whereas nausea and vomiting during the first trimester of pregnancy (up to 12-14 weeks gestation) is seen to be a normal physiological process, the symptoms appear to worsen and then escalate into HG.

The onset of HG is always within the first trimester, as early as 5-6 weeks and may continue up until 20-22 weeks or even in some cases for the duration of the entire pregnancy.

In most cases treatment of HG can prove difficult. It may be only when the vomiting persists and the woman is unable to maintain adequate hydration and nutrition which requires hospital admission and investigations that a diagnosis is made. It is not uncommon for some women to vomit upto 20 times a day. Constant nausea and ptyalism (excess salivation), ketosis and dehydration, resulting in weight loss rather than gain accompany this.

Whilst it has been documented that nausea and vomiting in pregnancy affects up to 50% of pregnancies (Nelson-Piercy, 1997), only a small percentage of women present with HG. The true incidence continues to be unknown, but having examined the literature it varies from between 0.3% to 3%.

Aetiology

The aetiology of HG remains unknown, with limited research available and very few randomised trials being carried out. There have been links made to hormonal levels, thyroid dysfunction, helicobacter pylori, psychosomatic factors, abnormal liver function and adrenocortical deficit (Vellacott, Cooke & James, 1998; Eliakim, Abulafia & Sherer, 2000) Many authors identify risk factors such as previous pregnancies with HG, a history of travel sickness, migraine headaches and a pre-gestational high saturated fat diet (Signorello, Harlow, Wamg et al, 1998).

It was Fairweather who managed to put a spanner in the works with his rather uncontrolled study relating to HG and various psychosocial factors (Fairweather, 1968). His results proved to be biased and somewhat flawed. I will argue that in most cases depression and psychological morbidity almost certainly develop after the condition has manifested itself and not before. McCall (2000) wrote about the rejection of psychosomatic disorder as an explanation for HG. She stated that anyone who readily subscribes to the idea that HG is a neurosis is doing the sufferers an injustice. HG is an illness, not a state of mind!

In reality it is not known what causes some women to become so desperate during their pregnancy as a result of HG, that terminating often much wanted pregnancies seems to be their only means of escape from sheer hell.

Management

Many women may be able to manage their condition at home with various remedies to prevent them from having to be hospitalised. These range from taking small regular meals, never eating and drinking together, avoiding fatty foods and caffeine-based drinks and sucking on small sweets, which may help with excessive saliva.

It is essential that midwives have a basic understanding of the condition, as well as ensuring that there is an up-to-date written protocol for the management of women who present with severe HG in hospital. These must be evidence-based, including the most effective treatments presently available, until hopefully there is a gradual improvement as the pregnancy progresses.

It has been stated that a request for a termination must not be assumed to indicate that the pregnancy was not wanted or unplanned. It may simply be an indication of the degree of desperation felt by the patient (Nelson-Piercy, 1997).

As health professionals, it is our duty to maintain confidentiality during these sensitive periods, as well as encouraging expression of thoughts and building a trusting relationship with the woman and those close to her.

A personal viewpoint

Like Charlotte Brontë, I also wrote down my experiences in a diary. I wrote constantly about the effects that hyperemesis was having upon my husband, my family and myself. Looking back, I wrote with great bitterness and contempt for the condition that had made me a shadow of my former self.

Hyperemesis made me very lonely and depressed. I would cry uncontrollably for what seemed to be hours, but I didn't even have the strength to produce tears.

Movement makes the condition worse, so I found myself spending days upon days lying still in bed, unable to make even the slightest movement for fear of vomiting. The only time the nausea left me was when I slept. I couldn't even tolerate my husband sitting on the bed beside me and I would scream for him to move. Even the smell of him would make me vomit.

At 13 weeks gestation I was at an all time low, having lost 2 stones in weight. I pleaded with my family to help me to terminate my pregnancy. At the time it seemed to be my only option. I needed to be normal again. How could I have even contemplated such a thing? But hyperemesis makes you think irrationally. I would have given anything for the nausea to subside.

If it wasn't for the love from my family, and my eternal hope that it would eventually ease, things might have been very different.

The nausea and vomiting carried on relentlessly for another 9 weeks. I spent most of this time in hospital and was able to go home only for short periods. Colleagues would pass me by, not recognising me, upsetting me all the more.

The management of my condition continued to be very difficult. There is no miracle cure for HG, no single treatment seems to be effective. My own treatment included anti-emetics, antacids, supplements, vitamins, corticosteroids, acupuncture and homoeopathy!

Eventually the nausea did subside. At 24 weeks I was able to manage small meals as well as keeping fluids down. But I never ate and drank at the same time. Even though I continued to be weak I was now able to function relatively normally. Though the vomiting ceased, my husband and I lived in fear of its return.

On 6th February 1999 Daniel James Jakeway arrived by emergency lower segment caesarean section. He weighed in at 8lb 10oz. Amazing when you think what he put his mother through. It just goes to show that even though you are going through hell, it is only in very severe cases that a baby may be born with a lower than average birth weight.

Looking back

Two and a half years on, the effects of HG on me are still apparent. Even now, certain smells or foods will bring that feeling of nausea back. I would love one day to have the courage to have another pregnancy, but HG has and will continue to prevent this from happening for a very long time – if ever!

Luckily, I have managed to cope with it all relatively well. I know that other sufferers have experienced post traumatic stress disorder, overwhelming fears of nausea and vomiting, and sexual difficulties.

Conclusion

Although HG continues to be a very difficult condition to manage, as midwives we must ensure that these women receive adequate emotional support and as much reassurance about their condition as possible. This, in combination with the most appropriate evidence-based treatment for that individual, may help sufferers to have a have a relatively normal pregnant life. The sooner that people realise HG needs more than ginger biscuits and sea-bands the better!

I am the first to admit that before my pregnancy I knew very little about HG, and so found it quite difficult to identify with such women in my workplace.

However, now as a survivor of HG and a midwife I can utilise this knowledge and past experience to give the necessary emotional support to women, their families and my colleagues.

Blooming awful

No one who has been affected by Hyperemesis Gravidarum will ever forget it. Women need to know that they are not alone and consequently those feelings of desperation may be lessened. That is the main reason why I have become involved with the new Internet-based support group Blooming Awful – the UK Hyperemesis Gravidarum Awareness Group.

Blooming Awful was 'conceived' by two women in the Hampshire area who met on an Internet discussion forum for pregnancy complications. Both were on the lookout for anyone who might have HG and a shoulder to cry on.

All our volunteers are survivors of the condition in one or more pregnancies and are committed to raising awareness and recognition of HG as well as providing practical advice and much-needed support to women and those close to them. Only a HG survivor will understand how that person is feeling, only they can truly empathise. One of the worst things about HG (apart from the nausea) can be the loneliness, so Blooming Awful is here to help.

Our website www.hyperemesis.org.uk is packed with information. You can also e-mail us at info@hyperemesis.org.uk

Or if you would prefer to speak directly to someone you can call 07050 655 094.

REFERENCES

Eliakim R, Abulafia O, Sherer DM. 2000. Hyperemesis Gravidarum: A current review. American Journal of Perinatology 17(4), 207-18

Fairweather DVI. 1968. Nausea and vomiting in pregnancy. Am Jour Obst and Gynaec 102, 135-175

Long P, Russell L. 1993. Hyperemesis gravidarum. J Perinatal Neonatal Nursing 6(4), 21

McCall AE. 2000. An HG sufferer speaks out. The Birthkit, 10

Nelson-Piercy C. 1997. Hyperemesis gravidarum. Current Obstetrics and Gynaecology 7, 98-103

Signorello LB, Harlow BL, Wamg S, Erik MA. 1998. Saturated fat intake and the risk of severe hyperemesis gravidarum. Epidemiology, 9, 636-40

Vellacott ID, Cooke EJA, James CE. 1988. Nausea and vomiting in early pregnancy. Intl Journ of Gynae Obstet 277, 57-62

Much ado about nothing?

Diagnosis and management of obstetric cholestasis

Emily McDermott

Cholestasis is a high-risk obstetric complication, which affects certain women, usually after the 28th week of pregnancy.[1] The prevalence of obstetric cholestasis (OC) is still unknown due to various factors such as small numbers of proven cases, and it is a condition which has only recently been acknowledged, so few studies have been undertaken with conclusive findings.

It is important for midwives to be familiar with this complication, as it has a negative outcome for both the mother and her baby. There are no long-term consequences for the mother, as the condition ceases after 1-2 weeks postpartum.[2] However, the woman can suffer physiologically, psychologically, emotionally and socially owing to the demoralising side-effects OC can cause. There have been some suggestions that prolonged cases can increase the incidence of gallstones and primary biliary cirrhosis.[3,4] The risks to the fetus are far more detrimental (Table 2.5.1).

Detection

The midwife may be the first person to suspect a woman to be suffering from OC. This includes both community and hospital based midwives, as they are the first contact person in antenatal care.[9] Midwives need to be aware of the appropriate care and know their role in carrying out the management of women with OC.

Jenny Chambers, who is currently generating awareness of OC, has spoken about her own very distressing experience of suffering two stillbirths due to OC (p33).[10] She had symptoms, but health professionals were unaware of the consequences of ignoring tests that showed signs of OC, even though she told them it wasn't right! This could be the case with many women suffering from stillbirth, who are unaware of OC. It is therefore imperative that health professionals are aware of symptoms associated with OC, as the outcome can be more desirable if it is diagnosed early, and intervention is used in needy circumstances.[6,11,12]

Table 2.5.1 Increased risks to the fetus due to OC[5-8]

Meconium stained liquor
Abnormal intrapartum fetal heart rates
Spontaneous premature labour
Intracranial haemorrhage
Perinatal mortality
Stillbirth

Table 2.5.2 Symptoms of OC[9-14]

Pruritus
Lack of sleep
Exhaustion
Generally feeling unwell
Pale stools
Jaundice (in severe cases)
Lowered appetite
Nausea and vomiting
Lethargy
Epigastric pain
Hypertension (in severe cases)
Disseminated intravascular coagulation (in severe cases)

Symptoms

There are many different symptoms of OC, which are diverse (Table 2.5.2). It presents with widespread pruritus (itching) of the body, in almost every woman.[9] Midwives unaware of this condition could mistake pruritus for itching caused by normal pregnancy stretching of the skin. However, this would only occur over the abdomen, whereas OC affects the limbs, the soles of the hands and feet and the trunk.[13] There is no visible rash with OC, suggesting that the cause could be the increased bile salts collecting in the bloodstream.[2]

Table 2.5.3 Conditions associated with OC symptoms[3,14,23]

Pre-eclampsia
HELLP (Haemolysis elevated liver enzymes and low platelets)
Acute fatty liver of pregnancy
Hepatitis
Gallstones
Primary biliary cirrhosis
Primary sclerosing cholangitis
Drug induced reactions
Toxoplasmosis
Cytomegalovirus
Epstein-Barr virus

Table 2.5.4 Liver enzymes that could be raised[7]

Aspartate aminotransferase (AST)
Alanine aminotransterase (ALT)
Alkaline phosphatase
Gamma-glutamate transpeptidase
Bilirubin

In up to 50% of cases, urinary tract infections (UTIs) can coincide with the manifestation of OC.[15] Symptoms could recur, though less severely, in the months following delivery, during menstruation and when taking the combined oral contraceptive pill.[12,16]

Aetiology

The cause of OC and stillbirth has still not been identified. However, there are various theories. One theory suggests that the liver cannot cope with high oestrogen levels, and that this interferes with biochemical activity.[11] This in turn elevates bile acid levels in the blood and liver, which causes pruritus.[1,2] However, if this were the case, why doesn't every pregnant woman suffer from OC? It could be due to placental dysfunction, as OC diminishes after delivery. However, as symptoms can recur with contraceptive therapy, it is likely that hormones play a role. Some investigations suggest that bile acids have a role in the cause of preterm delivery.[3] It is possible that OC sufferers have to experience different predisposing factors enabling this condition to take hold. Other theories are explained in full elsewhere.[3]

Risk factors

There is a tendency for OC to occur during the winter season, with levels at their highest in November.[3] The incidence varies between different countries.[11,17] Further pregnancies are susceptible to OC, manifesting earlier and more severely, especially if jaundice developed during the first pregnancy.[1,3] The rate is extremely high, at over 75%.[18] Multiple pregnancies carry a greater risk of the condition than singleton ones.[19] There have been suggestions that OC can be passed from father to daughter genetically with a dominant trait.[20,21] Vitamin K is a component in the clotting mechanism; therefore there is a risk of primary postpartum haemorrhage if fat-soluble vitamin K is not absorbed into the intestine.[17,21,22]

Diagnosis and management

A community midwife is usually the first person to be suspicious of OC. Antenatal visits could be increased during winter months or during the third trimester, so possible OC sufferers can be identified. The woman should be admitted to hospital for diagnostic tests. Some women will be discharged and monitored antenatally, having to return to hospital for regular tests. Those with more severe symptoms should be admitted until delivery. The management of OC should be undertaken with the involvement of specialists who have a good working knowledge of the condition.[1] The condition cannot be diagnosed using a single test. It is diagnosed via symptoms and exclusion of other conditions.[11,12] (Table 2.5.3) However, some conditions can co-exist with OC.

The condition should be monitored regularly, however no single test proves the state of the condition or the fetus.[6,11,24] The aim is to sustain the pregnancy with good maternal and fetal wellbeing until induction of labour (IOL) can be undertaken at 37-38 weeks gestation.[7] This ensures that the fetus has a better chance of survival outside the womb with enhanced lung maturation. IOL reduces the risk of perinatal mortality, however the resultant rates are still above that of the general population.[3]

Liver function tests (LFTs) should be undertaken; these show elevated liver enzymes that are present in liver cell destruction.[13] Table 2.5.4 shows the possible liver enzymes which could be raised. However, detecting the levels of serum bile acids (SBAs) in the blood is more likely to indicate OC than LFTs.[2,13] The level of SBAs indicative of OC differs between laboratories, therefore midwives need to seek this information from their local area. If levels are normal then retesting needs to be done 7 days later.[13]

Bile acids increase 100 times more in OC, and this can occur before the manifestation of pruritus.[22,25] The levels also increase earlier than liver enzymes, therefore testing SBAs has greater reliability.[21] Sometimes raised bile acids are the only biochemical abnormality seen.[7] Liver function tests should be performed regularly if the SBA or aspartate aminotransferase (AST) levels are raised.[21] Pancreatitis should be excluded as a possibility, by measuring the serum amylase.[3] Clotting studies should be undertaken, in case the woman needs administration of vitamin K on one or more occasions during the pregnancy.[11,13,21] Irrespective of prothrombin ratios, 10mg vitamin K should be given intramuscularly weekly beginning at 36 weeks gestation.[18] It is advised that both the woman and fetus have prophylactic vitamin K after delivery. This can prevent the woman from suffering a postpartum haemorrhage and the fetus from an intracranial haemorrhage.[11]

Blood pressure should be taken according to severity and treatment initiated. Urinalysis should show existing bilirubin, suggesting raised bile acids, or protein, suggesting a urinary tract infection.[3,18]

Fetal movements should be measured daily, indicating fetal wellbeing.[6] Regular cardiotocography (CTG) should be done to ascertain fetal compromise.[8,13] Regular ultrasound scans (USS) and biophysical profiles (BPP) can be performed to show fetal growth and wellbeing.[8,13] Topical relief from pruritus could include aqueous cream, and oil calamine lotion.[18]

All affected women should receive an ultrasound scan of the biliary tract to eliminate the possibility of biliary stones being present.[18] The biochemical state should be monitored until it has returned to normal levels.[18] Women should be counselled because of the possible emotional trauma sustained during the pregnancy. The possibility of recurrence in the next pregnancy should be included.[18]

It has been postulated that levels of maternal bile acids may not correspond with perinatal outcome.[26,27] Fetal distress cannot be reliably indicated using a CTG, during the intrapartum period.[6]

The management of cholestasis is still not satisfactory, as tests cannot show definitive answers. The severity of the symptoms and biochemical activity is not always a predictor of the fetal condition.[7] However, active management has been shown to improve perinatal outcome.[6,11,12]

Treatment

There have been no conclusive findings for the treatment of OC. However, there are various drugs that have had an impact on OC. One study showed that dexamethazone was effective.[28] It reduces oestrogen levels and bile acid levels, which in turn reduces pruritus. It also has two positive effects upon the baby. Firstly, reducing bile acids could reduce the risk of stillbirth. Secondly, if preterm delivery did occur then there would be better lung maturation, to help sustain life. The study did not show any adverse reactions to the treatment. However, only 10 participants were involved, therefore further studies should be undertaken to support the findings.

One study found that a combination of ursodeoxycholic acid and S-adenosylmethionine had positive effects upon reducing pruritus, bilirubin levels, bile salts and alkaline phosphatase.[29] It has been suggested that bile acids crossing over into the fetal system is the cause of fetal compromise.[14] These two drugs may have positive effects upon perinatal outcome. This was supported in another study, with deliveries occurring at or near term, with thriving, adequate birthweight babies in comparison to preterm deliveries with one stillbirth under the placebo management.[30]

Role of the midwife

Midwives have to be able to identify OC sufferers. To do this they must know the symptoms, risk factors and management necessary, so that the women receive optimum care. Once a history has been taken of symptoms and recent drug therapy, they must ensure that the woman receives the necessary diagnostic testing and management. They should ensure that all blood tests, USS, CTGs, BPP and general observations are undertaken and not ignored. Midwives must be familiar with blood values and when they become abnormal. Awareness of local policies and procedures should be a priority, as different areas may lack resources or manage OC differently. However, these are only guidelines; every woman and case is an individual one and should be managed accordingly.

Midwives must be able to support the woman, as this is a very distressing and debilitating condition, which could affect a woman in many different ways. The women suffers physiologically through pruritus, increase in blood pressure and fatigue. The midwife can help by suggesting ways of minimising the irritation, such as using topical creams, wearing loose cotton clothing, having cold baths and having short nails to avoid scratching the skin. The woman should be offered analgesia and antihistamines for relief. However, antihistamines in a preterm baby can elevate respiratory difficulties, by causing sedation.[11] Administration may have to be assessed if induction of labour is impending. If the woman is suffering from sleep deprivation, due to pruritus being worse at night, then anxiolytics could be offered.

The midwife should try to allay fears. Women can be reassured that the outlook is generally good.[16] Support groups are available, and the midwife should be able to facilitate access to these. The woman may suffer emotionally as she is entering an unknown passage, which can be frightening. She may suffer socially, as she may have to be admitted to hospital leaving other children at home. Family members should be included, consulted, and supported, as they count too! Some women suffer so much from the pruritus that it prevents them from going out socially.

If preterm delivery is foreseen then the midwife should organise a visit for the woman to see the neonatal unit and speak to staff, so that she will know what to expect, and be familiar with the environment.

Women must be involved in both their own and their baby's care. They should be informed at each stage and informed consent obtained. Informed choice is also paramount. Decisions should be made with the woman, otherwise psychological consequences could ensue. The woman may start to resent the pregnancy for making her endure the agonising pruritus. The midwife must be a proficient listener and answer any questions with recent research evidence.[9]

Continuity of care and carer would be most desirable, as the woman will feel more at ease and people involved will know the case history so information is less likely to be overlooked. Good involvement with other health professionals will mean that this is also less likely to occur. If continuity is not available then the midwife should ensure, as in all cases, that record keeping is of the highest quality.

When advising women about contraception, midwives should advise women to avoid the combined contraceptive pill in case symptoms recur.[7] Midwives should always try and focus on the normality of pregnancy, as OC sufferers may not enjoy or reap satisfaction in this very important time of their life, due to intervention and persisting symptoms.

Conclusion

There are still differences of opinion in the aetiology and management of OC. Further studies need to be undertaken to remedy this problem. The aetiology, diagnosis, management and treatment need to be identified and enhanced, enabling greater benefit to OC sufferers. It is imperative that midwives and other health professionals remain vigilant to this condition, as they are very involved in the care of these women. Their awareness can ensure that fetal demise is reduced.

Midwives should draw upon their midwifery skills and be 'with woman', in an obstetrically led pregnancy. Woman-centred care should be provided at all times. This condition is a serious one, and not 'much ado about nothing!' As this is a condition which is now being recognised, hopefully all cases will be identified and action taken.

REFERENCES

1 Chambers J. Obstetric cholestasis – A cause of unexplained stillbirth? Changing Childbirth Update 1996; 5: 4.

2 Redfearn J. Obstetric cholestasis. Midwifery Matters 1994; 62: 14.

3 Raine-Fenning N, Kilby M. Obstetric cholestasis. British Liver Trust factsheet. Ipswich: British Liver Trust.

4 Leevy C, Koneru B, Klein K. Recurrent familial prolonged intrahepatic cholestasis of pregnancy associated with chronic liver disease. Gastroenterology 1997; 113(3): 966-72.

5 Fisk N, Storey B. Fetal outcome in obstetric cholestasis. Br J Obstet Gynaecol 1988; 95(11): 1137-43.

6 Rioseco AJ, Ivankovic MB, Manzur A et al. Intrahepatic cholestasis of pregnancy: A retrospective case-control study of perinatal outcome. Am J Obstet Gynaecol 1994; 170(3): 890-5.

7 Nelson-Piercy C. Handbook of obstetric medicine. Oxford: Isis Medical Media, 1997.

8 Beischer N, Mackay EV, Colditz PB. Obstetrics and the newborn – An illustrated textbook. 3rd Edn. London: WB Saunders Ltd, 1997.

9 Redfearn J, Chambers J. Itching in pregnancy? Midwives must be alert. Midwives 1996; 109(1297): 36.

10 Redfearn J, Chambers J. Obstetric cholestasis. New Generation 1994; 13(1): 4-5.

11 Fagan E. Intrahepatic cholestasis of pregnancy. BMJ 1994; 309(6964): 1243-4.

12 Coombes J. Cholestasis in pregnancy: A challenging disorder. BMJ 2000; 8(9): 565-70.

13 British Liver Trust Information Service. What is obstetric cholestasis? [online] http://www.britishlivertrust.org.uk/publications/obstetric_cholestasis.html [03/12/00].

14 Floreani A, Paternoster D, Grella V, Sacco S, Gangemi M, Chiaramonte M. Ursodeoxycholic acid in intrahepatic cholestasis of pregnancy. Br J Obstet Gynaecol 1994; 101(1): 64-5.

15 Reyes H. The spectrum of liver and gastrointestinal disease seen in cholestasis of pregnancy. Gastroenterol Clin North Am 1992; 21(4): 905-21.

16 Fagan E. Disorders of the liver biliary system and pancreas. In: Swiet M (ed). Medical disorders in obstetric practice. 3rd Edn. Oxford: Blackwell Science Ltd, 1995.

17 Price S. Obstetric Cholestasis. Nursing Times 1995; 91(48): 57-8.

18 Walters BNJ. Hepatic and gastrointestinal disease. In: James DK, Steer PJ, Weiner CP, Gonik B (eds). High-risk pregnancy – Management options. London: WB Saunders Ltd, 1999.

19 Gonzalez MC, Reyes H, Arrese M et al. Intrahepatic cholestasis of pregnancy in twin pregnancies. J Hepatol 1989; 9(1): 84-90.

20 Holzbach RT, Sivak DA et al. Familial recurrent intrahepatic cholestasis of pregnancy: A genetic study providing evidence for transmission of a sex-linked dominant trait. Gastroenterology 1983; 85(1): 175-9.

21 Warwick K. Diagnosis and treatment for cholestasis in pregnancy. Midwives 1996; 109(1297): 37-8.

22 Axten S. Obstetric cholestasis. Modern Midwife 1996; 6(4): 32-3.

23 Olsson R, Tysk C, Aldenborg F et al. Prolonged postpartum course of intrahepatic cholestasis of pregnancy. Gastroenterology 1993; 105(1): 267-71.

24 Reid R, Ivey KJ, Rencoret RH et al. Fetal complications of obstetric cholestasis. BMJ 1976; 1: 870-2.

25 Schoor-Lesnick B, Lebovics E et al Liver disease unique to pregnancy. Am J Gastroenterol 1991; 86(6): 659-62.

26 Laatikainen T, Ikonen E. Serum bile acids in cholestasis of pregnancy. Obstet Gynaecol 1977; 50(3): 313-8.

27 Laatikainen T, Tulenheimo A. Maternal serum bile acid levels and fetal distress in cholestasis of pregnancy. Int J Gynaecol Obstet 1984; 22(2): 91-4.

28 Hirvioja M, Tuimala R, Vuori J. The treatment of intrahepatic cholestasis of pregnancy by dexamethazone. Br J Obstet Gynaecol 1992; 99(2): 109-11.

29 Nicastri PL, Diaferia A, Tartagni M et al. A randomised placebo-controlled trial of ursodeoxycholic acid and S-adenosylmethionine in the treatment of intrahepatic cholestasis of pregnancy. Br J Obstet Gynaecol 1998; 105(11): 1205-7.

30 Palma J, Reyes H, Ribalta J et al. Ursodeoxycholic acid in the treatment of cholestasis of pregnancy: A randomised double-blind study controlled with placebo. J Hepatol; 27(6): 1022-8. http://www.munksgaard.dk/hepatology/abs/he270610.html [03/12/00].

Obstetric cholestasis

A mother's experience

Jenny Chambers

I was a Building Society manager in 1986 when I was first pregnant. I had a good career, Richard, my husband, was doing well in his work and we had just moved into a new house. Everything seemed to be going just the way I had planned it.

From an obstetric point of view the pregnancy was textbook but at around 30 weeks I started itching. Nothing horrendous; it only seemed to be on my hands and feet and didn't keep me awake at night. At 36 weeks I saw my obstetrician for my final check up. He asked me if I had had any problems and I mentioned the itching. He reassured me that itching in pregnancy was normal, pronounced me to be fit and healthy and I went home.

The next day I went into labour and 24 hours later delivered our daughter, Victoria. She was dead. A post mortem revealed that she was 'just one of those things' – an unexplained stillbirth. We were devastated.

I blamed myself. I gave up work and became obsessed with conceiving again. Eventually, after a year I became pregnant but at ten weeks I miscarried. I finally learnt that there are some things in life that you simply cannot control. Seven weeks later my period still hadn't materialised – I was pregnant.

At around 28 weeks two things happened. I began itching again and I broke my knee cap. I remained in hospital but was allowed home at weekends. I mentioned the itching and the doctors said they would do some blood tests. I was told that they were normal and that the itching was just 'one of those things'. At night I would draw the curtains around my bed, strip off, and try to cool down. I was limited in how much I could walk because of the plaster cast and would lie on the bed crying with frustration, literally tearing at my arms and legs. I obtained a knitting needle to slip inside the plaster cast so that I could scratch. Finally, thankfully, at 38 weeks I was induced and Alexander was delivered. We were ecstatic.

In 1990 I was pregnant once more. Yet again the pregnancy was textbook. Once again the itching returned. We told the doctors and midwives who reassured us that there was nothing wrong. I was extremely concerned. My gut feeling was that there was something wrong but I didn't know what. I had more blood tests and was told they were normal. We asked for an early delivery but were told that there was no reason to; I was 'normal' now. I found that hard to accept. I argued that how could I be with a previous unexplained stillbirth? I was told to stop worrying, it couldn't happen again. Still the itching got worse. It would seem to arrive early evening and not leave until dawn, making me constantly scratch and forcing to me to walk endlessly around the house because to sit still was unbearable. Richard moved into the spare room. The hospital staff seemed to stop listening. I felt completely alone.

Finally it was agreed that I could be induced at 39 weeks. Two days before the induction date I went to the community midwife to be checked over. We listened to the fetal heartbeat, it was strong and steady. Two hours later I went into labour. We arrived at the unit full of anticipation. We left the next day, empty-handed. My worst nightmare had come true; our baby had been stillborn – another little girl. We called her Olivia.

We were referred to a different consultant at the hospital who advised us that I had obstetric cholestasis. The blood tests I'd had done in my previous pregnancies were in fact liver function tests and they were abnormal. They had been ignored because I hadn't been jaundiced. The consultant broke the news that I should have been delivered by no later than 38 weeks.

After the initial anger we decided that we wanted to try and prevent what had happened to us from happening to other parents. I started a Helpline, worked to raise awareness of the condition and helped to form a research group within the hospital. Collaboration with a London hospital took place in 1997 and our research has been growing steadily since then.

With the encouragement of my new consultant and hepatologist I went on to have Timothy and finally I began to heal. It has been a long, painful, strangely enriching, often frustrating journey but I wouldn't want to change a thing. I am the mother of four children and very proud to be so.

Is folic acid the best thing in sliced bread?

Judith Ockenden

Biology is complex, messy and richly various, like real life.
Peter Medawar, Nobel Laureate in Medicine, 1968

Biology altered by disease is even more messy, and our discovery of it sometimes progresses in unforeseen ways.
John Hoey, Editor in Chief of the Canadian Medical Association Journal, 1998

Twenty years ago, as a student of biochemistry, I learned that tetrahydrofolate is one of the B vitamins (sometimes called B9). It is needed in small amounts to facilitate many of the chemical reactions inside us that lead to growth and development – the pathways making the amino acids which form proteins and the nucleic acids which make DNA. We can't make it ourselves, so we rely on supplies from our diet or from the microorganisms in our gut that make it.

Five years ago, as a student of childbirth education, I heard that folate deficiency was one factor in the defective development of the neural tube in unborn babies – causing spina bifida and anencephaly. In fact, this possibility had first been raised as early as 1964. Following the publication of evidence supporting this theory in the early 1980s, the Medical Research Council launched a large trial involving around 1800 women who had already had an affected pregnancy, in 33 centres in seven countries. They were allocated randomly to groups either taking or not taking folic acid, with or without multivitamins.[1]

The trial was stopped early when the evidence was judged to be conclusive: folic acid supplementation could prevent 72% of neural tube defects in women previously affected. These women have a risk ten times that of the general population of having another affected pregnancy, and so have more to gain from supplementation, BUT 95% of babies with neural tube defects are conceived to first-time mothers. The MRC study said 'it is implausible that serial occurrences of the same event

have separate causes'. In other words, if it helps women known to be at risk, it must also help prevent these abnormalities in the general population.

Natural folate is found particularly in leafy green vegetables, potatoes, pulses and yeast extract. Cooking and storage reduce the amount of folic acid in food, and there is great variability in the level of consumption of different foods, but on average, people get about 0.2 milligrams (mg, equivalent to 200 micrograms) from their diet. This is not enough to prevent neural tube defects (NTDs); this is thought to require 0.4-0.6 mg (see later). The Department of Health recommended, therefore, that women planning to have a baby should take folic acid supplements daily from the time they start trying to conceive until 12 weeks after conception:

- women who already had an affected child should take 5 mg, and
- unaffected women should take 0.4 mg.

The problem with this, of course, is that about half of all pregnancies are unplanned, and by the time the pregnancy is confirmed, the timespan in which folic acid does any good has passed. In addition, a recent Mori Poll for the Charity, Action Research, found that only 56% of women aged 15-55 were aware that folic acid can prevent birth defects, and only 15% of women with babies or young children had followed Department of Health advice on supplementation. More than 70% were in favour of fortifying flour with folic acid – but would they still be pro-fortification if they were given more information?

The benefits of supplementation

Folic acid supplement is a synthetic form that is approximately twice as easy for the body to use as the natural form.[2,3] In the UK, in 1996, it was already added to 50% of breakfast cereals and about 10% of bread. In

1998, in the US, all grain products started to be fortified with folic acid. In practice, this meant that 274 million people were being exposed to extra folic acid in order to prevent 2000 neural tube defects per year.[4]

Soon, however, another benefit was confirmed: folic acid reduces the amount of an amino acid called homocysteine in the serum, a high level of which is associated with cardiovascular disease. And there is also some evidence that folic acid can help to prevent colon and rectal cancers, orofacial clefts in babies and mental health problems in the elderly.[5]

So, isn't supplementation of staple foods a very good idea? It certainly seems it is for those groups of people affected. But what about the rest of the population?

The doubts about supplementation

Folic acid is water-soluble and so readily excreted, and is not known to be toxic. However, no long-term studies on the effects of folic acid supplementation have been carried out. It is possible to think of many therapeutic chemicals that can be toxic at higher concentration: paracetamol, for example is safe (even in pregnancy) in the recommended doses – but an overdose can lead to irreversible liver failure. Oxygen (21% of air) is vital for life, but caused blindness when given pure to premature babies in the 1950s. Vitamin A, vital for growth and repair of cells, has been found to cause birth defects if consumed in excess in the first trimester of pregnancy. For this reason, pregnant women are advised not to eat liver – a rich source of vitamin A and folic acid!

A recent study[3] has shown that giving pregnant rats the amount of folic acid equivalent to 4 mg per day in humans (the level recommended for the prevention of NTD recurrence), throughout their pregnancy resulted in a significant reduction in the weight and length of the newborn rats. They suggested that these levels of folic acid are impairing the use of dietary protein. Another study[6] found that people given more than 0.3 mg folic acid per day for 5 days had non-metabolised folic acid in their serum. The long-term effects of this are unknown.

The Federal Drug Administration (FDA) in the US recommends, for adults, a daily dose of 0.4 mg, and a safe upper limit of no more than 1 mg. The recommended dose to prevent neural tube defects is 0.6 mg. At present food is supplemented at a level that will give, on average, an extra 0.1mg per day. Natural dietary sources account for about 0.2 mg, and anyone taking multivitamins or folic acid supplements will get another 0.4 mg. This gives a total of 0.7 mg. It has been found, however, that some food products contain up to double the amount of folic acid claimed on the label,[4] possibly increasing this 'average total' to 0.8 mg. This is still less

than 1 mg – but remember this is an average value. The wide variation in intake from all sources means that some people will consume more than the recommended daily limit.

There are now calls in the US to double the amount of fortification, to give an extra 0.2 mg per day, to give added protection to those not taking supplements. The UK Food Standards Agency has just finished consulting on a proposal to fortify wheat flour at a level to achieve 0.2 mg per day.[7] A Government decision is awaited.

It can be seen that, if these proposals are adopted, it will not be too hard for anyone to exceed the recommended 0.4 mg per day dose, and for more people to exceed the maximum recommended dose of 1 mg.[4,6] Remember too that children often eat large quantities of fortified cereal products: bread, flour, pasta, rice, breakfast cereals. The US Institute of Medicine recommends that children aged 1-3 years take 0.3mg per day, and those aged 4-8 take 0.4 mg per day.[4]

Do we yet know enough about the effects of increased folic acid to support calls to fortify foods at these levels or should we be concentrating our efforts on targeting those people at risk?

Known risks of supplementation

One drawback of supplementation is well known. Pernicious anaemia is a serious condition that causes neurological damage resulting from a deficiency of vitamin B12. Folic acid can alleviate the symptoms of this disease, which is great if you know you've got it, but bad news if you don't. While the symptoms don't show, the nerve damage continues, often irreversibly. At present it is not known how much folic acid you have to take before the anaemia symptoms are masked – indeed, available evidence suggests it varies in different people. The people most at risk of this condition are the elderly.

There is also concern by the US Institute of Medicine about the effects of high folic acid on people treated with anticonvulsants and methotrexate.[4,5]

Can less be best?

The reason that most women are advised to take 0.4 mg is based on observational studies in which women took multivitamins containing this amount of folic acid – the recommended daily allowance of the FDA.[4,8]

What is the lowest level, then, that could prevent the estimated 50% of NTDs that are related to folate metabolism? Mills[4] has conducted studies that suggest an extra 0.2 mg is enough to prevent 41% of NTDs. This is supported by observations in Adelaide, Australia.[9] Coincidentally, this also seems to be the amount that protects against cardiovascular disease.[2]

Thus, the current US level of fortification (equivalent to an extra 0.1mg) may be enough to take care of the health concerns, particularly as folate stores rise to a higher level with increased intake over time.

Before increasing levels of supplementation, we must have more evidence of how neural tube defect rates are being affected, and of how supplementation affects the rest of the population. In fact, supplementation makes it very difficult to conduct randomised control trials, because the whole population is being exposed to higher levels of folic acid.

Outstanding questions

As well as issues surrounding the effects of supplementation, there are a number of fundamental questions about the link between folic acid and neural tube defects that remain to be answered. For example:

- The UK has one of the highest NTD rates but is unlikely to be particularly deficient in folic acid.[1]
- The rate of fall in NTDs is decreasing.[8]
- Low risk populations have not shown the same relationship between supplementation and occurrence of malformations.[8]

There is little doubt that extra folic acid is of enormous benefit to some people in some situations. Whether it is beneficial to those same people in different circumstances, or to the population as a whole, is surely still under question. For now, I would argue that we should be cautious about food fortification, but passionate about educating everyone, from an early age, about how and when folic acid can benefit themselves and their babies.

Acknowledgement

I would like to thank Rosie Dodds for her helpful comments on this article.

REFERENCES

1 MRC Vitamin Study Research Group. Prevention of neural tube defects: Results of the Medical Research Council Vitamin Study. Lancet 1991; 338(8760): 131-7.
2 Oakley GP. Eat right and take a multivitamin. New England Journal of Medicine 1998; 338(15): 1060-1.
3 Achon M, Reyes L, Alonso-Aperte E, Ubeda N, Varela-Moreiras G. High dietary folate supplementation affects gestational development and dietary protein utilization in rats. Journal of Nutrition 1999; 129: 1204-8.
4 Mills JL. Fortification of foods with folic acid: How much is enough? New England Journal of Medicine 2000; 342: 1442-5.
5 Clarkson C. Folic acid: Should there be mandatory fortification? New Digest 1999; June: 19-20. (Available from The National Childbirth Trust, Alexandra House, Oldham Terrace, Acton, London W3 6NH.)
6 Kelly P, McPartlin J, Goggins M, Weir DG and Scott JM. Unmetabolized folic acid in serum: Acute studies in subjects consuming fortified foods and supplements. American Journal of Clinical Nutrition 1997; 65: 1790-5.
7 Barrowclough D, Ford F. Folic acid fortification: Proposed UK recommendations. The Practising Midwife 2000; 3(6): 32-3.
8 Mason J, McNabb M. Folic acid supplementation: Is it a safe option? British Journal of Midwifery 2000; 8(9): 581-6.
9 Halliday JL, Merilyn R. Letter to the Editor. New England Journal of Medicine 2000; 343(13): 970.

Massage in pregnancy

Mario-Paul Cassar

Massage therapy can be of great benefit during the prenatal period, in labour and post-partum. The more common effects it can offer are to relieve some of the discomforts associated with pregnancy, to maintain the overall function of the body and to provide emotional support. It is increasingly being sought by pregnant women and progressively practised by health carers such as nurses and midwives.

General effects

Hormonal changes, added weight and postural changes are some of the aetiological factors behind the back pain often endured during pregnancy.[1,2] One of the main applications of massage, particularly during the later months of pregnancy is to alleviate the pain in the lumbar area, and in some cases that of sciatica which is often connected with tightness of the lumbar muscles or the piriformis.

The hypotonicity in the peripheral blood vessels (caused by the increased production of progesterone) and the pressure of the uterine weight on the pelvic vessels are contributory factors to a sluggish circulation, leg oedema and varicose veins. The slow venous return in the iliac, femoral and saphenous veins can also increase the body's susceptibility to blood clot formation. Massage movements like effleurage[3] can be preventative in this aspect, as they help to create the 'back-pressure' needed to maintain the blood flow in the pelvic and peripheral vessels.

Massage has a number of beneficial effects on the other systems of the body. For example, glandular secretions are improved and consequently hormone levels and their overall effects are 'normalised'. By improving the systemic circulation massage also increases the supply of nutrients to the placenta. With the improved circulation the haemoglobin content of the blood increases. This in turn prevents (or lowers) the severity of anaemia; it also reduces fatigue. Another benefit of massage is the improved function of organs. An enhanced liver function, for instance, leads to the elimination of toxins and subsequently to an elevation of the energy levels.

Anxiety and mood swings can be a feature of pregnancy and massage is an excellent way of providing relaxation and support. The calming effect of massage can also be seen as extending to the baby in utero. Relaxing massage can be applied throughout pregnancy. Through its effect on the parasympathetic nervous system[4] it can stimulate the production of the body's natural endorphins and decrease blood pressure.

Reduced peristaltic activity and constipation are often present during pregnancy. Abdominal and colon massage is normally used to reflexively improve peristalsis and mechanically drain the colon. However, as pressure on the abdomen is best avoided, massage is applied on 'reflex areas' to the digestive system;[5] these include the thighs, the buttocks and the feet (reflex zones).

To an extent all of the massage movements help to maintain tissue pliability, particularly with the use of an appropriate body cream or oil, and can therefore prevent the likelihood of stretch marks. Massage to the abdomen however is best avoided except very lightly for the purpose of applying lotions and then only carried out with a flat palm of the hand. The perineum too can be massaged during pregnancy to maintain the flexibility and elasticity in the tissues thereby lessening the need for an episiotomy during childbirth. As it is not ethical for the massage therapist to carry this out, instructions can be given to the pregnant woman or her partner.

The first trimester

Massage is unlikely to harm the fetus or disturb the natural processes. However, being such a delicate and important time for the expectant mother it is advisable that any possible complications are avoided. Massage on the abdominal area is specifically not recommended during this phase and systemically contraindicated whilst there is still morning sickness or vomiting. Relaxing massage movements are otherwise of benefit.

Second and third trimesters

Studies have shown that 48-56 per cent of all pregnant women experience backache during pregnancy, mostly in the sacro-iliac region but also in the lumbar and thoracic spine.[6] The additional weight that is carried anteriorly, in the breasts and abdomen, alters the centre of gravity and consequently the pregnant woman's postural integrity. Fluid retention and a systemic increase in body weight add to the stress on the structure. The imbalance is compounded further by the pregnancy hormone relaxin, which softens the ligaments, fascia and tendons and, in so doing, causes a slight instability of the lumbar and pelvic structures.

In an attempt to steady her posture, the pregnant woman tends to laterally rotate her hips and walks with a waddle. This leads to a malfunction of the iliopsoas and piriformis muscles on both sides. The calf muscles are additionally susceptible to cramping, most likely related to the pregnant woman having to hyperextend the knees in order to counterbalance the weight at the front. These imbalances create a strain on the majority of the postural muscles. Those of the back and neck, for example, become overworked, fatigued, nodular and likely to house trigger points (hypersensitive zones which are the source of radiating pain to other regions). Understandably there is an exacerbation of discomfort, particularly in the pelvic area, during the last few months of pregnancy. Some studies indicate that the most uncomfortable period is between the fifth and ninth month.[6] During the second and third trimesters massage to the back and legs is perhaps the most needed of all movements as it helps to ease the pain of overworked and fatigued muscles and to reduce trigger points.

Contraindications

It is an essential precaution that all massage movements are carried out without causing pain to the pregnant woman. Adrenal stress hormones, released as a response to pain, have the effect of elevating blood pressure, respiration rate and heart rate; the immune function is also lowered and blood flow to the uterus is impaired.[7] It is feasible to imagine how these same negative effects of the stress hormones can also diffuse into the fetal circulation through the placenta.

As indicated earlier, massage on the pregnant abdomen is avoided other than very superficially for the purpose of applying creams or lotions. Compression is also avoided in the inguinal region as it can generate pressure on the iliac and femoral veins.

Systemic massage is also contraindicated if complications arise during the pregnancy particularly when there is a risk of increased intrauterine pressure. A case in point is an abnormality of the placenta (detachment or dysfunction) or irregularities in the uterus or cervix. Equally significant are disorders that can influence the blood supply to the fetus such as high blood pressure and multiple fetuses. A further contraindication is pain in the abdomen when it is not related to the later stage of pregnancy. Other precautions relate to persistent diarrhoea and gestational diabetes. Itching without the presence of a skin rash may be indicative of obstetric cholestasis and is a further contraindication to massage.

During the middle and later months of pregnancy, massage with the subject lying supine is best avoided as in this position the weight of the fetus presses on the major blood vessels like the inferior vena cava. Massage in the prone position should be avoided after the twelfth week of gestation or much earlier in the case of multiple fetuses. Even with the use of special cushions or equipment, the prone position may increase the intrauterine pressure and will inevitably intensify the tension on the over-strained uterine and lumbar ligaments. Due to the laxity in the ligaments, traction on any of the joints is contraindicated. Persistent or severe backache may need referral to a 'manipulation therapist' such as an osteopath or craniosacral practitioner.

Massage techniques

The massage movements can be carried out with the subject sitting on a chair or stool and supporting their arms, head and shoulders on a table in front of them. They can also be carried out with the subject side-lying on the massage couch. Cushions and bolsters are necessary to help support the pregnant woman and ensure comfort and safety. It is equally important for the operator to adopt a relaxed and comfortable posture whilst applying the massage. The principal objectives of the massage techniques are to induce relaxation, improve the circulation and ease muscle tension. It is also very effective in reducing pain.[8] The frequently-used massage movements are effleurage (stroking with the palms, the thumbs or the fisted hand), petrissage and kneading. Percussive-type movements such as tapotments are not applicable. Examples of the massage techniques for the back and the legs are described here.

Massage techniques: subject sitting

The lower and upper regions of the back can be massaged with the recipient sitting on a stool or chair, and with her arms resting on the treatment table.

She can either adopt a more upright posture (Figure 2.8.1) or lean forward to rest the weight of the head and shoulders onto the table (Figure 2.8.2). Cushions, folded towels and bolsters can all be used for additional support and comfort.

1. Effleurage to the back can be carried out with the massage practitioner kneeling on one or both knees. The effleurage is applied on the lumbar and thoracic regions, moving in a cephalad direction, using one hand at a time or both hands simultaneously. (Figure 2.8.2)

2. A slightly deeper and more local stroking on the muscles can be applied with the thumbs, placed one on each side of the spine. The effleurage is then carried out as short strokes (5cm) in a cephalad direction, and repeated several times on the same area. The thumb effleurage can be applied to both sides of the spine simultaneously, or on one side at a time. To facilitate an easier movement the whole hand can be moved upward whilst the pressure is mostly applied with the thumb. This technique is similar to the one described with the recipient in a side-lying position.

3. Stretching of the lumbar muscles and fascia can be achieved by using the effleurage du poing technique (Figure 2.8.3). The hands are held in a 'fisted' position and a stroking action is carried out from the upper lumbar area in a caudad direction, covering also the sacral area.

4. The upper region of the back, the neck and upper shoulders can be treated with the thumb effleurage. A kneading movement can also be utilised (Figure 2.8.4); it combines compression with the thumbs as well as a cross-fibre stretch. Compression is applied with the thumbs (lying flat to the skin surface) whilst a counter-pressure is exerted by the fingers on the anterior aspect of the trapezius and levator scapulae muscles. The tissues

are held in this grip as the muscles fibres are rolled forward with the thumbs and stretched transversely, pinching of the tissues being avoided. The grip is then released and the sequence repeated.

Massage techniques: subject side-lying

When the subject is in the side-lying position cushions and bolsters are needed to prop her up and prevent her from rolling onto her abdomen. The uppermost leg should be supported in a horizontal alignment with the hip, in order to avoid excessive side bending or rotation of the spine. A further consideration is that the side-lying patient may also require support underneath her trunk to prevent excessive scoliosis. Treatment procedures are planned so that the subject does not have to change position too often; this minimises any painful stretching of the softened ligaments, for instance those of the symphysis pubis.

Effleurage is used to increase the local circulation, to reduce muscle tightness and to apply a longitudinal stretch to the muscles fibres and the lumbar fascia. Although a firm pressure is applied with these strokes the massage is nonetheless relaxing and should not cause any discomfort. The movements are carried out very slowly, allowing about six seconds to complete each stroke. The thoracic, upper back and cervical areas are also massaged in this side-lying position, using effleurage and petrissage kneading techniques.

1. Palm effleurage movements are applied over the lumbar area and may also extend to the thoracic region. One hand is used to apply the massage whilst the other hand stabilises the pelvis. The direction of the movement is cephalad, commencing in the sacral region (Figure 2.8.5).

2. An additional palm effleurage can be applied from the lower thoracic area in a caudad direction over the lumbar and sacrum in order to stretch the lumbar tissues.

3. Effleurage du poing (fist massage) can be used

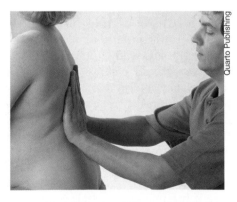

Figure 2.8.1 Massage can be applied with the subject sitting upright on a chair or stool

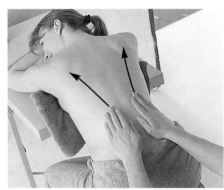

Figure 2.8.2 Palm effleurage to the back in a cephalad direction

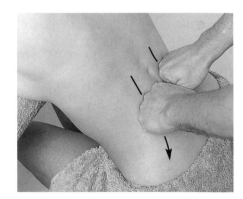

Figure 2.8.3 Effleurage du poing is applied over lumbar tissues and sacral region

instead of the palm effleurage, either to increase the pressure or to facilitate an easier stroking action. It is also ideally suited to stretch the lumbar and sacral fascia as well as the muscles, thereby easing the stress of lordosis. In this case it is applied in a caudad direction (Figure 2.8.6). Effleurage du poing is applied with the hand in a fist. However the fingers are straight, with the fingertips resting on the 'heel' of the hand. The stroke is carried out with the flat surface of the phalanges and not with the knuckles.

4. Thumb effleurage strokes are also carried out on either side of the spine to further release the paravertebral muscles. Thumb pressure is applied very slowly along the muscle fibres and the stroke repeated several times over the same region. (Figure 2.8.7)

5. In addition to the effleurage strokes and some kneading movements, gentle passive stretching of the piriformis muscle can also be applied in this side-lying position. Because of the laxity of the pelvic ligaments however, passive stretching should be kept to a minimum. Post isometric relaxation – where an isometric contraction is carried out against a resistance offered by the operator – may produce sufficient subsequent relaxation without the need of a passive stretch.

6. A passive stretch to the psoas muscle, whilst the patient is in the side-lying position, can help relieve some of the lumbar pain. The operator stands behind the pregnant woman and places a hand underneath the uppermost knee to support the weight of the leg. The subject's knee is held in a flexed position with the foot of the same leg resting against the operator's thigh or pelvis. The operator's other hand is used to stabilise the pelvis thereby reducing any lumbar lordosis; this is important bearing in mind the laxity of the pelvic structures. By taking the uppermost leg into extension, the operator can apply a gentle passive stretch to the psoas muscle on the same side. This can be repeated if the patient lies on the other side.

Massage techniques: lower limbs

In this side-lying position the massage movements are carried out on the lowermost leg, which rests on the treatment couch. If desired, effleurage and petrissage movement can also be applied to the uppermost leg in a similar manner, without the subject having to turn over.

As well as being very relaxing, effleurage massage movements to the lower limbs assist the venous flow and reduce the build-up of fluid. The movements are generally carried out very slowly and with minimal weight. Sustained or deep pressure should be avoided at all times and in particular on the medial aspect of the thigh (bearing in mind the risk of blood clots in the great saphenous and femoral veins). Decreasing the congestion in the lower limbs lessens the possibility of varicose veins even though the effleurage is omitted on areas where these have already developed. Effleurage and gentle kneading movements are also applied to the legs to ease cramps in the calf muscles. Passive movements of the hip joints can be carried out, to maintain the suppleness which would be of benefit during labour. It is vital to bear in mind however that, due to the laxity in the ligaments caused by the relaxin hormone, all joints can be potentially unstable. Any mobilising technique therefore should only be carried out within the range of movement.

1. Draining effleurage movements are applied firstly to the thigh in order to improve the venous return in this region; they are then repeated on the lower leg. Palm effleurage is mostly used and is perhaps the easiest of techniques. One method is for the operator to apply the stroking with one hand on the posterior-medial aspect of the thigh whilst exerting a slight counter-pressure on the anterior-medial aspect with the other hand (Figure 2.8.8). A similar pressure/counter-pressure is used to effleurage the anterior-medial region of the thigh.

2. Petrissage or kneading is carried out on the calf

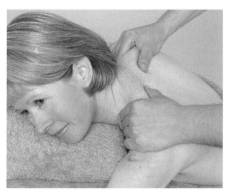

Figure 2.8.4 Kneading – compression and rolling forward of the tissues with thumbs and fingers

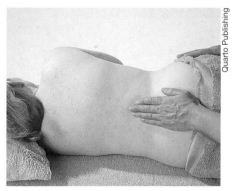

Figure 2.8.5 Effleurage in the side-lying position is applied on either side of the spine

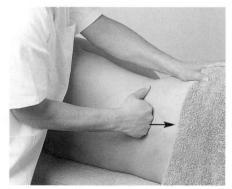

Figure 2.8.6 Effleurage du poing in a caudad direction over the lumbar and sacral tissues

Quarto Publishing

muscles. The operator stands on one side of the massage couch and reaches across to the lowermost leg, in this case the right leg with the subject lying on her right side. Compression of the muscles is applied with the fingers of the right hand exerting pressure against the thumb of the left hand. A slight twisting action is then applied in a clockwise direction, which has the effect of stretching the fibres transversely and breaks up adhesions (Figure 2.8.9). The muscles are then released and the same manoeuvre is repeated but with the hands' position reversed so that the pressure is applied with the fingers of the left hand against the thumb pressure of the right hand.

Labour

During this stage massage is used first and foremost to reduce the anxiety and apprehension associated with labour and parturition. Relaxation promotes the release of the opiates (endorphins and encephalins) whilst limiting the production of adrenalin. Massage also helps relieve the pain of contractions, eases muscular tension and alleviates cramps.[9] Relaxing techniques are also used in between contractions, to enhance relaxation and recovery.

Massage techniques are not pre-planned but applied according to the needs of the recipient. Sometimes she may prefer deep pressure, other times only light stroking is requested; or no massage at all but assistance with the breathing.

The areas where massage is applied can also vary. In the first stage of labour it may be the back, the neck and the legs (especially the thighs). Firm stroking is applied to the site of contraction or pain, or as indicated by the subject. Slow and rhythmic movements are mostly used, applied with the heel of the hand or with the distal phalanges held flat to the skin surface. Pressure can also be applied to the sacrum and buttock and is generally very effective in relieving the pain of contractions.

However the massage is applied wherever it is needed, even on the abdomen.

In the second and transition stage the subject may not want to be touched on the back at all, in which case soothing strokes to the forehead may be more appropriate. Massage to the feet is very relaxing and very useful when other regions are not available.

Finding the best position to carry out the massage may prove difficult. Lying on the side is one choice, with the recipient supported on cushions or a beanbag. Sitting astride a stool is also a useful arrangement, with the recipient also leaning forward on a beanbag or cushions.

Post-partum

Provided that no complications occur, massage can safely be applied during the puerperal period. Systemic massage is carried out to enhance the general circulation and the elimination of excess fluids. Energy levels are renewed and, emotionally, massage helps the mother to relax and adjust to her new role in life. Reducing stress levels is also instrumental in stimulating the production of milk.

Due to the stretching and weakening of the abdominal muscles during pregnancy, the abdominal tissues must not be stretched further during this postnatal period; stroking to these tissues is therefore carried out from a lateral to a medial direction only. Gentle colon and iliac colon techniques can be included if constipation persists.

Massage is said to encourage the involution of the uterus if it is applied every four hours, in a clockwise direction on the abdomen. As this can be a very painful procedure however it can only be carried out with the recipient's comprehension and consent. If there has been a caesarean birth, however, massage techniques on the abdomen are contraindicated until scar tissues are completely healed.

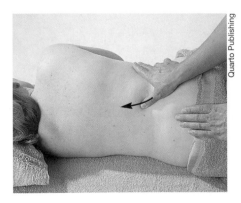

Figure 2.8.7 Short stroking movements with the thumb apply deep local pressure

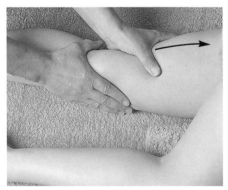

Figure 2.8.8 Effleurage on the posterior-medial aspect – counter-pressure on the anterior aspect

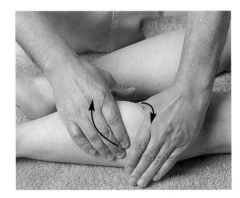

Figure 2.8.9 Petrissage – thumb of left hand pressing against fingers of the right

Back pain may persist for some time following childbirth so treatment to this area is continued using deep thumb effleurage and effleurage du poing. Effleurage and kneading movements are also carried out to the lower limbs, in order to reduce cramps. Massage is continued over the following weeks to help the subject regain muscle tonicity and structural balance.

Conclusion

The relaxation and emotional support offered by massage as well as the benefits it has on the circulation, the lymph system, on muscles, fascia, glands and other organs makes it a very useful aid in the care of the pregnant woman. It can also contribute tremendously towards an enjoyable pregnancy.

Adapted from Handbook of Clinical Massage published by Churchill Livingstone (in press).

REFERENCES

1 Cailliet R. Low Back Pain Syndrome. FA Davis Company, 1995.
2 Hart F (Ed). French's Index of Differential Diagnosis. John Wright & Sons Ltd, 1985.
3 Dubrovsky V. Changes in muscles and venous blood flow after massage. Teoriya i Praktika Fizicheskoi Kultury 1982; 4: 56-7.
4 Tovar MK, Cassmere VL. Touch – the beneficial effects for the surgical patient. AORN Journal 1989; 49: 1356-61.
5 Cassar M-P. Handbook of Massage Therapy. Butterworth-Heinemann, 1999.
6 Ostgaard HC, Andersson GBJ et al. Prevalence of back pain in pregnancy. Spine 1992; 17(1): 53-5.
7 Gorsuch R, Key M. Abnormalities of pregnancy as a function of anxiety and life stress. Psychosomatic Medicine 1974; 36: 353.
8 Jacob M. Massage for the relief of pain; Anatomical and physiological considerations. Physical Therapy Review 1960; 40: 93-8.
9 Chamberlain et al. Pain and its relief in childbirth – the results of a national survey conducted by the National Birth Trust. Churchill Livingstone, 1993.

Reflecting on pregnancy

- Although Gemma Purrett's article draws on a wide variety of research around the area of estimating date of birth, her tool has not yet been tested. Midwives may like to use the tool to work out dates with women in practice in order to assess whether this is – in reality – more accurate than current measures used. (You can contact Gemma via email through www.withwoman. co.uk)

- What is the prevailing attitude towards hyperemesis in your workplace? I'm sure I am not alone in having worked in places where hyperemesis is still seen as more of a psychological than a physical condition. Where this is the case, what can we do to change attitudes about this condition and provide the support that women clearly need?

- Following on from this, if there is a psychological element in conditions encountered in pregnancy (and we are always striving to remember that the mind and spirit are just as much a part of the experience as the body), how can we work towards ways of helping women address this factor without blame or judgement entering the equation?

- What do you do when women tell you that they are feeling 'itchy' in pregnancy? How can we best differentiate conditions such as obstetric cholestasis from other conditions (for example excema or psoriasis), which can also cause itching? How can we work to ensure that we do 'pick up' women who have symptoms which may be indicative of a condition such as this (or may be a sign of something less potentially harmful)? Is it a case of referring everybody who may have a problem to another specialist, or can we use midwifery judgement to discern who really needs obstetric or other help?

- Is it possible that we could incorporate pregnancy massage into midwifery practice, or at least facilitate groups of women who might like to offer massages to each other?

Focus on:
Domestic violence

SECTION CONTENTS

Domestic violence in pregnancy

How can midwives make a difference?

Sally Price, Kathleen Baird

This article outlines the prevalence of domestic violence, and indicates the link between domestic violence and pregnancy outcomes. It acknowledges that midwives in the UK are reluctant to routinely screen for domestic violence in pregnancy because they feel ill-equipped to do so. By the implementation of various multi-professional training programmes and with support from managers and supervisors of midwives, North Bristol Trust has been able to introduce guidelines for dealing with domestic violence. Evaluation demonstrates that a majority of midwives in the Trust now have the necessary skills and knowledge required to screen for domestic violence in pregnancy.

Domestic violence is an issue that affects both users and professionals providing maternity services. The Government has recognised the need to raise the awareness, recognition and understanding of domestic violence, to encourage victims to come forward.[1,2] However, research has shown that midwives do not feel adequately prepared to deal with victims of domestic violence, and that a gap in knowledge and practice experience requires education and support.[3]

Background

Domestic violence is a major public health issue. It could be suggested it has reached epidemic proportions, with one in four women experiencing violence in the home at some point in their lives.[4] This is likely to be an underestimate, with on average a woman being assaulted 35 times before reporting it to the police.[5] The health problems experienced by victims are widely varied and include psychological as well as physical effects. Victims also have an increased risk of overuse of alcohol, cigarettes, and prescribed and illegal drugs,[6] using these drugs of solace as a form of coping mechanism. Violence occurs in all social groups, highlighting social inequalities in power within a patriarchal society.[7] Research has

demonstrated the links between domestic violence and child protection issues. Where women are abused, children are more likely to be also abused. Domestic violence forms 25 per cent of all crime reported to the police and where mothers are subject to violence in the home, it is reported that their children witness 45 per cent of incidents.[4]

The evidence related to domestic violence shows that pregnancy is far from being a time of safety for women. For some women the pregnancy may act to trigger violence, for others it may result in an increase in existing patterns of abuse, possibly related to jealousy or anger towards the unborn child, or simply just 'business as usual'.[8] The Confidential Enquiry into Maternal Deaths (1994-1996) revealed that six women were murdered by their partner.[9] The pregnancy outcomes for women experiencing violence in the home demonstrate an increase in the incidence of miscarriage, stillbirth, prematurity and low birth weight. Other significant factors include gynaecological problems such as vaginal or urinary tract infections and removal of perineal sutures by the perpetrator to enable sexual intercourse.[6,10]

The need for the maternity services to provide an effective, co-coordinated approach to the issues of domestic violence seems apparent. Government recommendations are that if an effective healthcare response is to be promoted, purchaser and provider units should take into account the needs of victims when planning the purchase and delivery of services.[1] Those working within the primary healthcare field, such as community midwives, may be the first to whom a woman needing help may present. However, there is evidence demonstrating that the majority of women seeking help do not reveal that they are experiencing domestic violence.[5]

The Government recognises the need for help and continued support for women experiencing violence at home.[2] The Royal College of Midwives recommends that every midwife should assume a role in the detection and management of domestic abuse, by providing affected women with care, support, information and referral to appropriate services. Integral to this is a systematic and structured framework to facilitate the midwife's role.[6]

In order to achieve this, midwives at North Bristol NHS Trust initiated and developed policies and guidelines for practice and introduced effective training programmes. The support of managers and supervisors of midwives was sought, and the skills to liaise and work in partnership with other agencies were encouraged.

Planning the strategy

The first task was to ascertain what was currently available within the Trust. It became apparent that although there were policies in place for caring for vulnerable adults, there was no existing structure in place to deal with domestic abuse in relation to the maternity services. Current research and literature on domestic abuse in pregnancy was reviewed. Contact was made with professional groups who had successfully implemented strategies to address domestic violence within other Trusts. With the available evidence acquired, a working group of midwives and survivors of domestic violence created a strategy to present to the directorate's management and clinical teams.

It was decided that one of the key aspects should be a multi-disciplinary approach, with a large emphasis on support for staff and mechanisms to address challenges that individual practitioners may experience. Midwives could not and should not be asked to take on any role for which they felt unprepared. However, it was firmly believed that with support and training midwives could make a difference to victims of domestic violence.

Draft guidelines for practice were developed, based on present Government policy, professional guidelines,[6] and recent evidence-based literature.[3,8] These were circulated for consultation to the clinical teams and a wide range of professional groups and voluntary organisations, receiving a positive response. Central to the successful implementation of the guidelines was a programme of multi-professional training sessions for staff. It was decided that a multi-layered structure, with diverse training forums to target different issues and barriers to change would be a more effective approach than a single intervention.[11]

Mandatory child protection training was based around domestic violence, facilitated by the Trust's Community Training Officer with a member of the working group very active in the planning and provision. It is clear from the research that those women who are themselves victims are not in a position to protect their children from the perpetrator. With all the available

---

Box 1 The learning objectives of workshops

To improve awareness and understanding of domestic violence

To be able to recognise and to increase sensitivity to potential signs of abuse

To ensure an appropriate response to identified abuse; this was to include documentation and record keeping

To ensure awareness of local specialist services and resources

To increase confidence amongst healthcare workers in their ability to provide support and facilitate inter-agency liaison

---

Box 2 Five-stage plan

Recognition of the abuse

Provision of private environment

Identification of abuse

Documentation of abuse

Provision of information, resources and options

---

evidence it was vital that the strong link between domestic violence and child abuse was emphasised to midwives attending the workshops.

Midwives need to appreciate the importance of the protection and wellbeing of the children as well as the mother in any violent relationship.

An experienced trainer facilitated counselling study days, and workshops on dealing with violence and aggression are now established as a rolling programme, within in the Directorate. Equipping staff with the knowledge and skills to deal with difficult situations is imperative when dealing with domestic violence. Members of the working group facilitated workshops on domestic violence. The workshops were planned to ensure that the learning objectives would be met (see Box 1) and that a multi-disciplinary audience would be reached. Many health professionals were targeted including midwives, health visitors, GPs, nurses, accident and emergency staff, obstetricians, police, social services, voluntary sector workers. The workshops were held mainly in the community at local health centres and GP surgeries, but were also held in the hospitals for hospital-based staff. It was considered vital that delivery suite, antenatal, and postnatal ward staff are also aware of the signs of domestic violence and feel equipped and able to offer necessary support. New doctors arriving on the unit are also asked to attend the workshops.

Guidelines

As part of the training every midwife was made aware of the guidelines. The guidelines followed a five-stage plan.[6] (See Box 2)

A flow chart was developed to give clear guidance on the role of the practitioner and the action to be taken in a

Figure 3.1.1 Domestic violence flow chart

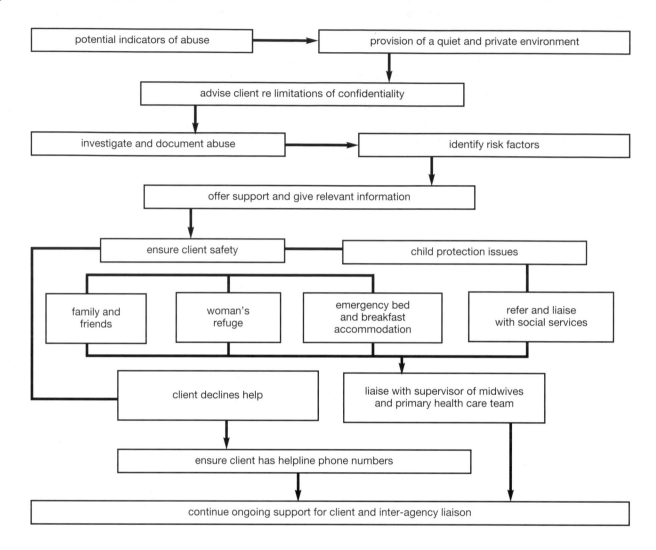

variety of situations related to the client's individual needs (see Figure 3.1.1). A database of multi-agency services has also been created.

The most important contribution midwives can make to ending the abuse is to identify and acknowledge that the abuse is happening. When a woman does disclose her abuse to a health professional at North Bristol Trust, she is asked to consider what action she wishes to take. Some women choose to do nothing at that particular stage, other than to speak freely and in confidence to someone they trust. Some simply want a place of safety to think and consider their options, whilst others will decide to leave their abuser. Part of the Trust's strategy has been to consider how a woman's choices can be facilitated; for example, women who require a place of safety can be admitted to the ward, if family or friends, or a woman's refuge cannot accommodate them.

Midwives can make appropriate referrals with the woman's consent, to the relevant agencies, since tackling domestic violence is never a single agency issue. Other responsibilities include providing sensitive support, clearly and safely documenting the abuse (never in hand-held notes for the woman's safety). Optimal care for any victim of domestic abuse will often depend on the health professional's knowledge of local resources which can provide safety and support.[3] Access to telephone numbers of national and local agencies is readily available.

Evaluation

Domestic violence training at North Bristol Trust has received a positive response by health professionals who attended the workshops. Midwives within the Trust have reported that they now feel more confident and able to screen and tackle the issue of domestic violence in pregnancy. Following a period of reflection, workshops for practitioners were held to discuss professional and practice issues and to refine the strategy.

The necessity for professional support has been addressed by all North Bristol Trust supervisors of midwives who are offering their skills and support if required to any midwife who is giving care to a client experiencing domestic abuse in pregnancy. The obligation to offer support to members of staff who themselves are victims or survivors of domestic violence has also been addressed. Confidential support and advice is available through supervisors of midwives, members of the working group, occupational health and the hospital chaplaincy.

The next step is to evaluate what impact screening for domestic violence in pregnancy has on the victims and survivors. Research into this sensitive area will require ethical approval. A research proposal is being written and sources of funding are being explored.

Conclusion

It is acknowledged that nationally some midwives have taken up the challenge of confronting the issue of domestic violence and its effects in pregnancy. However, the vast majority of midwives, although ideally placed to identify abused women, feel unable to tackle such a major issue without a legitimate and conversed role. At North Bristol NHS Trust a culture has been created where it is safe for woman to disclose their experience of abuse, secure in the knowledge that practical and emotional support is available from well-informed health professionals.

Without screening for domestic violence in pregnancy, many victims will remain undetected. Midwives must feel able to ask the woman if she has experienced physical or mental abuse. This would allow the midwife to be aware of an 'at risk' pregnancy which may otherwise have gone unnoticed. The midwife could then offer support and inaugurate measures which may help prevent further abuse. Learning how to ask the question and then to be able to listen is not easy, because often the explicit details are shocking. However, failing to ask the question when all the signs are there can only be seen as collusion on behalf of the perpetrator. Are midwives really prepared to do nothing, rather than tackle an issue which is contributing to the death of one woman every three days?[4]

The authors would like to acknowledge the contribution of Vicky Carne and Nicola Bruton in the planning and implementation of the Domestic Violence Strategy at North Bristol NHS Trust.

REFERENCES

1 Home Office. Inter-agency circular: Inter-agency co-ordination to tackle domestic violence. London: Home Office and Welsh Office, 1995.

2 Home Office. Domestic Violence: Break the chains. Inter-departmental guidance for agencies dealing with domestic violence. London: Home Office, 1999.

3 Scobie J, McGuire M. The Silent Enemy: Domestic violence in pregnancy. British Journal of Midwifery 1999; 7(4): 259-62.

4 Home Office. Domestic violence: Findings from a new British crime survey self-completion questionnaire. Home Office Research Studies. London: Home Office, 1999.

5 Department of Health. Domestic Violence: A resource manual for healthcare professionals. London: DoH, 2000.

6 Royal College of Midwives. Position Paper 19: Domestic abuse in pregnancy. RCM Journal 1999; 2(3): 84-5.

7 Hunt S, Martin A. Pregnant Women, Violent Men: What midwives need to know. Oxford: Books for Midwives, 2001.

8 Mezey G, Bewley S. Domestic violence and pregnancy. British Journal of Obstetrics and Gynaecology 1997; 104: 528-31.

9 Department of Health. Why Mothers Die. Report on the confidential enquiries into maternal deaths in the UK 1994-1996. London: HMSO, 1998.

10 Steen M. Personal communication. 3/5/01.

11 NHS Centre for Reviews and Dissemination and University of York. Getting evidence into practice. Effective Health Care 1999; 5(1).

Identifying a cry for help

A case study describing a proactive approach towards tackling domestic violence

Sue Cripps

I have been a midwife in the community for over seven years. I have often suspected domestic violence or child protection issues, and there have been many times when women have disclosed abuse to me. My midwifery training did not include domestic violence issues. My early child protection training did not discuss multiple victims or the fact that domestic violence and child protection are intrinsically linked. But times have changed. Domestic violence is out in the open, and it is no longer acceptable. Research has identified risk factors and potential indicators that can minimise harm. Action can be taken in partnership with other agencies to work together with victims to find solutions. Led by Government, the issues of domestic violence are openly debated. Front-line workers are receiving training and a multi-agency approach is being encouraged.[1]

Case study

Mrs X has come for her booking. It is her third pregnancy, but her previous two ended in miscarriages. She is 29; her husband, who is present at the appointment, is 9 years older. Mrs X is reserved and quiet, admits to smoking heavily but denies alcohol.

Her husband appears protective, keen to talk for her, and expresses great concern about this pregnancy. He asks for a scan for reassurance due to her previous history. She is now 11/40 and although there is no history of bleeding and her LMP is known I arrange a viability scan for the following week. It is common for partners to accompany their wives on their booking appointment, but this makes it difficult to ask intimate questions about the relationship. However, a simple question such as 'are you both looking forward to becoming parents?' or 'how are you both getting along at the moment?' can give parents permission to reveal difficult issues. If the woman comes for booking alone then I ask 'how are things between the two of you?' and

'have there been times when you have felt vulnerable?'

In the antenatal period Mr X accompanies his wife to every appointment. Mrs X consistently remains quiet and reserved and allows her husband to take the lead. Mrs X's pregnancy progresses normally, although there is concern about fetal growth and she is encouraged to reduce her smoking habit.

A regular pattern of contact with Mrs X via the pager emerges, and she reports a variety of vague symptoms such as abdominal pain, feeling unwell, urinary symptoms and reduced fetal movements. We become concerned and suspect relationship tensions. On each occasion of investigation nothing of note is diagnosed. Mr X is always present.

At our next team meeting we set out an action plan. We will ask the GPs and health visitors at the next practice meeting for any background information. We will try and see Mrs X alone and ask more probing questions, and we will document our cause for concern in our client update folder. The GPs disclose that there are financial problems and that Mrs X has been to see the GP on more than one occasion feeling unwell and worried about mounting debts. The health visitor has no knowledge of the couple, and Social Services have not been involved.

No major incidents occur and Mrs X has a normal delivery of a little boy at term. There are no visible causes for concern in the postnatal period, but over the next 18 months events intensify. The police are called to an incident: the couple are fighting in the street. No charges are made. Shortly after, Mrs X drops into the health visitors' base, clearly distressed, but the health visitor was not immediately available and Mrs X left without explanation.

Mrs X always attends her child's health checks but discloses nothing. The child is thriving and meets all his milestones. The couple move house but stay within the area. Mrs X falls pregnant again. Again, Mr X is clearly in control and usually present for appointments. Mrs X has a heavy early bleed and is admitted to hospital at 19/40. In hospital Mr X displays anger and anxiety: he is concerned that his wife may miscarry. Mrs X is scanned and reassured. She is offered hospitalisation for observation but is anxious to go home to look after her little boy as her husband works such long hours: he is not used to being the sole carer and 'isn't very patient'. It is not thought appropriate to question her further at that time. When she is next alone for her antenatal appointment she denies there are any problems. She states that now they have moved house she and her husband have more space and things are a lot better. At this time it is made explicit to her that she can contact us via our pager at any time and we are here if she wants to talk.

At approximately 36 weeks Mrs X misses her antenatal appointment. This is unusual. She contacts us later that day and explains she is staying with a relative out of the area. We arrange to meet at another base, which is easier for her to get to, on another day.

Mrs X comes alone. She discloses domestic violence and asks for help. She is anxious about her own safety and that of her unborn child, disclosing physical and emotional abuse. She has fled to a relative who is looking after her little boy. She is worried that her husband will guess where she is staying.

I make an immediate referral to Social Services and give her contact numbers for Women's Aid, Victim Support, and the police domestic violence unit. Our multi-agency approach to her care involves the primary healthcare team, social services, and the police domestic violence unit. At a case conference it is decided to work with the family including anger management and debt advice. Mrs X moves back to her home; Mr X has limited supervised access. Mrs X is helped to become financially independent. Mr X finds alternative accommodation.

Conclusion

Clear guidelines and multi-professional training have improved my practice. I now have increased awareness of potential signs of abuse, and improved listening and questioning skills. I have clearer knowledge about documentation and where this should be placed. Finally, I have more confidence about how to respond to a request for help.

REFERENCES

1   Department of Health. Domestic Violence: A resource manual for healthcare professionals. London: DoH, 2000.

Addressing domestic violence through maternity services: policy and practice

Sally Marchant, Leslie L Davidson, Jo Garcia, Jacqueline E Parsons

Objective: to explore current policies and practices in maternity units that aim to identify, assess and support women experiencing domestic violence.

Design and setting: a postal survey, conducted between June and October 1999, of all NHS Trusts in England and Wales that provided maternity services.

Participants: Heads of Midwifery or the midwife with expertise or interest in domestic violence in each Trust.

Main outcome measures: use of written policies and agreed practices for identifying and referring women experiencing domestic violence, such as availability of information, routine questioning of all women and offering women an appointment without their partner.

Results: 87% (183) of the 211 NHS Trusts providing maternity care participated in the survey. Twelve per cent of units had written policies for identifying women experiencing domestic violence, and a further 30% had some form of agreed practice. Less than half of maternity units routinely offered women an appointment without their partner, and just over half displayed material about domestic violence in places where women receive maternity care. Only three units had undertaken audit on their domestic violence practices.

Conclusions: there is considerable variability around England and Wales in policies and practices related to domestic violence. It is evident that clear guidelines for identification and referral, training, audit and the integration of domestic violence policies with child protection and other policies are necessary to fully address the issues.

Background

The extent to which women are subjected to episodes of domestic violence in the UK is not known, but domestic violence is cited as a frequent cause of injury and emotional trauma to women (Mooney 1993, Acierno et al. 1997, Mezey & Bewley 1997a, Richardson & Feder 1997). The 1996 British Crime Survey reported that 44% of all violent crimes against women were domestic violence incidents (BMA 1998), while the Confidential Enquiry into Maternal Deaths reported that between one in three and one in ten women experience domestic violence at some stage (Department of Health et al. 1998). It is possible, though not conclusively proven, that pregnancy and the postpartum period are associated both with the initiation of violence within a relationship or with an increase in the severity or frequency of domestic violence (Mezey & Bewley 1997b, Campbell 1998). Domestic violence affecting pregnant women may also affect the health of the fetus (Bullock & McFarlane 1989, Berenson et al. 1991, Dye et al. 1995, McFarlane et al. 1996).

Recognition by the Health Services of the importance of domestic violence has increased substantially in the UK over the past decade, and in July 2000, the Home Office announced £7 million grants for projects in a range of settings including health, aimed at tackling domestic violence, rape and sexual assault. Women experiencing domestic violence frequently present to health services requiring intervention from a wide variety of healthcare professionals (Schei & Bakkesteig 1989, Bergman et al. 1992, Plichta 1992, Drossman 1995, Collins et al. 1999). Maternity services are a universal point of contact for childbearing women and, therefore, potentially an important setting for providing assistance to those women experiencing violence (Bewley et al. 1997). However, current maternity policies encouraging partners to be present when women receive maternity care, and for women to carry their own maternity notes, may impede the potential for women to seek help with violence (Bewley et al. 1997).

Research evidence makes it clear that women expect health professionals to include domestic violence as a healthcare issue and expect to be asked about it, and to be offered support and appropriate referral and advice (Rodriguez 1996, Hayden 1997, Caralis & Musialowski 1997, Henderson 1997, Sleutel 1998). Although there is a vast literature about screening for domestic violence from the USA (for example Hamberger et al. 1992, McFarlane et al. 1991, Norton et al. 1995), there are few studies addressing the impact of systematically identifying women through the health services on later outcome (Chalk & King 1998, Davidson et al. 2000).

The World Health Organization (WHO) recommends that a health worker can at a minimum 'where feasible, routinely ask all clients about their experience of abuse ... provide appropriate medical care refer and patients to available community resources' (WHO 2000). In England, the most recent triennial Confidential Enquiries into Maternal Deaths (CEMD) 1994-1996 (DoH 1998) has highlighted violence as a cause of maternal death and made a series of recommendations, broadly based on those of the publications of the Royal College of Obstetricians and Gynaecologists, the Royal College of Midwives and the British Medical Association (RCM 1997, RCOG 1997, BMA 1998). It supported:

- The responsibility of all health professionals to be aware of the importance of domestic violence.
- The development of local strategies and guidelines for the identifcation and support of women victims, including multi-agency working.
- The provision of information in clinics about sources of help for victims.
- That routine questions about violence be included in asking about social problems and that obstetricians and gynaecologists should ask all women about violence.
- That all women are seen on their own at least once during their antenatal care.
- That routine questioning must be accompanied by training for professionals and provisions for referral.
- That an interpreter should be provided if needed who should not be a partner, friend or family member.

In the light of such recommendations, a survey of current policies and practices in maternity care in all NHS Trusts in England and Wales was undertaken in 1999 to measure the extent to which current practices matched the guidelines. Information was also sought about the resources and training available both within the Trust or from other agencies and the relationship to child protection. Because it might not be reliably answered, the survey did not include questions about the provision of interpreters.

Methods

After piloting, questionnaires were sent by post in June 1999 to maternity units in England and Wales. The questionnaire focused on provision of information, strategies for referral, liaison with other disciplines and opportunities for training. Domestic violence was defined in the questionnaire as violence taken in its widest form to include women who are being abused psychologically as well as physically or sexually. Respondents were also asked to comment on written policies and agreed common practice which did not include written documentation. A letter to the Head of Midwifery or the appropriate Senior Midwife accompanied each questionnaire and contained an explanation of the aims of the survey and overall approach of the questionnaire. They were asked to forward the questionnaire to the most appropriate midwife with responsibility for, or with expertise in, domestic violence issues. Non-respondents were re-contacted twice to increase the response rate.

Findings

A total of 211 maternity units in England and Wales were sent a questionnaire. The overall response rate was 87% (*n*=183), however, there was regional variation with the lowest response rate in Wales (66%, 10/15) and the highest in Trent and the West Midlands (100%, 18/18 and 19/19 respectively).

Information available to women with regard to domestic violence

Maternity units were asked if there was any printed material, such as leaflets, pamphlets or posters about domestic violence on display where women received care. Only just over half of the units had printed material on display (Table 3.3.1). Other locations mentioned included community health centres and general practitioner (GP) surgeries, accident and emergency departments, public reception areas, gynaecological wards and outpatient areas, social work waiting areas and paediatric wards.

The information available was produced by a small number of agencies; the national (31%, 32/104) and local (28%, 29/104) branches of the Women's Aid organisation; the NSPCC (8%, 8/104) and Government departments (29%, 30/104; multiple responses allowed).

Identifying women at risk of or experiencing domestic violence

Units were asked if they had formal written policies or commonly agreed practice regarding identification of women experiencing domestic violence, the results are shown in Table 3.3.2. Units were also asked if they routinely screened all women by asking specific questions about domestic violence. Twelve per cent of units (21/183) routinely screened for domestic violence in this way. The practices in relation to the CEMD recommendation, that maternity units offer women an appointment to see a healthcare professional unaccompanied by her partner, are shown in Table 3.3.3.

Free-text responses in the questionnaire highlighted some difficult aspects of identifying women at risk of or experiencing domestic violence.

Often the women are accompanied by the violent partner. Their controlling influence is extremely strong. Therefore disclosure is difficult for the woman.

Supporting and referring women who are identified as at risk of or experiencing domestic violence

Where women were identified as experiencing domestic violence, midwives would routinely advise or notify a range of professionals with the woman's permission. Over two-thirds of units would notify the woman's GP (127/183) and health visitor (136/183), while over half would notify the supervisor of midwives (107/183), consultant obstetrician (110/183), social worker (110/183) and the child protection team (100/183). Less than one quarter would notify police (33/183) or the community paediatrician (13/183), while 5% (9/183) notified none of these. Over one-third of units (64/183) also reported that they would notify certain health professionals without the woman's permission, most often the child protection team, supervisor of midwives, social services and health visitors. Many Trusts reported that they would notify these professionals without the woman's permission only if it was felt necessary and decisions were made on an individual basis. There was emphasis on women being informed of these notifications even if they were not asked for permission.

Units were asked if the co-ordination of referrals was undertaken solely by the individual midwife or if there was a designated person at Trust or district level to do this. Forty-three per cent of respondents (75/177) knew of a designated person at Trust level, while only 19% (25/129) knew of a designated person at district level. However, 54 units did not answer the question about district co-ordination. Of those who responded to both of these questions (n=129), more than half (74/129) knew of no designated person at either Trust or district level,

Table 3.3.1 Availability of printed information about domestic violence where maternity services given

Printed material available	n	%
No	79	43
Yes	104	57
Location:		
main antenatal clinic	85	82
postnatal area	60	58
toilets	55	53
delivery suite area	21	20
neonatal area	14	14
other	34	33

Multiple responses allowed

Table 3.3.2 Proportion of maternity units with written policies for identifying women at risk of, or experiencing domestic violence

	n	%
No written policy or agreed practice	103	57
No written policy but agreed practice	54	30
Written policies	22	12
Written policies under development	2	1

Note: 2 missing

Table 3.3.3 Proportion of units that offer women an appointment without partner

	n	%
No	91	51
No plans to introduce a separate appointment	35	20
Has been formally raised and is being discussed	44	25
Policy document is under discussion	12	7
Yes	88	49
On informal basis according to midwives	73	41
Not written policy but offered in some antenatal clinics	11	6
Formal policy offered in all antenatal clinics	4	2

Note: 4 missing

while 14% (18/129) knew of a designated person at both Trust and district level. Some midwives reported cases where there had been difficulty in providing support and referral where it was needed but the woman would not receive it. The woman wouldn't have social service help due to fear of her children being taken into care. She did not want her husband challenged.

Table 3.3.4 Knowledge of local agencies with specific services for women experiencing domestic violence

Agency	n	%
Refuges or shelters	147	84
Telephone advice/support	105	60
Voluntary services	85	49
Social services	73	42
Women only counselling	55	31
Legal aid	34	19
Health services for abused women	24	14
Other	16	9
Don't know	19	11

Note: 8 missing

Record keeping

In most Trusts women hold the NHS records for their pregnancy. However, this practice raises issues about access and maintenance of confidentiality. To overcome this, it would appear that many of the units maintain two records, one which is kept as a hospital record and one which the woman retains. Eighty-seven per cent (155/179) of Trusts recorded information about disclosure of violence in hospital records.

Knowledge of services for women

Respondents were asked if they knew of local agencies which offered services for women experiencing domestic violence. The findings are presented in Table 3.3.4. Thirty-four per cent of units (60/178) reported midwife involvement with inter-agency groups about domestic violence. Of these units, five were in the initial stages of development and seven were within a group where domestic violence could be raised, but was not the primary focus.

Audit of practices or policies related to domestic violence

Only three units had undertaken any form of audit or review of practices around domestic violence initiatives. Two units that had conducted an audit did so as part of studies by midwives and health visitors with a special interest in domestic violence; the third was the evaluation of a pilot project.

Relationship to child protection issues

Respondents were asked if, when the Trust or district Child Protection Team were informed about a newborn baby who was at risk of, or was believed to have been abused, any investigations were undertaken to assess whether the mother might also be at risk of domestic violence. Over half of the respondents (54%, 98/183) considered that some exploration of the mother's situation would certainly or probably take place. Thirty-three per cent (61/183) of respondents did not know.

Units were asked if a woman with existing children was identified as being either at risk of, or currently experiencing domestic violence, this information would be passed on to the Child Protection Team at Trust and/or district level. Seventy-two per cent (132/183) of units reported that this would happen, 20% (36/183) reported it would happen on an occasional basis and 4% (7/183) would not pass on this information.

Training opportunities

Midwives from nearly three-quarters (135/183) of units had been offered training days or specific sessions that informed or raised awareness about domestic violence in the healthcare setting. Nearly half (46%, 84/183) had been offered sessions within their Trust, while 24% (44/183) had been offered training at local level and nearly one-third (56/183) at national level.

The questionnaire revealed a need for better training and support for midwives so that cases could be dealt with appropriately:

I didn't know what to do and I didn't want to draw attention to my observations in case I made the situation worse for the woman.

I felt inadequate because I could not offer the solutions to her problems at the time.

Did not know how to ask questions/respond.

Relationships between policies and recommendations

The data were analysed using chi square tests to see if any associations existed between units which had written policies or agreed practices and some of the recommendations of the key professional bodies. Findings are presented in Table 3.3.5. Trusts which reported that they were in the process of writing policies ($n=2$) were included with Trusts with written policies and agreed practices for the purposes of this analysis.

Having a written policy or agreed practice was statistically significantly associated with the implementation of three of the four recommendations listed in Table 3.3.5. The fourth, asking routine questions of all women, approached significance ($P=0.064$) for Trusts with written policies or agreed practices compared to Trusts with no agreed policies or practices. In looking more closely at this relationship, Trusts with written policies were significantly more likely than both Trusts with agreed practices ($x^2=6.93$, df–1, $P=0.008$) and Trusts

Table 3.3.5 Associations between policy status and other practices related to domestic violence

	Trusts with written policies or agreed practices		Trusts with no policies or agreed practices		Chi square tests
	$n=78$	%	$n=103$	%	df=1
Routinely question all women on domestic violence	13	16.7	8	7.8	$x^2=3.42$ $P=0.064$
Routinely offer women an appointment without her partner	46	59.7	41	41.0	$x^2=6.11$ $P=0.013$
Participated in internal, local or national study and training days	63	82.9	71	69.6	$x^2=4.13$ $P=0.042$
Display material about domestic violence	55	70.5	48	46.6	$x^2=10.35$ $P=0.001$

with no policies or practices ($x^2=11.55$, df=1, $P=0.0007$) to routinely question all women about domestic violence.

Discussion

This study showed that, although there is considerable activity in maternity services around the identification and referral of women experiencing domestic violence, there is substantial variation in the extent to which maternity units around England and Wales have implemented the policies recommended by the Department of Health and the professional organisations.

This descriptive survey establishes a representative baseline measure of activity in England and Wales in 1999 around the time of publication of the recommendations (1997-1999). It is limited in that it is based on responses from the lead midwife commenting on unit-wide practices, which is not as accurate as measuring the occurrence of actual practices. However, the survey reveals some important findings about the current policies and practices of midwives in relation to domestic violence.

The finding that only just over half the maternity units had printed information associated with domestic violence on display in the maternity area was surprising. Only half of those maternity units that did display material (only one quarter overall) did so in the toilets, which might be considered the best place to reach a woman safely and effectively with information on how to get help. Only a small proportion of units in this survey were routinely screening. Two contradictions emerge in current recommendations for maternity policy. Over the last decade, maternity policies have recommended that partners be included in all aspects of maternity care, while new recommendations aimed at identifying women experiencing domestic violence require women to be seen alone (Bewley et al. 1997, DoH et al. 1998). Secondly, policies that advocate that all women hold their own notes create challenges in intra professional communication regarding domestic violence, as careful attention to confidentiality is needed in order not to put the woman at risk. While most maternity units have their own ways of dealing with this issue, there are no national guidelines to inform best practice.

Despite there being little evidence about the risks or benefits of routine questioning of all pregnant women about domestic violence (Davidson et al. 2000), the RCOG, the BMA and the CEMD have recommended it (RCOG 1997, BMA 1998, DoH et al. 1998). The impact of universal screening needs to be assessed in a trial to provide the evidence for the benefits and risks resulting from these recommendations. The importance of training in supporting health sector programmes is clear from the literature (Davidson et al. 2000), however, the survey reveals a relative lack of training available to midwives in the UK. There is clearly much work to be done to ensure best practice. The study into the training of midwives to take on the task of universal screening recently conducted at Guy's and St Thomas's will provide more information on midwife practices and the experiences of women accessing maternity services (Lorraine Bacchus, personal communication).

It is well recognised that domestic violence and child protection are closely entwined (Warshaw 1994, McKay 1994, Hall & Lynch 1998). However, it appears in practice that often protocols regarding disclosure of domestic violence to child protection authorities do not exist, or if they do, they do not give clear guidance. The publication from the Department of Health, 'Working together to safeguard children' gives some guidance in how to approach these issues (DoH 1999). However, recent model job descriptions issued by the Royal College of Paediatrics and Child Health (2000) for named doctors for child protection do not mention domestic violence. This survey revealed inconsistencies regarding referral and disclosure to Area Child Protection Committees and the Trust named doctor and nurse for child protection, especially in relation to the circumstances under which disclosure occurs and whether the woman has given permission. The Department of Health publication 'Child Protection: Messages from Research' emphasises the necessity to support mothers, but does not address approaches to integrating intervention in domestic violence and child abuse (DoH 1995). Policy development and research are required to unravel these issues so that expected practices and referral patterns are clear, and midwives know where they can turn for support. This will require further input from women, midwives, child protection teams, social services, voluntary organisations, paediatricians and the Department of Health.

Finally, it is apparent that midwives may be inappropriately isolated from other agencies and services, given that they are expected to play a greater role in identifying and supporting women experiencing domestic violence. Written policies and protocols, clear guidelines for identification and referral, adequate training, and audit of practices are required to ensure that maternity units can play their part in reducing the impact of domestic violence. The integration of policies addressing domestic violence, child protection and other relevant areas is essential to maximise the capability of maternity services to fully address the issues.

Acknowledgements

This work was supported by the BMA Rose Dawkins Fellowship and the Department of Health Research and Policy Programme grant to the NPEU. We are very grateful to the midwives who completed the questionnaires and who gave us additional information. Thanks also to Hazel Ashurst, Sarah Ayers, Lynne Roberts, Lyn Pilcher, Lorraine Bacchus, Sheila Hunt and Jo Richardson for their help with the questionnaire.

REFERENCES

Acierno R, Resnick HS, Kilpatrick D 1997 Health impact of inter-personal violence 1: prevalence rates, case identification and risk factors for sexual assault, physical assault and domestic violence in men and women. Behavioural Medicine 23(2): 53-64

Berenson AB, Stiglich NJ, Wilkinson GS et al. 1991 Drug abuse and other risk factors for physical abuse in pregnancy among white non-Hispanic, black and Hispanic women. American Journal of Obstetrics and Gynecology 164: 1491-1499

Bergman B, Brismar B, Nordin C 1992 Utilisation of medical care by abused women. British Medical Journal 305(6844): 27-28

Bewley S, Friend JR, MezeyGC eds 1997 Violence against women. RCOG Press, London

British Medical Association 1998 Domestic violence: a health care issue? BMA, London

Bullock LF, McFarlane J 1989 The birth-weight/battering connection. American Journal of Nursing 89(9): 1153-1155

Campbell JC 1998 Abuse during pregnancy: progress, policy and potential. (Editorial). American Journal of Public Health 88: 185-186

Caralis PV, Musialowski R 1997 Women's experiences with domestic violence and their attitudes and expectations regarding medical care of abuse victims. Southern Medical Journal 90(11): 1075-1080

Chalk R, King P 1998 Assessing family violence interventions. American Journal of Preventive Medicine 14(4): 289-292

Collins KS, Schoen C, Joseph S et al. 1999 Health concerns across a woman's lifespan: the Commonwealth Fund 1998 survey of women's health. The Commonwealth Fund, New York

Davidson LL, King V, Garcia J et al. 2000 Health services in: reducing domestic violence... What works? Briefing Notes, Home Office, London

Department of Health 1995 Child protection: messages from research. DoH, London

Department of Health 1999 Working together to safeguard children. The Stationery Office, London.

Department of Health, Welsh Office, Scottish Office Department of Health, Department of Health and Social Services Northern Ireland 1998 Why mothers die: report on confidential enquiries into maternal deaths in the United Kingdom 1994-1996. The Stationery Office, London

Drossman DA 1995 Sexual and physical abuse and gastrointestinal illness: review and recommendations. Annals of Internal Medicine 123(10): 782-794

Dye TD, Tollivert NJ, Lee RV et al. 1995 Violence, pregnancy and birth outcome in Appalachia. Paediatric and Perinatal Epidemiology 9(1): 35-47

Hall D, Lynch MA 1998 Violence begins at home. Domestic strife has lifelong effects on children. British Medical Journal 316(7144): 1551

Hamberger LK, Saunders DG, Hovey M 1992 Prevalence of domestic violence in community practice and rate of physician inquiry. Family Medicine 24(4): 283-287

Hayden SR 1997 Domestic violence in the emergency department: how do women prefer to disclose and discuss the issues? Journal of Emergency Medicine 15(4): 447-451

Henderson S 1997 Service provision to women experiencing domestic violence in Scotland. Scottish Office Central Research Unit, Edinburgh

McFarlane J, Christoffel K, Bateman L et al. 1991 Assessing for abuse: self-report versus nurse interview. Public Health Nursing 8(4): 245-250

McFarlane J, Parker B, Soeken K 1996 Abuse during pregnancy: associations with maternal health and infant birth weight. Nursing Research 45(1): 37-42

McKay MM 1994 The link between domestic violence and child abuse: assessment and treatment considerations. Child Welfare 73(1): 29-39

Mezey GC, Bewley S 1997a Domestic violence and pregnancy. British Journal of Obstetrics and Gynaecology 104(5): 528-531

Mezey GC, Bewley S 1997b Domestic violence and pregnancy. British Medical Journal 314: 1295

Mooney J 1993 The hidden figure: domestic violence in North London. Islington Council, London

Norton LB, Peipert JF, Zierler S et al. 1995 Battering in pregnancy: an assessment of two screening methods. Obstetrics and Gynecology 85(3): 321-325

Plichta S 1992 The effects of woman abuse on health care utilization and health status: a literature review. Women's Health Issues 2(3): 154-163

Richardson J, Feder G 1997 How can we help? – the role of general practice. In: Bewley S, Friend JR, Mezey GC (eds) Violence against women. RCOG Press, London

Rodriguez MA 1996 Breaking the silence: battered women's perspectives on medical care. Archives of Family Medicine 5(3): 153-158

Royal College of Midwives 1997 Domestic abuse in pregnancy (Position Paper No.19). RCM, London

Royal College of Obstetricians and Gynaecologists 1997 Recommendations arising from the Study Group on Violence Against Women. Accessed at www.rcog.org.uk/study/violence on 20/7/00

Royal College of Paediatrics and Child Health 2000 Model job description: Health Authority designated doctor for child protection and NHS Trust named paediatrician for child protection. RCPCH, London

Schei B, Bakkesteig LS 1989 Gynaecological impact of sexual and physical abuse by spouse: a study of a random sample of Norwegian women. British Journal of Obstetrics and Gynaecology 96: 1379-1383

Sleutel MR 1998 Women's experiences of abuse: a review of qualitative research. Issues in Mental Health Nursing 19(6): 525-539

Warshaw C 1994 Domestic Violence: challenges to medical practice in Dan AJ (ed) Reframing women's health. Sage, London

World Health Organization 2000 Violence against women. A priority health issue. What health workers can do. Accessed at: http://www.who.int/violence_injury_prevention/vaw/infopack. htm on 29.11.00.

Women's responses to screening for domestic violence in a healthcare setting

Joan Webster, Susan M Stratigos, Kerry M Grimes

Background: interest in the health impact of domestic violence is increasing and routine screening for violence in health settings has been recommended. However, there are limited data about how women feel about such screening.

Aim: to investigate women's responses to being screened for domestic violence during a routine clinic visit.

Method: a cross-sectional cohort study. Women (1500) from five Queensland hospitals were asked to complete a self-report questionnaire during the visit following the consultation at which they had been screened for domestic violence. Sealable envelopes and a 'posting box' were provided to ensure anonymity of returned envelopes.

Findings: of the 1313 respondents, 98% believed it was a 'good idea' to screen for domestic violence. Over 96% felt 'OK' during the process and 77% of the 30 women who felt uncomfortable still agreed that it was a good idea to screen. Women from rural and remote areas of Queensland had similar responses to those of their city counterparts.

Conclusion: women in Queensland found screening for domestic violence acceptable and, where health providers are suitably educated, it should be included when taking a routine health history.

Introduction

The effect of domestic violence on women's health is receiving increased attention from local and international policy makers (WHO 1997, Queensland Government 1999) and from the healthcare community (Warshaw 1997, Rodriguez et al. 1999). This is partly due to an increased awareness of the prevalence of abuse (Gazmararian et al. 1996) and also because more is now known about the impact of domestic violence on health (Roberts et al. 1998, Letourneau et al. 1999, WHO 2000). Injury is an obvious manifestation but it accounts for only a small proportion of adverse health outcomes. Recent reports indicate that a wide range of conditions are associated with domestic violence including urinary tract infection, vaginitis (Muelleman et al. 1998), sexually transmitted diseases (Martin et al. 1999), asthma, epilepsy, miscarriage (Webster et al. 1996), gastrointestinal disorders (Drossman et al. 1995), severe depression (Scholle et al. 1998), carotid artery dissection (Malek et al. 1999) and other somatic complaints (Koss & Heslet 1992). Suicide and homicide are also more prevalent amongst women who have experienced domestic violence (Hillard 1985, Wadman & Muelleman 1999).

Healthcare providers have an important role in identifying the women at higher risk for these adverse outcomes. However, it is well known that most health carers find it difficult to ask about domestic violence; they feel inadequately trained to do so, believe it is not their core business or that they do not have the skills to deal with a positive response (Hamberger et al. 1992, Sugg & Inui 1992). To make this easier, screening guidelines have been developed that include suggested ways to ask about domestic violence which are non-judgemental, professional and sensitive to women's feelings (Flitcraft et al. 1992). Despite this, it is still rare for women to be screened for domestic violence when they visit a primary or tertiary health care setting (Isaac & Sanchez 1994) and it is unusual for women to say that they are experiencing domestic violence unless specifically asked (Gerbert et al. 1999).

Pregnancy is an ideal time to screen for domestic violence. Midwives and doctors are in recurring contact with women who would not normally enter the healthcare system. In Australia, where rates of domestic violence are not unlike those from other Western countries (Webster et al. 1994) approximately half of all confinements occur within the public system. This means that women receive all of their prenatal care in a hospital clinic or 'share care' between the hospital and their general practitioner. Opportunities to introduce healthcare initiatives are made easier because of this system. In 1999, the Queensland Health Department supported a project to develop, test and evaluate a system to routinely screen all women attending either a public prenatal clinic or an emergency department (Queensland Government 1999). Five Queensland hospitals (two based in the capital city, one in a large regional centre, one in rural Queensland and one in a remote setting) agreed to participate in phase 1 of the Domestic Violence Initiative (DVI). Representatives from each of the participating hospitals were invited to join the DVI Reference Group and meetings were held monthly through video conference links. This provided an opportunity for input from the 'coal face' and for support and feed back to midwives who would be involved in screening. Following a literature review, the domestic violence screening questions were developed and endorsed by the Reference Committee (Appendix). In line with recommended practice, questions were to be asked directly, in a conversational way, as part of the routine 'booking in' history. Before screening began, all staff who would be asking about domestic violence attended a four-hour inservice education session. Sessions were led by midwives and social workers with backgrounds in domestic violence education. Role-play, using the domestic violence questions, was an important component of the education and training, and so was making sure that participants were aware of referral options in their local community. Staff safety and safety of the women were emphasised. Follow-up education and training has continued at regular intervals to make certain that new staff are educated and trained and that the momentum does not wane amongst those already screening.

Evaluation of the first year of the Initiative included: (i) an investigation of staff responses using focus groups, (ii) a record review at all sites to establish the rate of screening and (iii) an assessment of the training programme. We also surveyed women's responses to being asked about domestic violence to make sure that they did not object to being screened. The aim of the present paper is to report on the quantifiable aspects of these responses.

Methods

The evaluation commenced three months after screening had started and included all women attending the prenatal clinic at participating sites. Approval to incorporate questions about domestic violence into the prenatal history was obtained from each facility at the beginning of the Initiative. As we were evaluating a change to routine practice, written consent was not required. However, the purpose of the study was explained to the women and verbal consent obtained. Those who could not read or write English were excluded, unless they had responded to the original questions through an interpreter and an interpreter was available to assist with the evaluation. A target number of women to be surveyed, based on the annual expected birth rate for each site, was set for each hospital ($n=1500$). Data collection continued until the target number had been achieved. At the beginning of the visit following the booking in visit, the woman's pregnancy health record was checked to make sure that the domestic violence screening questions had been asked. Where evidence existed, she was asked to complete a short, self-administered questionnaire. The questionnaire, developed for the study and tested on several women and members of the reference group for readability and relevance, could be completed in approximately two minutes and included both open-ended and closed choice items (Box 1). No names were required and a sealable envelope and 'posting box' were provided to ensure anonymity. As with the screening questions, care was taken to make certain the woman was safe by giving her the questionnaire when she was alone. For statistical analyses SPSS version 10.0 (SPSS 10.0 for Windows 1999) was used.

Findings

Of the 1500 questionnaires distributed 1313 (87.5%) were returned. This represents 13.2% of the annual birth rate of all hospitals included in the study. Most of the respondents, 1263 (98%), believed it was a good idea to ask women about domestic violence when visiting a hospital. There were no difference in the responses from either rural, remote or inner city sites (range 98.6-95.5%, $x^2=7.38$, df 4, $P=0.117$). Nor were there differences between sites in terms of how women felt when asked domestic violence questions ($x^2=8.68$, df 8, $P=0.37$). Three responses were possible: 1197 (96.1%) felt OK about being asked, 18 (1.4%) felt relieved to be able to talk to

Box 1 Domestic Violence Initiative Evaluation

Reason for this survey

At your first antenatal visit, we asked you some questions about anyone at home who hurt you physically or emotionally or who threatened to hurt you. We asked these questions because emotional or physical abuse may affect your health and possibly the health of your baby. What we don't know, is how women feel when talking about these issues with health care providers. It would help us and other women having babies, if you would answer the following questions

(Please tick box)

1. Did you attend antenatal clinic at:

The Royal Women's Hospital ❑

The Mater Hospital ❑

Kirwan Hospital ❑

Cairns Base Hospital ❑

Mt Isa Hospital ❑

2. Do you remember being asked questions about domestic violence at your first hospital antenatal clinic visit?

Yes, I was asked questions ❑

No, I wasn't asked questions ❑

No, I wasn't asked, probably because

my partner/husband was with me ❑

I can't remember whether I was asked or not ❑

3. Please tick how you felt when you were asked questions about domestic violence.

I felt OK about being asked ❑

I felt relieved to be able to talk about my problems ❑

I felt uncomfortable about being asked ❑

Not applicable ❑

Other feelings (please comment).

....

....

4. Do you think it is a good idea to ask women about domestic violence when they are pregnant?

Yes ❑   No ❑

Why

....

....

5. Who do you think should ask questions about domestic violence? (You may tick more than one box)

My own GP ❑

Hospital clinic doctor ❑

The midwife in clinic ❑

A social worker ❑

No-one ❑

Other (please list name/s)

....

....

6. Is there a better way to ask these questions? (You may use the back of the form if you wish)

....

....

....

7. Is there anything else we should ask about?

....

....

8. Did anyone help you to complete this form?

Yes ❑   No ❑

9. If 'yes' who helped?

....

....

Thank you for answering these questions.

Please place the form in the envelope and leave it in the box in the clinic.

Your name is not required; your answers are anonymous

someone about their problem and 30 (2.4%) felt uncomfortable. Twenty-three (76.7%) of the women who felt uncomfortable, still agreed that it was a good idea to ask about domestic violence. When asked about which health carers should screen for domestic violence, multiple responses were possible: 1068 (64.9%) of the women nominated midwives, 1055 (64.1%) nominated general practitioners, 809 (49.2%) selected social workers and 771 (46.9%) selected hospital doctors. Only 42 (2%) thought no one should ask. A number of women wrote comments such as 'anyone who cares should ask'. When analysed by hospital, respondents from the remote area site were less likely to select the hospital midwife (x^2=17.2, df 4, P=0.002) or the general practitioner (x^2=18.2, df 4, P=0.001) than those from either rural or city hospitals. Of those responding, 122 (9.4%) stated that they were not asked the questions at their first visit, a further 5 (0.4%) indicated that they were probably not asked because their partner was present and 52 women (4.0%) stated that they could not remember whether they had been asked about domestic violence or not.

Discussion

Little information exists about pregnant women's views of screening for domestic violence (Stenson et al. 2001). Our study was restricted to one Australian State and only included women within the public hospital system. This means that privately insured women were not screened so findings may be biased towards the views of those from a lower socio-economic group. Despite these limitations, findings of our study reinforce earlier work, which quite clearly indicates that women do not mind being asked about domestic violence, in fact they welcome it (Caralis & Musialowski 1997, Stenson et al. 2001). The rate of agreement with the statement 'do you think it is a good idea to ask about domestic violence' was higher than has previously been reported. When McNutt et al. (1999) asked a comparable question only 75% of respondents thought screening was appropriate. This may reflect a different client population. Women in the McNutt study were of reproductive age but not necessarily pregnant. Similarly, 80% of Swedish women responding to an open-ended question about violence screening in antenatal clinic found it acceptable (Stenson et al. 2001). However, looked at another way, only 3% of these women found such screening unacceptable, a result consistent with our findings. It seems probable that protecting the baby may be a strong motivator in women's endorsement for domestic violence screening.

Our study was also larger and had a higher response rate than has been previously reported. Of those approached, only 13% did not return the evaluation form. At two of the hospitals the response rate was close to 100%. Women from these hospitals held views that were no different to those from other sites, further confirming the validity of our findings. This convincing support from women provides a persuasive mandate for universal screening for domestic violence when taking a routine history. Of course some women will choose not to disclose at the time of screening, but it is important for women to know that, when they are ready, they will be listened to and their experience validated. Being asked about domestic violence may also raise the woman's awareness of the seriousness of the problem and act as a catalyst for change (Gerbert 1999).

The high rate of support for screening suggests that women believe the healthcare setting is a safe place to respond openly to questions about domestic violence. It also implies a belief that healthcare providers may be able to help. Unfortunately, evidence shows that this is often not the case. Insensitive responses and an inability to provide assistance or useful information at the time of disclosure have been reported (McNutt 1999). In these situations women maybe left wondering why they were asked and reduce the likelihood of telling other professionals about partner violence again. Because midwifery and medical education rarely includes information about how to support women experiencing domestic violence (Rodriguez et al. 1999) and because the consequences of disclosure, without a suitable response may be devastating we believe that screening should not occur unless staff have received appropriate education. We found that careful preparation, including the four-hour training session, development of simple resources and a clear understanding of referral options help to make screening easier for staff. Role-play and practising direct questioning techniques are important in developing the skills and confidence needed to screen for domestic violence (Bates & Brown 1998). A further strength of the study was that it tested the opinions of women from inner city, rural and remote areas of Queensland. There is some evidence that domestic violence is more hidden in rural and remote areas because women are more isolated and because they want to protect their partners in communities where members are well known to each other (Alston 1997). To some extent, our data support this view. Women from the remote site in this study were certainly less likely to select their local midwife or general practitioner to screen for domestic violence, and this may be because the respondents knew them. On the other hand, these women agreed with their rural and city counterparts that screening for domestic violence was an appropriate part of health care; they were also prepared to reveal experiencing domestic violence at a similar rate to other women. Results from a related part of the evaluation showed that the rate of disclosure at the remote hospital was 10.5% compared with an average of

Appendix Domestic Violence Initiative Screening Questions

(Questions below can be introduced in a conversational style.)

In this hospital we are concerned about your health and safety, so we ask *all women* a few questions. Whatever you reply will remain strictly confidential (Please circle answer)

1. Are you ever afraid of your partner?

Yes ❑   No ❑

2. In the last year, has anyone at home hit, kicked, punched or otherwise hurt you?

Yes ❑   No ❑

3. In the last year, has anyone at home often put you down, humiliated you or tried to control what you can do?

Yes ❑   No ❑

4. In the last year, has anyone at home threatened to hurt you?

Yes ❑   No ❑

5. (If any answers are yes) Would you like help with any of this now?

Yes ❑   No ❑

6. This could be important information for your health care. May we send a copy of this form to your own doctor?

Yes ❑   No ❑

Name of Doctor:

....

Signature of client

....

Address

....

....

Post code..

Date ....

Action:

Woman declined assistance at this time ❑

Referred to Social Work Department ❑

Referral to other agency/program ❑

Other – please indicate

....

....

....

....

Information:

Woman declined information at this time ❑

No information required ❑

Help line number ❑

Information about domestic violence ❑

Other – please indicate

....

....

....

....

Print name

....

Date

....

Position

....

Signature

....

7.3% for all hospitals surveyed (Queensland Health 2000). Screening may be particularly important in parts of the country where few services are available, especially if the healthcare provider has had some education and training in counselling for domestic violence. Even providing minimal help, such as ensuring that the woman knows the domestic violence help-line number so she can call when she is ready and when it is safe to do so, may be vital.

The finding that most of the women who felt uncomfortable when asked about domestic violence still believed it to be a good idea is not surprising. Questions may have aroused unpleasant memories or feelings, yet they still wanted to be asked. Barbara Gerbert discusses the same ambivalence when she talks about the 'dance of disclosure' and the emotions associated with domestic violence being raised in a healthcare context (Gerbert 1999). Understandably, if the woman's partner was nearby she may have been fearful or concerned that the disclosure would not be kept confidential. Some women may believe that it is not the business of healthcare providers, they may be embarrassed or worried that they would be judged for staying in the relationship. Another concern for many women experiencing violence is that their children maybe removed.

It is difficult to explain why 122 of the women surveyed stated that they were not asked questions about domestic violence during their booking in visit, even though evidence of questions being asked was part of the inclusion criteria. Midwives in the clinic were responsible for identifying eligible women. Relief and agency staff are often employed in the area, so some midwives may have been unaware that not all women were to be included. It is even harder to understand why 52 women did not remember if they had been asked about violence at all. The questions would have been quite unexpected and confronting so the finding is quite surprising. We did consider not including these responses in the analysis, however, responses to other questions were relevant.

Screening for domestic violence in pregnancy demonstrates to women that midwives and doctors are concerned about the potential health impact of domestic violence on her and her unborn child. Moreover, it has been shown that asking women about violence and acknowledging the issue can be a positive intervention in itself (Parker et al. 1999). Any overt expression that domestic violence is taken seriously may help the women to feel more confident about disclosing and seeking help. A workforce familiar with the prevalence and impact of domestic abuse and comfortable about discussing associated issues may also help to reduce the shame some women feel about their situation and assist in the efforts to make violence a public rather than a private problem.

Acknowledgements

We wish to acknowledge the input of members of the Evaluation Committee – Gwen Roberts, Marilyn Harris and Anne McMurray. We would also like to thank the DVI Reference Group, staff at the pilot sites and the women who participated in the survey.

REFERENCES

Alston M 1997 Violence against women in a rural context. Australian Social Work 50(1): 15 -21

Bates L, Brown W 1998 Domestic violence: examining nurses' and doctors' management, attitudes and knowledge in an accident and emergency setting. Journal of Advanced Nursing 15: 15-22

Caralis P, Musialowski R 1997 Women's experiences with domestic violence and their attitudes and expectations regarding medical care of abuse victims. Medical Care and Domestic Violence 90: 1075-1080

Drossman DA, Talley NJ, Leserman J et al. 1995 Sexual and physical abuse and gastrointestinal illness. Review and recommendations. Annals of Internal Medicine 123: 782-794

Flitcraft AH, Hadley SM, Hendricks-Matthews MK et al. 1992 American Medical Association diagnostic and treatment guidelines on domestic violence. Archives of Family Medicine 1: 3947

Gazmararian JA, Lazorick S, Spitz AM et al. 1996 Prevalence of violence against pregnant women. Journal of the American Medical Association 275(24): 1915-1920

Gerbert B, Abercrombie P, Caspers N et al. 1999 How health care providers help battered women: the survivor's perspective. Women Health 29: 115-135

Hamberger LK, Saunders DG, Hovey M 1992 Prevalence of domestic violence in community practice and rate of physician inquiry. Family Medicine 24:283-287

Hillard PJA 1985 Physical abuse in pregnancy. Obstetrics and Gynecology 66(2): 185-190

Isaac NE, Sanchez RL 1994 Emergency department response to battered women in Massachusetts. Annals of Emergency Medicine 23(4): 855-858

Koss MP, Heslet L 1992 Somatic consequences of violence against women. Archives of Family Medicine 1: 53-59

Letourneau E, Holmes M, Chasedunn-Roark J 1999 Gynecologic Health Consequences to Victims of Interpersonal Violence. Womens Health Issues 9(2):115-120

Malek AM, Higashida RT, Phatouros CC et al. 1999 A strangled wife. Lancet 353: 1324

Martin SL, Matza LS, Kupper LL et al. 1999 Domestic violence and sexually transmitted diseases: the experience of prenatal care patients. Public Health Reports 114: 262

McNutt L, Carlson BE, Gagen D et al. 1999 Reproductive violence screening in primary care: perspectives and experiences of patients and battered women. Journal of the American Medical Women's Association 54:85-90

Muelleman RL, Lenaghan PA, Pakieser RA 1998 Non-battering presentations to the ED of women in physically abusive relationships. American Journal of Emergency Medicine 16: 128-131

Parker B, McFarlane J, Soeken K et al. 1999 Testing an intervention to prevent further abuse to pregnant women. Research in Nursing and Health 22: 59-66

Queensland Government 1999 Queensland Health 1999-2000 Corporate Plan. Queensland Health, Brisbane

Queensland Health 2000 Initiative to combat the health impact of domestic violence against women. Stage 1 Evaluation Report. Queensland Health, Brisbane

Roberts GL, Lawrence JM, Williams GM et al. 1998 The impact of domestic violence on women's health. Australian and New Zealand Journal of Public Health 22: 796-801

Rodriguez MA, Bauer HM, McLoughlin E et al. 1999 Screening and intervention for intimate partner abuse. Practices and attitudes of primary care physicians. JAMA 282(5): 468-474

Scholle SH, Rost KM, Golding JM 1998 Physical abuse among depressed women. Journal of General Internal Medicine 13: 607-613

SPSS 10.0 for Windows 1999 SPSS Inc., Chicago, Illinois

Stenson K, Saarinem H, Heimer G et al. 2001 Women's attitudes to being asked about exposure to violence. Midwifery 17(1): 2-10

Sugg NK, Inui T 1992 Primary care physicians' response to domestic violence. JAMA 267(23): 3157-3160

Wadman MC, Muelleman RL 1999 Domestic violence homicides: ED use before victimization. American Journal of Emergency Medicine 17: 689-691

Warshaw C 1997 Intimate partner abuse: developing a framework for change in medical education. Academic Medicine 72(1 Suppl): S26-S37

Webster J, Sweett S, Stolz TA 1994 Domestic violence in pregnancy. A prevalence study. Medical Journal of Australia 161: 466-470

Webster J, Chandler J, Battistutta D 1996 Pregnancy outcomes and health care use: Effects of abuse. American Journal of Obstetrics and Gynecology 174:760- 767

World Health Organization (WHO) 1997 Elimination of violence against women http://www.who.int/violence_injury prevention/vaw/endvaw.htm

World Health Organization (WHO) 2000 Violence against women. Fact Sheet No 239 http://www.who.int/inf-fs/en/fact239.html

Being with women

The term 'midwife' comes from the old English 'mid wyf', meaning 'with woman'. Which is, as we all know, why male midwives are still called midwives and not 'midhusbands'. But what does 'being with' women really entail? Why is it so difficult to achieve today? Why do so many women feel that no-one is really 'with' them at all? This is perhaps one of the most important issues to explore within midwifery today, as we face continual pressures on our time, resources, role and practice.

It is an interesting challenge to practise midwifery in the age of information, where often the women you are with know more about a subject than you do. There is so much to know nowadays about any given topic that we can strive either to know a bit about a lot of things, or a lot about a few. Either way, it is not uncommon to meet women who know more than you do about a given subject, particularly where this subject is a health-related condition, such as diabetes, which they have experienced for many years. With the combination of published and web-based information (albeit not always the most accurate, or empowering) available to anybody who has a computer and a phone line, the existence of midwifery and medical knowledge as the sole property of professionals is, perhaps thankfully, a thing of the past. But what information do we offer women, especially when there is so much around, yet often so little time to discuss and share it?

Hannah Hulme Hunter explores this further in looking at how we can be with women in relation to offering information upon which they can base decisions. Crucially, she differentiates information from advice and begins to unpick some of the issues that have confused us for years, as to why women simultaneously report that they are given too much, and too little, information by midwives. This is a topic that is also considered by Helen Davies, who looks at the ways in which we can explore our own decision-making processes within the current culture of maternity services, in enabling the empowerment not just of childbearing women, but of ourselves as well. We also need to keep up-to-date in order to be able to be with the different groups of women who make up our multicultural society. Two of the articles in this section address birth practices in non-Western cultures. Christine Grabowska offers an insight into midwifery in China, while Aziz Sheikh and A R Gatrad's article will help midwives increase their knowledge of Muslim birth practices, and gives ideas about how we can better 'be with' Muslim women and families.

Cecily Begley's research explored the feelings and views of student midwives in Southern Ireland, highlighting ways in which staff shortages and systemic constraints impacted both on the students' experience of learning and women's experiences of birth. While it is depressing that the experiences of the students parallel those of factory workers, and that the prevailing model seems to have moved on from the medical to the economic, this kind of study can make real the experiences of those 'at the coalface' and inform change as a result.

The final article in this section, Shona Hamilton's exploration of maternal mental illness and maternal suicide, may not be comfortable reading for everybody. But it highlights an area that has been particularly neglected and, as she points out, is one of the leading causes of maternal mortality today. In asking how we can be with women, it is important to remember that this is not only about finding time to listen, helping women to solve the minor problems, or choose from the menu of labour options, but sometimes can be about dealing with the stark reality of the choices surrounding death, just as with the choices surrounding life.

Ways and means...

Of giving information

Hannah Hulme Hunter

I don't usually read the parents' pages in The Times (been there, done that) but a recent article caught my eye. 'YOU ARE THE ONLY EXPERT!' shouted the headline. A quote will set the scene:

...first time parents are encouraged to turn to the experts. And even if they don't seek it, the advice is provided anyway – on feeding, bathing, clothing, putting to bed, comforters, toys, immunisation [etc. – you get the idea]. At first sight this seems 'empowering'. In reality, however, it is the opposite. Too often parents are made to feel like incompetent fools... [1]

The writer is a Dr Frank Furedi, a sociologist and father. He certainly struck a chord with me. Which is ironic – because I spend most of my working life doling out information to childbearing women, either face-to-face on hospital wards, on the telephone, or via websites, books, and articles.

Most of the time I feel good about what I do. Survey after survey[2,3] tells us that new mothers feel they are not receiving enough information, for heaven's sake! At the same time, I do think Dr Furedi has a point. If a Professor of Sociology can be made to feel an 'incompetent fool' by the intrusive advice of healthcare professionals, what harm must we be doing to less confident, less well-educated, less analytic parents?

Recent surveys give us some insight:

...they [the midwives] didn't treat me like I knew anything... [3]

One advises you to do one thing, the other sees you and tells you off like a naughty school child... [2]

I am... normally a confident person and cannot believe how I allowed her [the midwife] to act as she did. [3]

Conflicting advice from different midwives about breastfeeding made me feel guilty and inadequate. [3]

Conflicting advice is a constant theme in surveys into postnatal care. Over a decade ago, some 40% of new mothers complained about this.[4] Today's estimate is nearer 60%.[3] Not doing very well, are we?

Conflicting advice contributes to low self-esteem and emotional distress in new mothers.[4] Women who lack confidence are more likely to blame themselves when things go wrong. And so the spiral to despair can begin.

On one hand, not enough information. On the other, too much. And the poor old midwife, as usual, stuck in the middle feeling more and more persecuted. (Apparently Frank Furedi has just published a book called *Paranoid Parenting*.[6] So look out for my new title – The Paranoid Midwife...).

Would you like a few pointers for dealing with this? I don't pretend, for even one minute, to have all the answers – but I have thought about this a lot, and I do try hard.

Don't give advice – give information

It's so simple, you're probably insulted. The words may be often be used interchangeably, but 'information' is not the same as 'advice'. Skim back through the last few paragraphs. From Dr Furedi down, the word 'advice' has negative connotations.

Advice is rarely empowering. Receiving advice beholds you to your advisor. If the advice works, you feel grateful – but belittled. If it doesn't work, it's either because you didn't do it right (your fault) or your advisor is flawed (and if she got this wrong, what else will she get wrong?).

Don't set yourself up to fail. Give information, outline options, step back. Let somebody else make the decisions for once.

Make sure the information you give is of impeccable pedigree

Giving information is not so easy as giving advice. You have to know your facts. There is no room for glib answers, vagueness, or pet theories. Dr Furedi again:

Most parents don't realise that the advice they receive is usually nothing more than someone's individual opinion... rarely supported by robust evidence. [1]

In the last ten days, I have come across midwives advising grated carrot for sore nipples, pineapple for unripe cervices, and cabbage leaves for engorged breasts. The last I can just about live with (one small randomised controlled trial). However, I search in vain for 'robust evidence' on carrots or pineapples. Just because it's edible, doesn't mean it's effective, safe, or even agreeable to use.

Two bits of advice (oops!):

- Be aware where on the hierarchy of evidence your pet theory sits. Top is randomised, controlled trials (preferably multi-centre, multi-this, and multi-that). Bottom is opinion and observation. All the rest lie in between. Start at the top and work down. There's nothing wrong with giving a woman a piece of information that belongs in the 'opinion and observation' category – just make sure she knows its lowly status.

- Know your physiology inside out. Physiology Rules Okay. It's official. It says so in *A Guide to Effective Care in Pregnancy and Childbirth* on page 486.[5] If the information you give supports physiology, you can't go too far wrong. And remember: basic physiology doesn't need the backing of a randomised controlled trial. One can take these things too far. (Hmm... can pineapple be physiological if you live in Iceland?)

One of my regular jobs is 'resident midwife' to a UK parenting website. When I reply to women's emails, I write with two people in mind. One is a lonely, frightened pregnant woman. The other is a consultant obstetrician who hates midwives and has a barrister for a brother.

No wonder I'm a slow writer.

Use more conditionals

People who write on occasion for the National Childbirth Trust (as I do) get very good at this, sometimes to an irritating degree. 'You may like to try...', 'This might work...', 'That could be helpful...', 'Some women find...'. (NB: not 'most women' – if it doesn't work for you, you feel a deviant.) Other useful phrases include 'Research shows...', 'However...' and 'On the other hand...'. Corny and rather time-consuming – but oddly effective.

You might like to try this next time a new mother asks you what to do with her crying baby. Or you could tell her he's hungry and needs a top-up.

Ask one, or all of these questions:

- 'What do you want to do?'
- 'What feels right to you?'
- 'What do you think you should do?'

Her answer will help you get straight to the heart of her problem – rather than wasting time pontificating on what you perceive her problem to be. Plus, she'll probably have the answer, too – if you give her half the chance to work it through.

One word of warning: when you ask one of these questions, be prepared for the mother to hesitate and give a little start of surprise – as in 'What do I think?!'

Chances are, nobody else has asked her opinion recently.

REFERENCES

1 Furedi F. You are the only expert. Times 2 (supplement to The Times), March 12 2001, 8-9.

2 Garcia J, Redshaw M et al. First Class Delivery: A national survey of women's views of maternity care. London: Audit Commission, 1988.

3 Singh D, Newburn M (Eds). Access to Maternity Information and Support: Women's needs and experiences before and after giving birth. London: National Childbirth Trust, 2000.

4 Ball J. Postnatal care and adjustment to motherhood. In: Robinson S, Thomson AM (Eds). Midwives, Research and Childbirth (Volume 1). London: Chapman and Hall, 1989.

5 Enkin M, Keirse MJNC et al. A Guide to Effective Care in Pregnancy and Childbirth. Oxford: Oxford University Press, 1995.

6 Furedi F. Paranoid Parenting. London: Allen Lane/The Penguin Press, 2001.

Client-centred midwifery: no easy option

The role of conscious decision making in empowering practitioner and client

Helen Davies

Much has been said of the benefits of client-centred care, particularly for women using maternity services. Some midwives have found it relatively easy to practise in this way and others have found it difficult. The ease with which the individual can make decisions for herself, and is able to facilitate this process in others, is at the heart of the challenge that is client-centred care.

What does it mean to make a decision? The dictionary definition is 'to determine the result of; to make up one's mind about'.[1] This implies awareness and action intertwined but does this reflect our everyday reality? We all make countless decisions the majority of which are made on 'automatic pilot'. Our unconscious decision-making processes take over. A driving analogy demonstrates this: when we begin to learn to drive we have to consciously decide when and how to change gear. As we become more skilled we begin to change gear automatically, only becoming aware of the process when something occurs which makes the action critical, needing to avoid a pedestrian for example. Transactional Analysis calls this the 'Adult Ego State' which frees us from the 'necessity of making innumerable trivial decisions'[2] thus giving us mental capacity to deal with more complex tasks. How does this concept of 'the adult' as performer of routine experiences relate to the work of the experienced practitioner? Benner's work describes the route by which new skills are acquired, initially following strict instructions then gradually moving along the continuum to the expert or 'intuitive' practitioner where one is freed from conscious thought 'without wasteful consideration of a large range of unfruitful, alternative diagnoses and solutions'.[3]

Superficially this would appear to be of great benefit: we can 'take as read' certain tasks and actions. This has few consequences if we are involved in a routine mechanical task, other than perpetuating the 'how we do it here' culture which tends to limit improvements. The danger for midwives working intimately with others is that application of skill, without active engagement with ourselves, colleagues or clients may lead to unthinking assumptions about the best course of action. Over time the sphere covered by 'implicit practice' tends to grow. Information shared with clients and colleagues may be pre-selected, preferred course of action may be indicated, direction may be given about what the client should do next. As a consequence the possibility of informed choice is removed. 'Intuitive practice' therefore needs to be regulated by challenging reflective practice to ensure that we are not unconsciously making decisions for others, removing the possibility of them taking actions and decisions for themselves.

In more complex situations we define the situation, what led up to it, and identify possible options and the consequences of them before we make a decision. Even here there are subdivisions about what is important, for example they could range from 'deciding' to find time to listen to a woman at an antenatal clinic to a decision to call in medical assistance during a labour. The latter has to be dealt with immediately. The former may be difficult to find time for; there is a woman waiting in the next room; urgent work on the desk for after clinic; a meeting that has already started; missed lunch again! All are automatically put into the equation, set against the needs of the women and the demands of the midwifery role. Is it any wonder that sometimes we feel that our heads are completely full and we are totally incapable of making any decisions!

Yet the imperative remains, decision-making is at the heart of informed choice. Midwives cannot effectively offer informed choice unless they are aware of the complexity of factors that affect both themselves and the women that they care for. A multiplicity of factors affect the way in which we make decisions and the conclusions that are 'available' to us. This is to a large extent controlled by our personal and social context and our experiential learning. Identifying these factors is an

Figure 4.2.1 Factors which affect the decisions we make

Education

Upbringing

Relationships

Experiences – both personal and professional

How we feel about what is going on in our life today

Our reactions to decisions we have taken in the past

Culture of the workplace

   – protocols and policies

   – hierarchical structure

   – power balance/imbalance

   – involvement in decision making

   – client expectations

   – expectations of workplace

essential first step (Figure 4.2.1).

The logical next stage would be to take each of the bullet points and make notes about how each affects the way in which you take decisions. Consider for a moment education. Think about not only the level of your education but the ways in which you were taught to make decisions, the implicit messages about women, learning and jobs which you were exposed to. All of these get deep inside us. Remind yourself of a powerful memory from your days of formal education. If those around believed in you and your abilities then you too were likely to share this belief. The power of those beliefs was potent, building self-esteem and personal resilience, enabling you to set personally challenging goals without fearing failure. Sadly for many our educational experiences were less positive, perhaps we were made to feel inadequate, fearful of trying to achieve things in case we failed. The way in which powerful managers or teachers influence our performance Senge calls the 'Pygmalion effect'.[4] Feelings born out of past experiences remain powerful and can have profound effects in our adult life. On occasions a 'button' is pushed and those emotions positive or negative live again affecting our actions and reactions. Women you care for will have had these experiences too. They are moving out of their 'comfort zone' into someone else's territory where the professional is perceived to have all the power and authority. Moving into an environment of power imbalance, clients have to decide how much they are prepared to give up and conform to the behaviour the organisation and the practitioner expect.[5] 'A strong culture is a system of informal rules that spells out how people are to behave most of the time.'[6] Attempting to

make decisions which go against those rules can be extremely difficult. The challenge for midwives is to break through these barriers to begin building an effective relationship.

The culture of the NHS and the sub-cultures operating in the hospital trust, directorate, ward or team can be difficult to identify clearly. The view that the NHS is a hierarchical and still largely patriarchal culture is widely held. However the dominant culture of an organisation is often overlooked by those who have worked within it for any period of time: 'we just find ourselves feeling compelled to act in certain ways.'[6] The consequences of working within this culture are incredibly potent. The patriarchal, 'you must do because I say so' comes into direct conflict with the matriarchal 'I'll look after you'. Both disempower people who use the service and those who provide it. They encourage in women who are already feeling vulnerable a childlike acceptance of 'the rules'; in others they provoke an aggressive response. This makes it difficult to build a supportive relationship with them.

Operating in a patriarchal society tends to lead to centralised decision making. Important decisions are often taken several layers away from where those decisions become actions. The further removed practitioners are from the decision-making process the less responsible they feel for their actions and the less involved in the service they feel. This in turn leads to a culture of dependency where eventually many practitioners take fewer and fewer decisions for themselves, escalating decisions up through the structure.

The ability to take decisions can also be removed by the organisation particularly where a 'blame culture' operates. In the NHS this is both internal – you are blamed for your actions – and external – clients are looking for someone to blame when things don't go as they had wished. Errors are made and individuals should be held to account in such instances. However, when blame becomes the instant response it blocks the inquisitorial, reflective response which would engender learning from experience. Involving women and their partners effectively in making decisions about their care can help them to take appropriate responsibility for their actions and can help them to understand that childbirth, although very, very safe, carries no guarantees. Fostering dependency leaves the practitioner open to blame and does little to prepare the woman and her partner for the reality of parenthood.

'Learned helplessness', where the individual feels that they have little control is extremely destructive both of self esteem and ultimately of one's physical health.[7] The NHS has a culture where this is endemic. A blame culture in action works like this: an individual is blamed for an action she takes, she then feels guilty and the next

Figure 4.2.2 Behaviour loop

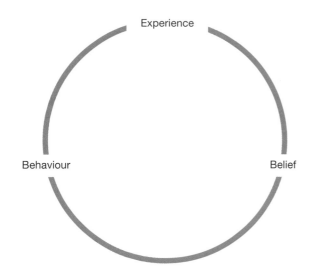

or feeling that your judgment is being called into question. Models of structured reflection can help you to 'see yourself in a particular situation and honestly observe how they have affected a situation and how the situation has affected them'.[8] Taken a step further it can help you to 'look inside and know who they are as they strive towards understanding'.[9]

If we feel powerless we learn behaviour to 'work the system', either to protect ourselves or the women in our care, or to avoid conflict and still get what we think of as important. For example we may behave submissively with certain powerful or senior colleagues, we may manipulate others or be aggressive to those we see as weak, we may work around hospital policies because we don't feel able to challenge them. This is a short term expedient which perpetuates the established culture, changing nothing. Only those strong enough to bend the rules can help either themselves or the women they care for.

Developing self-awareness then, helping the individual to understand her motives, is crucial to the provision of client-centred care. Significant factors which influence the question of 'self' are illustrated below. Some of these have already been touched on. Asking others about how honest they think you are, how you use your body in communication and where your 'buttons' are would be a very valuable exercise (Figure 4.2.3).

Raising self-awareness can be done in an issue- or task-based way. Considering the way in which you share information and present pathways of care to clients will yield information relevant to all of the factors shown in Figure 4.2.3. It will help you to understand both how you decide what to say and how to say it and how this affects the choices made by clients in your care. For example,

time she is called upon to make a decision she hesitates. Her own self belief begins to falter, confidence in her abilities declines. If this happens often enough, some people become unable to make decisions always deferring to their peers or more likely their superiors. She comes to BELIEVE that she can't do it; her belief affects her BEHAVIOUR – the way she attempts a task; this in turn affects her EXPERIENCE – what happens. Repeated often this leads to a dependency loop (Figure 4.2.2). Telltale signs of a dependency loop getting out of hand are the increasing need to seek permission from someone senior to you, increasing personal feelings of inadequacy

Figure 4.2.3

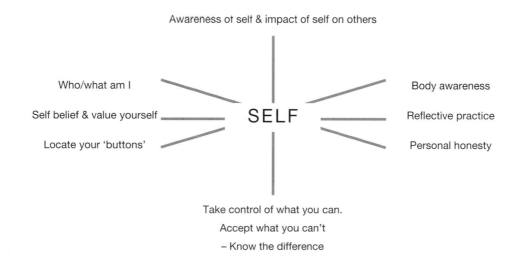

Figure 4.2.4 Sharing information to facilitate informed choice

Ask yourself...

– Why am I suggesting this procedure intervention

– Is it what I usually do? Is it hospital protocol?

– Am I indicating the response I would prefer? How?

Does the information I am sharing with the client cover...

– Why am I suggesting this course of action

– Advantages and disadvantages

– Possible consequences

– Effects on the woman and baby including side effects

– Changes in role of the partner

– Effect on the labour

– Alternatives including doing nothing at this point

– Medical reason for taking action now (not using euphemisms)

– How any intervention will be administered and who will do it

– Consequences of delay. Will this choice be available later?

you may know that in a particular set of circumstances 90% of women go on to use an epidural. Either consciously or unconsciously you may present information in a way weighted towards the choice of an epidural. This then perpetuates your view of events and validates your opinions, reinforcing your belief, behaviour, experience loop. You have also encouraged the client to become dependent on you and removed her access to informed choice.

Lorraine Sherr describes the difficulty of attempting to make decisions within a medical setting where 'it is rare for people to make decisions based on a complete rational examination of all options and pathways open to them'. She argues that this can be due to a number of factors including the way in which information is 'presented' and 'framed'.[10] Developing a mental script, which you change regularly to prevent over-familiarity, can help you to avoid some of these pitfalls. Figure 4.2.4 contains suggestions, based on questions that women and their partners regularly ask in antenatal classes, about how you can structure sharing information to help clients make informed decisions.

Like all reflective practice this article comes with a health warning. The more you develop your sense of self and your ability to reflect on and in practice, the more you will question things that you have always taken for granted. For example, differences in practice between yourself and colleagues, little quirks of 'how I do this' become far more significant as you begin to understand the effect these have on others working in the NHS and on those for whom you are caring. You become more aware of the often hidden messages in policies and protocols. Are you ready for the challenge?

REFERENCES

1 Collins English Dictionary. London: William Collins, 1974.
2 Berne E. Games People Play: The psychology of human relationships. London: Penguin, 1968.
3 Benner P, Tanner C. Clinical Judgement: How expert nurses use intuition. American Journal of Nursing 1987; 87(1): 23-31.
4 Senge PM. The Fifth Discipline: The Art and Practice of The Learning Organization. London: Random, 1990.
5 Handy C. Understanding Organisations. 4th Edition. London: Penguin, 1993.
6 Deal T, Kennedy A. Corporate Cultures: The rites and rituals of corporate life. London: Penguin, 1988.
7 Goleman D. Working with Emotional Intelligence. London: Bloomsbury, 1998.
8 Atkins S. Developing underlying skills in the move towards reflective practice. In: Burns S, Bulman C (eds). Reflective Practice in Nursing: The Growth of the Professional Practitioner. 2nd Edition. Oxford: Blackwell Science, 2000.
9 Johns C. Opening the door of perception. In: Johns C, Freshwater D (eds). Transforming Nursing through Reflective Practice. Oxford: Blackwell Science, 1998.
10 Sherr L. The Psychology of Pregnancy and Childbirth. Oxford: Blackwell Science, 1998.

Midwifery in China

Christine Grabowska

I was invited to spend a month teaching doctors and midwives in Beijing about practices in England. Nicky, the midwife who invited me, went to the International Conference for Midwives in Manila. There she met Chinese midwives who asked her if she could arrange for a midwife teacher, from England, to go and spend a month in China. When I got there I realised part of their reason for this was that they wanted to learn to speak English. Most of the group could read it, but had no idea of pronunciation. However, it was a fantastic month; I learned so much and absorbed some of the Chinese culture that has helped me to view people from China differently.

The way that midwives are trained is different from England. Midwives do a three year direct entry course and can enter from the age of 19 whilst nurses also do a three year course but there seems to be no mechanism for nurses to become midwives. In both courses the first two years are spent in the classroom and the final year is spent totally in practice. There are plans to start a diploma course in 2001.

I visited six maternity units in Beijing. An official visit would involve a hospital administrator showing me around. However, I was privileged to have Nicky with me. She knew some of the nurses and midwives in these hospitals and I was shown around unofficially. In some cases this caused discomfort; the nurses would not answer any questions because they were afraid that it might not be what would 'officially' be said.

Private hospitals

One of the hospitals I visited, Beijing United Family Hospital, was private. This could not be compared to the other five hospitals. It catered mainly for Westerners, who paid through insurance companies for their care. Local people could go there if they could pay. The doctors were all from abroad and the nurses and midwives needed to speak English fluently to be employed. Two of the midwives were from the USA and one trained in England. They had a total of 300 births a year; these were conducted in a bedroom-type, individual room. The cost for a full antenatal package was US$1,000, followed by the birth ($6,800 for a normal delivery, $8,800 for a caesarean, $10,000 for an emergency caesarean) and the daily in-patient stay cost $700-800 a night. This was the only hospital I visited that catered for multiparous women, because of the one child policy in China. If the mothers were from abroad the policy did not apply. This was also the only hospital I visited that had similarities with the way maternity care is organised in England: this is where the familiarity ended. I spent the first two weeks feeling shocked and critical of the systems of care I observed in the public hospitals.

Public hospitals

The public hospitals I visited were Union Hospital, Mi Yun County Women and Children's Hospital, Beijing Friendship Hospital, Beijing Maternity Hospital and the Chinese/Japanese Friendship Hospital. The hospitals were divided into District, City and Ministry levels. District was seen as the lowest status and Ministry as the highest, and this also affected the cost of care in these hospitals. District hospitals charged about £80 for a normal delivery and £180 for a caesarean. In city hospitals the cost of a normal birth was just under £200 and a caesarean just under £300. At ministry level the cost of a normal birth was about £300 and a caesarean just over £400. However, people who are employed by the state get the cost of their births reimbursed. This includes about 80% of the population.

Fathers are expected to pay an extra £10-30 to be present for the birth. One hospital said that they did not have the facilities for fathers but the mother could go out into the corridor to speak to him. They did not have a single delivery room – most rooms were multiple occupancy. In one hospital women could choose to stay in a six bed postnatal ward, with a nurse present in the room, for 24 hours if they paid 45p an hour. Alternatively, women could stay in a small two-bedded room using a call bell system for nurse availability.

All parents were expected to buy two sets of hospital baby clothes, and mothers wore hospital pyjamas. I was told that nothing would go missing this way. In fact, I was taken to the factory where these clothes were made for all the maternity units in and around Beijing. The owner suggested that I introduce the same system into hospitals in England!

The average age for having a baby was about 22-23. Reproductive technology was not available for anyone over the age of 45. Contraception consisted mainly of using the IUCD for about 60% of women in China. Oral contraception was used in 5% and Depo-provera was the other favourite.

Primigravid women made up 98% of all births. The multiparous 2% were made up of mothers who would have had an 'abnormal' baby (the doctor can 'allow' the mother a second child) or country people who can have a second child once the first one has reached the age of five. I was told that people from the countryside prefer boys. The orphanages contain mainly female children. The trade in female infants for adoption in the West is well known.

The maternity departments had family planning wards which were dealing with abortions to enforce the law. These wards also offered a pre-marital check-up, which amounted to genetic screening. Premature and sick babies were treated very differently from England. The general feeling was that it was better for the woman to have another baby, rather than care for this sick one. Their attitude towards care was often to support the dying process. The only equipment they had was PCO_2, apnoea and ECG monitors, and equipment for taking blood pressure.

Labour ward practices also varied from England. Staff had to wear flip-flops, a gown and a hat when on the labour ward. Labour wards seemed so relaxed. Staff stood around having private conversations and giggling. I never saw anyone rushing around. A junior doctor would give one-to-one labour care to a woman undergoing an induction of labour! All hospitals had a first stage of labour room, usually of six beds with just enough room for someone to stand between the beds. There was no privacy as no curtains or screens were available. Even vaginal examinations were conducted in front of the other room occupants. There seemed to be one CTG to a bay of six beds – this was not done routinely. Doppler ultrasound was used to monitor the fetal heart at regular intervals. Women were free to walk around, eat and drink and generally were stoical in dealing with their labours. I observed one labour aid, a tall zimmer frame into which women could lean when walking around. Labour wards had some aesthetic aids such as cassette players. TENS machines were readily available, but were applied to the abdomen rather than the back.

The episiotomy rate was 70-100% and this was said to be necessary because Chinese women are 'small'. Instrumental deliveries were mainly forceps – many hospitals did not use ventouse but at one hospital I found the midwives doing ventouse and the doctors performing forceps deliveries. Epidurals were not offered routinely in labour, with a rate of about 10%. However, this was the anaesthesia of choice for caesareans. Pethidine was used post-operatively and for 10% of labourers. Pain relief in labour consisted of massage, TENS, ear and body acupuncture. I saw an ear-piece that delivered electrical stimulation to acupuncture points being used for pain relief. It felt similar to the pulse that is emitted from a TENS machine. I observed an acupuncture point (Bladder 32), being injected bilaterally with 1% procaine, into the second sacral foramen – 10mls on each side. It really made a difference to the woman, who calmed down and started conversing. The analgesic effect lasted for about two hours, when the procedure could then be repeated.

The second stage took place in a very public room, with glass doors to the corridor. Two or three women were lined up, pushing, next to each other on plastic tables, in lithotomy position with no more than an incontinence pad and one pillow. The midwife would conduct all deliveries. I was told that the use of the lithotomy position and episiotomies was to avoid a third degree tear – midwives' careers would be threatened in the event of a third degree tear.

Caesarean with acupuncture

One of the most amazing things I witnessed was a caesarean with the use of acupuncture for anaesthesia. Electro-stimulation was applied to two needles inserted into the Spleen 6 and Stomach 36 points on the leg. The effect of this was so strong that the woman's leg muscles reacted violently. Two needles, that looked about six inches long, were inserted subcutaneously from each side of the umbilicus down to the pubis. These also had electro-stimulation applied but this was not as strong as the leg stimulation. Tape was used to keep the ends of the needles against the skin. The woman was given pre-medication of 50mg pethidine prior to the procedure and a local anaesthetic of 1% procaine was injected into the wound site prior to incision. A vertical incision was made between the two long needles. The woman seemed to feel the incision, the moment when the baby was removed and the stitching. She made no noise but contorted her face. She got just a glimpse of the baby before it was taken away for routine weighing, measuring and photograph taking. Acupuncture caesarean has been performed in China since 1966. The doctor commented that this provided good analgesia as the abdominal muscles were relaxed. Post-operatively the woman did not have further acupuncture or any other form of analgesia. She was mobile and there were no obvious adverse effects.

The caesarean rate is about 50% – I was told that this is because people are looking for perfection with the one child that they are allowed. August 8th was a very busy caesarean section day because eight is associated with luck in money and families wanted their babies born on a day when they could ensure that the child would be rich. Overall, the birthrate is decreasing, and some units may have to close. However, because this is the year of the Dragon (and considered lucky) many people had planned to have their one child this year – and therefore the overall decline in the birth rate was halted.

Antenatal and postnatal care

Doctors do all the antenatal checks. The clinic has more than one couch and more than one doctor in the room. A woman waiting to be checked would come into the examination room and walk around the tables watching what was happening to everyone else. She would get onto a couch whilst someone else was getting off. One of the antenatal wards had use of a blackboard to educate the mothers. The midwives would change the information every two weeks. But all of the hospitals displayed health education posters. This was considered essential. However, it was doctors that organised antenatal education and this took place in a formal classroom setting. Interaction was not expected.

All the hospitals I visited had Baby Friendly status. They all displayed breastfeeding promotion posters, but I also saw posters by Nestlé and Johnson and Johnson. The hospitals had breast milk in their freezers, which they said was pasteurised. There appeared to be no skin-to-skin contact – I was told they were too busy. The baby is taken from the mother at birth to perform routine tasks. Interestingly, Baby Friendly was asked by the Chinese government to train assessors from within China to award the status. The internal assessors have since awarded the status to many of the hospitals in China.

Routine tasks following labour included taking pictures and footprints (which will be set into glass or marble). The hospital charges for these mementoes. (Mementoes are not available following a stillbirth, which seems to be treated in a similar way to that in this country in the 1950s). The baby is weighed, tagged and the cord has iodine and an elastic band applied. Vitamin K is given. All babies will have a hepatitis and BCG vaccination before discharge. Some hospitals put the babies in the nursery at night and no special baby care units would allow the mother or any relative admission because of the infection risk. The mother could, however, send her expressed breastmilk. The babies' cots were attached over the end of the mother's bed. Babies are separated from mothers on the ward for a daily rinse, under a tap, and for routine screening. Bloods for hypothyroid were taken on day three.

Air-conditioning units were present in all the hospitals but rarely used. The average daily temperature was about 30°C during my visit in July/August. This appeared to be the women's choice. They were afraid that they would have an invasion of pathogenic wind and become sick. So I observed them sweating in bed with flasks of hot water on their lockers to make drinks. Visiting hours were limited to two hours daily with a maximum of two visitors at all the hospitals. Partners would stand by the bedside, or sit on the bed, as there was very little room between the beds.

My attitude changed as I started to absorb the culture. I understood that women's expectations were not the same as in England. Rather than being moralistic and preaching right or wrong, I found myself in a position, when asked by a labour ward sister what improvements could be made, of saying that the West has not got all the answers and nor is it always 'the best'. However, we did talk about the high episiotomy and caesarean section rates.

I was in a privileged position at the hospital in which I taught; the staff accepted me and I had a freedom in the hospital not afforded in the other units I visited. I received great hospitality in being shown the surrounding area of Beijing, being invited into people's homes, being given gifts, food and friendship. I can recommend this experience to anyone wanting to broaden their insight into another culture. It has broadened my perspective of life and given me the opportunity to see things differently.

Muslim birth practices

Aziz Sheikh and AR Gatrad

Over 20,000 Muslim babies are born annually in the UK.[1] Britain's Muslim population, estimated at two million, is largely composed of migrants from the Indian sub-continent; more recent Muslim migration has been from Western Africa and the Balkans.[2] Though ethnically heterogeneous, these diverse communities are tied by a religious narrative that has successfully permeated almost all aspects of Muslim culture.[3] In this paper we provide an introduction to Muslim birth practices. To the untutored eye, these may appear as excessive, unnecessarily rigid and prescriptive; for those within the tradition they are however viewed as deeply symbolic and coherent. Understanding, we believe, is the key to allow culturally competent and sensitive care to flourish, hence we aim to provide an 'insider's account' of issues of importance in the care of pregnant women and their infants. The information here presented should be seen as providing relevant background information to allow the individual patient-professional encounter to be accurately contextualised. Stereotyping – the process of indiscriminately assuming that cultural characteristics hold true for a particular individual – is not recommended.[4]

Antenatal care

Clinic attendance

Notions of structured proactive care are unfamiliar to many migrant communities; this perhaps explains why hospital attendance rates are on the whole lower for these communities than those observed in Caucasian patients.[5] Other possible factors include being offered clinic appointments at inconvenient times (such as religious holidays or at prayer times), socio-economic factors (the proportion of Muslim households living in poverty is much higher than that seen in the host population), and

concern that the care provided will be culturally insensitive.[6] Examples of the latter include inadequate access to interpreting services or clinicians of the same gender. In a study by Watson et al, the recollected waiting times in antenatal clinics were much longer for Bangladeshi women, though it was not clear whether this was due to lost case records, language difficulties, shyness or altered perception of time due to anxiety and confusion.[7]

Improving attendance for antenatal care in these populations is particularly important given the increased risks of congenital anomalies and prenatal mortality.[8] A recent study showed that significant improvements in hospital attendance rates can be achieved by taking steps to actively engage with minority communities through initiatives such as working with local religious organisations, use of link workers, and the incorporation of a multicultural calendar into the clinic booking template.[9,10]

Fasting during pregnancy

It is estimated that over 90% of adult British Muslims fast during Ramadan. Whilst this might come as a surprise to many, considering that the fast involves complete abstinence from food and drink during daylight hours, even more surprising is that most pregnant women will also choose to fast. Interestingly, such fasting has not been shown to affect the mean birth weights of babies at any stage of gestation.[11] Nonetheless, pregnant and lactating women are exempt from fasting, and are in fact strongly discouraged from doing so if medical advice is that the ritual may either harm the mother or the developing fetus. Whilst most mothers will readily comply with medical advice, if faced with a dissenting mother about whom one is particularly concerned, we would suggest that staff consider enlisting the help of a local religious leader.

Termination of pregnancy

Deliberate termination of pregnancy is contrary to the principles of Sacred Law,[12] although if continuation of pregnancy jeopardises the mother's life then all Muslim authorities agree that termination of pregnancy is justified. In such a situation, an existing life, with its responsibilities and ties, takes preference over a developing one. Serious congenital anomaly is regarded as grounds for termination by a minority of jurists, but only if this takes place prior to fetal ensoulment. Based on a Prophetic tradition, ensoulment is believed to occur 120 days after conception.[12] Advances in the use of first trimester chorionic villus biopsy as a screening tool are thus particularly welcome, allowing detection of fetal anomalies (and treatment or therapeutic abortion) prior to ensoulment.

Consanguinity, a known risk factor for congenital anomalies, is common amongst Muslims from Turkey, Pakistan and Arab countries.[13] Greater access to appropriate genetic counselling services, especially for couples with a personal or family history of birth defects, is urgently required considering Muslim sensitivities regarding termination of pregnancy.

Labour and postnatal care

Care during labour

There exists considerable variation in culturally acceptable behavioural responses to pain. There is however no scientific basis to the calumny that Asian women in labour have a lower pain threshold than the indigenous white community. Certainly, they require the same attention, support and sympathy that all labouring women require at this great turning point in their lives. Attending staff should be aware that unfamiliar surroundings and difficulties in communicating might lead to increased (but avoidable) anxiety. In addition, it may prove useful to be aware that maternal mortality rates remain very high in some of the countries of origin of migrant patients; many labouring mothers may thus have had first-hand experience of a death during labour, compounding their sense of apprehension regarding labour.

Gender segregation is an important feature of most Muslim cultures, such customs existing to minimise risks (perceived or actual) to the integrity of the family unit which forms the cornerstone of Muslim society.[13] These laws are relaxed somewhat if urgent medical attention is required. Muslims will nonetheless prefer to be attended by a clinician of the same gender, particularly if an intimate physical examination is required. Such sensitivities should be respected as far as is practicable; in cases where there is difficulty in attending to this request, it is best, we believe, for clinicians to adequately discuss the situation with the patient and their family. Such explanation is greatly valued and co-operation is typically forthcoming.

Labouring mothers may prefer to have an older female, such as their mother or mother-in-law in attendance rather than their husbands. The observation that males are infrequently in attendance has led to the abject charge by some that this represents a lack of paternal concern. Rather, it is indicative of a culture in which modesty, even between husband and wife, continues to be valued.

Postnatal care

Mothers will traditionally stay in bed for a few days, a practice that is quite distinct from the 'get up and go' culture now seen in many postnatal wards. Effective communication is again important, and with explanation that prolonged bed rest predisposes to deep vein thrombosis, most will quickly see the benefits of mobilising shortly after delivery.

When checking the baby after delivery, one needs to be vigilant in looking for cyanosis and jaundice as these conditions can easily be underestimated in babies with pigmented skins. Coloured babies often have a blue discoloration over their buttocks and back; these Mongolian blue spots are easily confused with bruising from non-accidental injury.

Custom dictates that many African and Asian nursing mothers will not leave their homes for about six weeks after delivery, some choosing to return to their parental homes for this time period. This may therefore affect attendance for postnatal examinations or infant assessments. It is possible that this custom originated as a way of reducing high rates of maternal and infant infection at a time when both are particularly vulnerable. Nursing mothers are often fed a high calorific diet typically comprising a mixture of nuts, ghee (purified butter) and natural herbs. It is commonly believed that this reduces the risks of infection, helps backache, improves milk flow and may even decrease postnatal discharge. Spices are often avoided as it is thought that these pass into breast milk and may give the baby colic and dysuria. In parts of Africa and the Indian sub-continent, warmed bricks are placed on the abdomen to help involution of the uterus, although in Britain a hot water bottle is more commonly used. Infants may be regularly massaged with oil such as almond oil in order to keep the skin supple. Mothers may take offence if such harmless customs are thoughtlessly criticised.

Birth customs

The Adhan

All children have the right to know their Lord, and hence it is considered essential that the first words to which the impressionable new life is exposed is the Testimony of Faith, the pole around which the rest of his/her life should pivot. Both these pronouncements are conveniently encapsulated within the Adhan or Call to Prayer. It is customary for the father, or a respected member of the local community, to whisper the Adhan into the baby's right ear shortly after birth. This simple ceremony takes only a few minutes, and it is generally appreciated if parents are offered a little privacy to perform this dignified rite.[14]

The Testimony of Faith

There is none worthy of worship except God, and Muhammad is God's Emissary.

Tahneek

Soon after birth, and preferably before being fed, a small piece of softened date or honey is gently rubbed into the infant's upper palate. A respected member of the family often performs this, in the hope that some of his or her positive attributes will be transmitted to the fledgling infant.

Taweez

The Taweez is a black piece of string with a small pouch containing a prayer, which is tied around the baby's wrist or neck. Believing that it protects the baby from ill health, this practice is particularly common amongst Muslims from the Indian sub-continent. For obvious reasons, it is important that the Taweez be handled with respect at all times.

Male circumcision

Islamic Law requires male infants to be circumcised. Personal hygiene is considered important, and once circumcised, there no longer exists concern that when the child matures, and begins to offer prayers, small amounts of urine held up in the foreskin may soil clothing, thereby nullifying the prayer. Circumcision is usually performed within a few weeks of birth. It is important to remind parents of jaundiced infants about the need to delay circumcision until after the jaundice has resolved because of the risks of prolonged bleeding. Circumcision also needs to be postponed in infants with hypospadias until after a surgical opinion has been sought, as the foreskin may be required for corrective surgery. Frequent nappy changes, together with liberal use of barrier creams, may minimise the risk of ammonical dermatitis and the associated risks of meatal stenosis and ulceration whilst wound healing occurs.[14]

Shaving the hair

Scalp hairs that grow in-utero are removed, traditionally on the seventh day of life, and an equivalent weight in silver is given to charity.

Muslim names

A good name is considered a fundamental human right. It is hoped that the name will both inspire self-respect and also give the child something to aspire towards in the years that lie ahead. It may be a few days before the infant is named, as it is usual to seek the advice, and approval, of members of the extended family. Each Muslim name has a meaning attached to it, for example Ahmed, a common boy's name, means 'Praiseworthy' and Salma, a popular female name, means 'Peaceful'.

Breastfeeding

Religious teachings recommend that mothers suckle their offspring for up to two years. Although many mothers may wish to breastfeed, the lack of adequate privacy offered by some postnatal wards is an important barrier to initiating breastfeeding. It is thus often deemed more convenient to bottle-feed whilst in hospital, although few mothers seem to appreciate that this may adversely affect later milk production.

There is a commonly held belief amongst some sections of the Muslim community that colostrum is either harmful to the baby, or that it has poor nutritional value.[15] Supplements of honey and water will often be used for the first few days of life. This represents an example of a cultural tradition that contradicts religious teaching, and this dissonance offers a very useful window for the development of educational campaigns directed towards Muslim mothers, with the support of religious leaders and Muslim organisations. Prolonged breastfeeding (greater than six months), combined with delayed weaning, is the norm amongst Bangladeshis.[16] Iron deficiency, anaemia and rickets may ensue if breastfeeding is not supplemented with an appropriately balanced diet. Most Asian families change from an infant formula to 'doorstep' milk at about five-six months, a practice that is contrary to the Department of Health's recommendation that states that reconstituted infant formulae should be continued beyond six months in order to prevent deficiencies of iron, and vitamins A, C and D.[17]

Stillbirth and neonatal death

Stillbirth

Even if stillborn, it is important that the baby be named before disposal. Although such babies are usually buried in the UK, religious law does not require a full funeral service and there is thus no absolute requirement for burial in a cemetery. In fact burial in non-consecrated grounds such as a garden is not unusual in the Indian subcontinent. Neither the ritual washing nor shrouding is necessary for stillbirths. Placental tissue is considered part of the human body and should therefore be buried and not incinerated as presently happens in the UK.

Neonatal death

If an infant is very ill, or death imminent, family members may wish the baby to be given water from the sacred well of Zam-Zam in Mecca, Saudi Arabia. Nursing and medical staff ought to be aware of the significance of the water so as to minimise the chances of causing undue offence if it is felt not to be in the infant's interests to receive the water on medical grounds. It is customary for the face of the dying to be turned towards Mecca (southeast in the UK); if this is impractical turning the head to the right will usually suffice.

On dying, the infant's arms and legs should be straightened and the eyes and mouth closed. It is a religious requirement for burial to take place as soon as possible after death. Problems may arise if there is delay in issuing a death certificate or if there is difficulty in registering the death as may occur at weekends or on public holidays. Post-mortems are generally considered taboo in Muslim culture and parents will thus very rarely allow such examinations unless they are legally required. The trend towards Magnetic Resonance Imaging necropsy may offer a more acceptable alternative to formal 'open' post-mortem examinations.[12]

Conclusions

Few UK trained clinicians will have received any formal training in the principles or application of transcultural medicine. Caring for patients with distinct cultural practices that are at times in sharp contrast with the dominant tradition is consequently challenging and at times difficult. In this paper we have attempted to provide an overview of key Muslim birth practices, and give insight into their meaning and significance. An appreciation of such customs offers unique insights into the lives of Muslim families; such insights, we believe, are important to the creation of an environment in which patient-professional dialogue can take place and genuine client-centred care flourish.

REFERENCES

1 Pharoah POD, Alberman ED. Annual statistical review. Arch Dis Child 1990; 65: 147-51.
2 Anwar M. Muslims in Britain: demographic and socio-economic position. In: Sheikh A, Gatrad AR (eds). Caring for Muslim patients. Oxford: Radcliffe Medical Press, 2000.
3 Winter TJ. The Muslim grand narrative. In: Sheikh A, Gatrad AR (eds). Caring for Muslim patients. Oxford: Radcliffe Medical Press, 2000.
4 Galanti GA. Caring for patients from different cultures. Philadelphia: University of Pennsylvania Press, 1997.
5 Gatrad AR. Comparison of Asian and English non-attenders at a hospital out-patient department. Arch Dis Child 1997; 77: 423-6.
6 Bowler I. 'They're not the same as us': Midwives' stereotypes of south Asian maternity patients. Social Health Illness 1993; 15: 157-78.
7 Watson E. Health of infants and use of health services by mothers of different ethnic groups in east London. Community Med 1984; 6: 127-35.
8 Sheikh A. Ethnicity and child health. In: Harnden A (ed). Child health promotion. London: RCGP, 2001 (in press).
9 Gould C, Rose D, Woodward P (eds). SHAP calendar of religious festivals. London: SHAP Working Party, 1999.
10 Gatrad AR. A completed audit to reduce hospital non-attendance rates. Arch Dis Child 2000; 82: 59-61.
11 Cross JH, Eminson J, Wharton BA. Ramadan and birth weight at full term in Asian Muslim pregnant women in Birmingham. Arch Dis Child 1990; 65: 1053-6.
12 Gatrad AR, Sheikh A. Medical ethics and Islam: Principles and practice. Arch Dis Child 2001; 84: 72-5.
13 Dhami S, Sheikh A. The Muslim family: Predicament and promise. WJM 2000; 173: 352-6.
14 Gatrad AR, Sheikh A. Muslim birth customs. Arch Dis Child 2001; 84: F6-8.
15 Lee E. Asian infant feeding. Nursing Mirror 1985; 160: S14-5.
16 Harries RJ, Armstrong D, Ali R, Loynes A. Nutritional survey of Bangladeshi children aged under 5 years in the London Borough of Tower Hamlets. Arch Dis Child 1983; 58: 428-32.
17 Gatrad AR, Sheikh A. Birth customs: Meaning and significance. In: Sheikh A, Gatrad AR (eds). Caring for Muslim patients. Oxford: Radcliffe Medical Press, 2000.

'Giving midwifery care'

Student midwives' views of their working role

Cecily M Begley

Objective: to explore the opinions, feelings and views of student midwives of their education as they progressed through their two-year programme in Ireland, with the intention of interpreting and understanding the working and learning world of the participants so that future students might be assisted to improve their educational experiences.

Design: using quantitative and qualitative methods. A phenomenological approach was used to guide the qualitative section of the study reported here.

Setting: all seven midwifery schools in Southern Ireland.

Participants: all students in the first intake of 1995 in every midwifery school in Ireland (*n*=125).

Data collection: individual and group interviews, diary-keeping and questionnaires.

Key conclusions: the endings presented here illustrate the students' views of their working role. The environment appeared to be one of work, rather than learning, and the students' status that of junior employee rather than 'learner'. They perceived themselves as 'thrown in the deep end' without much support from qualified staff. They were unsure of themselves and suffered from role conflict and loss of status. There appeared to be an acute shortage of staff and care given was seen to be the basic minimum, fulfilling women's physical needs but ignoring emotional ones. Care appeared to be planned according to routine and economic necessity rather than for sound midwifery, medical or social reasons.

Implications for practice: education needs to focus on the development of autonomous practice. Routines and non-research based care should be phased out. Students need to be assisted, with support from educated mentors, to plan care in a holistic way and develop their midwifery skills.

Introduction

Since the midwifery profession was legitimised in the UK and Ireland with the passing of the first Midwives' Act in 1902, there has been an increase in hospitalisation for normal births and a concomitant increase in the medicalisation of childbirth, which has led to a diminishing of the midwife's role (Donnison 1988, Wagner 1994, Murphy-Lawless 1998). In Ireland, studies of midwives' provision of care have not shown them to be executing their role in the fullest sense (Byrne 1989, Coleman 1989). It is notable that midwives in some hospitals in Ireland act more as obstetric nurses than as autonomous practitioners (Murphy-Lawless 1991), which may be due to the effectiveness or otherwise of their education or to the structure and organisation of the maternity services.

Literature review

An extensive review of the literature was under taken through Medline, CINAHL, ERIC and Cochrane databases, using the key words 'midwifery education' and 'nursing education'. A number of studies emerged which had examined the world of the student nurse (Melia 1981, Treacy 1987, Seed 1991), but it appeared that there was very little work into the lives of student midwives.

Davies' small qualitative study of student midwives as they went through the first three months of their education in the UK demonstrated that, although students were taught that midwives were 'practitioners in their own right', the reality they encountered on the wards was quite different (Davies & Atkinson 1991). A larger quantitative study of the quality of student midwives' education in the UK made recommendations for changing the content and delivery of the programme with the introduction of the new 18 month course

(Golden 1980). These studies were both carried out prior to the linking of midwifery education with third level establishments.

Aim of study

The study from which this small section of findings is taken (Begley 1997) was designed to explore the opinions, feelings and views of student midwives as they progressed through their two-year educational programme in Ireland. The main aim was to endeavour to interpret and understand the working and learning world of the participants with a view to assisting future students to improve their educational experiences.

Methods

The methods, instruments and conduct of this study have been described in detail in a previous paper (Begley 1999a), so only a brief synopsis is presented here. The technique of triangulation (Begley 1996) was employed in the full study in a number of ways as a means of ensuring confirmation and completeness of data. Quantitative and qualitative methods were used together; the quantitative section of the study used two questionnaires which were administered to the total population in their first week on the course and two to three months prior to completion respectively. The qualitative part of the study included diary-keeping, interviews and focus group interviews. A pilot study was carried out and all necessary changes made.

Population

Permission for the study to be carried out was granted by the matrons and principal tutors of all seven of the midwifery schools in Southern Ireland. The population included all students in the first intake of 1995 in every midwifery school in Ireland (n=125). All participants were female. The students all agreed to participate, following an information session on the purpose and proposed conduct of the study. Nineteen students chose to keep an unstructured diary and 31 volunteered to be interviewed. All students were included in the focus group interviews.

Instruments

The initial questionnaire concerned demographic details and future plans, and included some measures of assertiveness and self-esteem. It was administered to the whole population during the first week of their programme.

Nineteen volunteers were asked to keep unstructured diaries for the first 10 weeks of their clinical placement. Thirty-one students took part in unstructured interviews three times during their two-year course at four, 12 and 20 months.

The final questionnaire was administered to the whole population two to three months before the end of their programme when the students were in their last week in the classroom. The first section of the questionnaire repeated the measures of self-esteem and assertiveness in order to compare the respondents' views prior to and following completion of their midwifery programme. The main part of the final questionnaire was formed from questions derived from the qualitative data, using sequential triangulation (Field & Morse 1985), and the results of this section served to corroborate the qualitative reports of the volunteer group. Students' views of the adequacy of their clinical education were also sought and their opinion of the amount and quality of the theoretical course content was ascertained. The two questionnaires were pre-tested on a group of five midwives, prior to employing them in the pilot study of eleven student midwives.

Focus group interviews were conducted following the administration of the final questionnaire, when the students were 21 to 22 months into their programme.

Data collection

The first questionnaire was completed by all 122 of those present in class on the day of administration. The author carried out all interviews, the majority of which took place in the students' homes. The individual interviews lasted from 15 to 76 minutes with a mean of 35 minutes (S.D. 11); group interviews lasted between 30 and 70 minutes. All interviews were tape-recorded and, when transcribed, produced a total of 451 649 words.

The 19 diaries returned had been kept from three to ten weeks. They produced a total of 19 151 words between them, with the shortest diary having 254 words and the longest having 2638 words, a mean of 1008 (S.D. 768) words.

The final questionnaire was administered to the total population two to three months before the end of their programme and was completed by all 119 students left on the course.

Pseudonyms were used for the participants and identifying letters for the hospitals in order to keep all data strictly confidential.

Data analysis

The questionnaires were analysed using descriptive and inferential statistics. The complete interviews and diaries were transcribed, copied into the software programme 'Ethnograph' and introductory analysis took place, during which 163 codes were applied to the data. A phenomenological approach was used to guide data analysis, using the 'description and interpretation' system of the Dutch school (Holloway & Wheeler 1996) and eight themes were identified from the data obtained from the diaries and first interviews. A further four themes emerged from the data gathered from the second interviews.

The 'thick description' of these 12 themes was sent to the 50 students who had contributed to the qualitative section of the study and they were asked to read the explication of the selected quotes and to answer a verification questionnaire. Thirty-one students responded with reference to the preliminary findings of the first interview and diary data (62%) and 29 students responded in relation to the preliminary findings of the second interviews (58%). Between 23 (79%) and 31 (100%) of those who replied agreed that a particular theme was either 'very' or 'fairly' true to life. The final results were documented following further analysis. Three more themes were identified from the data emerging from the third and group interviews; as the students were by this time approaching their final examinations, verification of these themes was undertaken during the final questionnaire only.

The findings identified a number of areas where improvement in the structure of midwifery education in Ireland is required. The demographic details and findings in relation to students' views of their education have been presented in a previous paper (Begley 1999b). Another section of the findings is presented here to illustrate the students' views of their working role.

Findings and discussion

First interviews and diaries

The students were very enthusiastic participants in the interview process during these first interviews and needed little encouragement to continue talking. Eight themes were identified from the first interviews and diaries and were labelled: 'It's a whole new ball-game', 'Thrown in the deep end', 'Them and us', 'It's all routine', 'We're workers, not learners', 'Good days and bad days', 'They all have their moments' and 'Getting the hang of it'. Three of these applied specifically to the students' working role and are presented in this paper.

Verbatim quotes are used where suitable and the identifiers with each quote contain the pseudonym of the student, date of interview, number of interview and the identifying letter of the hospital. Words encased in parenthesis, thus < >, have been inserted by the author to improve understanding and those enclosed in ordinary

brackets, such as these ( ), indicate non verbal cues used by the respondents.

All student midwives in Ireland are employed in the maternity hospitals as part of the work force. At the time of this study, they were scheduled to have 13 weeks in the classroom and the remainder of their time was spent working in the clinical areas. The findings of this study demonstrated clearly that, for most student midwives, 'surviving' as employees in the work place was a task at least as important to them as learning new skills.

'Thrown in the deep end'

The students' overwhelming sense was that they had been thrust into a new domain, different entirely from the environment of nursing with which they were familiar. They were confused, bewildered and unprepared:

My first day was like my first day as a PTS. The nervousness was the same, the butterflies in my stomach, the fact that I was already a qualified general nurse with two years' experience as a staff nurse in an acute and extremely busy surgical unit was irrelevant. All my previous knowledge seemed to evaporate and counted for very little. +Linda, diary, G, 12-22

In Ireland, until 1 June 2000, all student midwives had to be registered general nurses first, although the EC Directives governing midwifery education state that a 'direct entry' programme is an acceptable method of midwife preparation (Council of the European Communities 1980). Midwifery education is referred to as a 'post-registration' course, which implies that it provides specialist education, which leads on from, and complements, the general education already received. This does not appear to be the case and begs the question: why waste three years undertaking education in the nursing care of ill males and females if one wishes solely to care for childbearing women and their babies?

Almost all the students stated that the one to two weeks of theoretical preparation they received did not give them sufficient knowledge to enable them to cope with the work expected of them in the clinical areas. Even when they gathered information to assist them in carrying out their duties, the students did not fully understand why they were to perform certain tasks:

One, I did not know what I was doing, I hadn't a bloody clue (very emphatically, chopping down with her hands). *All I knew was from what I had seen with the other girls, I knew but I didn't understand. I was doing things and I didn't know why I was doing them...*+Eleanor, 5th July 95, 1st int., A, 63-70

It has been postulated that the performance of midwifery tasks without knowing why one is doing them leads to dangerous practice (Fraser et al. 1998). Davies (1993) studied first-year undergraduate student nurses and found that knowledge discovered through observation of role models was related to what is done and how it is done, rather than to the theoretical reasons for action. This would also appear to accord with how student midwives learn, the only difference being that student midwives take as their role models the other, more senior students, as they do not appear to work closely with qualified staff (Begley 1999b). Observation which is not accompanied by explanation can be misleading (Chamberlain 1997), particularly if students observe other students who may make mistakes or take 'short-cuts' in a procedure.

Because they had so little knowledge, the students did not feel that they could contribute to the workload of the clinical area. This led to them feeling 'useless', a crime in the eyes of most nurses (Clarke 1978):

The worst day would be the worst day in delivery on your own with this person and you're told 'go in and do the breathing exercises'. How was I supposed to know what I'm supposed to be doing with breathing exercises? +Gertie, 11th July 95, 1st int., C, 382-388

C.B.: *How did you get on in pre-natal?*

Eva: *I just felt a waste of space, really, up there...*+Eva, 5th July 95, 1st int., A, 492-494

Davies' study of student midwives in the UK suggested that when under stress the students had recourse to using tried and tested nursing skills, such as 'doing the observations', which made them feel they were contributing to the work in the ward (Davies & Atkinson 1991). These students did not appear to find these tasks comforting, rather they were bored by them and felt that they were learning nothing new by repeating well-known skills:

C.B.: <re previous comments on the ante natal ward> *Was it just doing obs, doing work?*

Eleanor: *Doing obs, obs, obs yes. Obs have their place, we know why we have to do them but oh...no* (shaking head and making a face). +Eleanor, 5th July 95, 1st int., A, 448 453

A number of students spoke of how unsure they were that the care they gave to women and babies was good, or even safe:

... and then we were put with a patient <in labour> on a CTG machine and 'call me if anything goes wrong'. And you're saying, what is 'wrong' as such, you know? +Olive, 13th July 1995, 1st int., D, 71-75

These students are, officially, under the supervision of a qualified midwife, but, given the expressed low levels of staff (Begley 1999b), one wonders just how close that supervision can possibly be. The responsibility the students were expected to take on seemed, to them, to be enormous, especially as they were left to cope on their own. As one student wrote, in the first verification questionnaire:

Rebecca, D: *It was terrifying looking after a mother in labour not knowing what was normal and abnormal. It was negligence really.*

The mentorship or preceptorship system has been endorsed by a number of writers in the UK who have studied the benefits of both systems from the students' (Earnshaw 1995) and preceptors' (Coates & Gormley 1997) viewpoint. Two hospitals provided mentors for the students' first week in the wards, although in one hospital this service did not apply to, of all places, the labour ward, and if the workload increased these mentors had to become part of the ordinary workforce.

'It's a whole new ball-game'

Almost all the respondents expressed how difficult they found it to 'get used to working in midwifery' and many commented on the differences they found between general nursing and midwifery. In her study of new nursing students, Bradby (1990) found that they felt 'comfortable' in their first ward after two to four weeks, and in their second within two weeks. None of the students in this study felt 'settled' by the time of the first interviews. The change from being a 'staff nurse' to being a 'student' led to a perceived drop in status, an adjustment which many found difficult:

... you are a staff nurse, and yet you're not given the respect of being a staff nurse, you know, you're just back to being a student again. +Jo, 6th July 95, 1st int., A, 105-108

This reflects the hierarchical nature of nursing, where status is so hard-won that any slight drop is felt as a backward step. A loss of status and respect has been found to decrease job satisfaction in nurses (Seymour & Buscherhof 1991), so that some assistance with anticipatory socialisation and, in particular, some education in the area of conflict management (Shead 1991) may be helpful to prepare students for their new role.

While dealing with this emotional upheaval, the students also had to contend with the workload of the hospital. There were conflicting opinions on the amount of work, mainly due to different perceptions as to whether teaching and talking with women counted as 'work':

I still can't get over how light the workload is compared to general nursing. I think that's why I feel so useless as we are not doing a lot of manual work. +Kirsty, diary, A, 317-321

This supports the findings of other studies where the students had formed the impression that 'talking isn't working' (Melia 1981) and demonstrates that these qualified nurses had been socialised during their nursing programme to believe that such is the case.

Many students stated that the workload in their hospital was unreasonable mainly due, in their eyes, to low staffing levels. Excessive workloads mean that students (and staff) are working as hard as they can throughout the whole shift which leaves little or no time to teach or learn. Some students maintained that the work was the same as they had been doing in general nursing:

C.B.: *Is the work different?*

Eleanor: *Em...no, you still have to dress the beds, you still have to do the observations, you're still caring for your patient...I just think it's another area...you're still doing the basic things that a nurse does for anybody...* +Eleanor, 5th July 95, 1st int., A, 943-950

The emphasis on physical care is strong here, with little recognition of the midwife's role as counsellor and educator. Some students did acknowledge this role, although without much enthusiasm:

But I miss being a nurse. Here I'm more a teacher, even as I'm being taught. It's different, I'm not sure I like it yet. +Violet, diary, C, 327-330

'It's All Routine'

In general, the students spoke of the work as being monotonous and governed by routine. The work was described as consisting mainly of tasks, rather than the giving of holistic care, probably because they were assigned to give the routine, day-to-day care of women which they were capable of doing with little instruction and guidance:

... you've eighteen women and you're asking them all the same questions 'how are your breasts this morning' and 'are you sore', 'have you gone to the toilet', 'do you want Panadol' and, like, ultimately you know the answers, you know, (laughs), they're all going to be the same. +Heather, 10th July 95, 1st int., B, 408-415

This method of work allocation has been shown to be a quick and efficient way of training a transient population to care for patients and ensures that a minimum standard of care is given (Proctor 1989). The drawbacks of this are, firstly, that qualified staff also conform to the routine (Proctor 1989) and settle into a non-thinking way of giving care based on rituals. Secondly, the students learn to use routines and may not be helped to plan care in a holistic way that would be of use to them in the future. This also affects the women in their care, as women who are empowered and cared for in a holistic manner are then better able to care for their own babies and gain in self-confidence (Ball 1989).

The majority of the respondents thought that they did not have time to look after the women and babies properly, which may predispose to this routinisation of the work. Some of this pressure of time may have been artificial in that in at least four of the hospitals the importance of getting the work done by a certain time was stressed:

... you had to have every baby washed by half nine to...go to coffee and there was nothing (holding hands up, eyebrows raised) *to do the rest of the morning.* +Gertie, 11th July 95, 1st int., C, 98-102

Further pressure on time may come from the repetition of tasks that may not be useful or effective, such as frequent temperature-taking (Walsh & Ford 1989) and the daily bathing of babies. There did not appear to be an emphasis on using research-based practices in the various hospitals around Ireland, and some of the practices described had been shown by research to be useless, time-wasting or inadequate:

... it's just pure task orientated. You do the jobs whether they need to be done or not. There's no assessment of whether you could discontinue this, discontinue that. If they've had prolonged rupture of membranes or if they've had a section, they'll have obs here four-hourly until they go home. +Ruth, 13th July 95, 1st int., D, 754-762

Although all students were qualified nurses, over half of them reported that staff midwives often repeated observations that they had performed. Coxon (1990) maintains that nursing has developed a system of checking and counter-checking even the most simple of tasks so that qualified nurses are given no responsibility.

Some of the students liked the routine, in much the same way as the students in Davies' study (Davies & Atkinson 1991) used routine observations as a way of coping with the strangeness of the new situation. However, others did not and queried the meaning of all that they were doing:

... you find yourself nearly saying the same things, you know, all the time; how to bath the baby, how to...which is fine for the first while but after a few weeks of that you kind of say, God, is this what it's all about, you know. +Lilian, 7th July 95, 1st int., C, 737-742

The feelings of futility expressed here are similar in many respects to the views of young female workers in Pollert's (1981) study of factory workers' lives, who endured the tedious work for the sake of the weekly pay packet. When midwifery work is based on task allocation, the care given is administered routinely through a conveyor-belt approach more suited to industrial management.

Some students also felt that their learning and progress was impeded by the fact that they had to attend to the routine tasks:

... say you were on post natal checks in the morning, you were shown one, and then you were 'off you go', (pushing out with hands) *that was it, you know.* +Nancy, 13th July 95, 1st int., D, 58-62

The Council of the European Communities' Directive on midwifery education states unequivocally that students 'shall be taught the responsibilities involved in the activities of midwives' (Council of the European Communities 1980, p. 3). The teaching of psycho-motor skills such as carrying out postnatal 'checks' and abdominal palpations requires initial demonstration followed by practice, with feedback (Quinn 1995), under decreasing supervision. The majority of students in this study did not appear to receive much initial teaching and certainly did not have a lot of supervision or feedback. In her study of the clinical learning of student midwives Chamberlain (1997) also found that teaching by qualified staff was minimal and students were often left to fend for themselves after an initial demonstration.

Second interviews

The students were noticeably quieter and less enthusiastic than in the first interviews, and a number of them appeared slightly depressed. This may have been the normal reaction of many students when half-way through a course, but it was striking to see such a clear difference between their demeanour in this interview compared with their previous behaviour. Four themes were identified and named 'Knowing your place', 'Counting the days', 'It's a Do-It Yourself Course' and 'Gaining confidence and competence'. This last theme was the only one that related specifically to the students' working role.

'Gaining Confidence and Competence'

At the time of the second interviews, when students had been enrolled on the course for approximately one year, the majority felt confident in giving postnatal care. Antenatal and intranatal care was perceived by the students as more difficult to learn and the students who still felt under-confident were those who had not yet been allocated to these areas for a 'long stint' (i.e. six weeks or more).

With increasing seniority, the students were given increased responsibility, particularly on night duty, and this, in turn, gave them more confidence. Their greater understanding of the theory they had been learning over the past year assisted their increasing clinical competence. Many students, in common with those in other studies (Chamberlain 1997), identified opportunities to teach which the qualified staff missed:

...<in> antenatal we've asked would it be possible for a senior student to go every morning on the doctors' round because antenatal is very interesting but nobody would pull you aside and say 'right, come on'...all you do is make beds and boil urine...+Cecilia, 1st May 96, 2nd int., C, 452-459

Some students spoke, almost with awe, of midwives who had a superior knowledge and an 'instinct' for clinical decisions. Most qualified staff cannot explain why they make certain decisions and, in this example, Heather does not explain her 'gut feeling' either:

I'm pretty confident, like, dealing with patients and sort of... looking at the patients and saying 'well these six are all right, that woman looks a bit iffy'...+ Heather, 14th March

96, 2nd int., B, 637-642

It is interesting that some of these students were expressing their perceptions of developing intuition at this early stage (one year into the programme). In a longitudinal study of 17 Project 2000 students, Gray and Smith (1999) identified that intuition was demonstrated in some of the students from two years onwards. It is possible that experienced nurses, as all these student midwives were, are capable of developing intuition at an earlier stage than do pre-registration students.

Benner and Tanner (1987) maintain that it is hard to learn that sort of intuitive judgement, but skilled pattern recognition can be taught by encouraging students to focus on the whole situation and providing feedback as to the accuracy of their clinical judgements. Clinical reasoning exercises can also strengthen students' analytical ability (O'Neill 1999).

Third and group interviews

The students were talkative during the third interviews and some were enthusiastic, but the majority appeared to be just trying to survive until the course was completed and they could leave. Three themes were identified and were labelled: 'There's a definite hierarchy', 'Giving midwifery care' and 'Learning to be a midwife'. Only one related specifically to the students' working role and is presented here.

'Giving Midwifery Care'

At this stage of the programme, after 19 or 20 months' experience in midwifery, the students all expressed themselves as 'settled' in to the hospital and their role. Some of the students felt fully confident in their abilities in certain areas and enjoyed taking responsibility, but a number complained that they were not given credit for their knowledge and experience. For example, Ruth was recording a routine cardiotocograph tracing for a woman in the antenatal ward:

It was the worst CTG I'd heard in a long time and I really didn't like it. And my gut instinct told me there was something wrong, so I turned her on her right and left lateral and had wedges in and everything and ...I let the staff know, and she said: 'oh, it was fine the last one, the last one was just as bad, and he <the doctor> signed the last one'... and I said: 'it's not just loss of beat-to-beat it's just so flat, it's unbelievable and it sounds really flat' and she said: 'it's all right, and what would you know anyway' (sneering tone, making a face). <This woman had to have an emergency Caesarian section for fetal distress later that day>. +Ruth, 11th Dec. 96, 3rd int., D, 81-104

This aggressive type of behaviour from senior members of a group is characteristic of the 'horizontal violence' seen in oppressed groups as a result of the incapability of these members to rebel against their seniors (Roberts 1983). As they do not feel able to express their anger directly to their own oppressors, they take out their annoyance and frustration on their more junior colleagues. Such behaviour can be construed as a form of bullying in that the future midwife's professional ability is challenged in such a way as to upset her and shake her confidence (Royal College of Midwives 1996). A study of this issue carried out by the RCM showed that 43% of the 462 midwife respondents had been bullied at some time in their career. In 51% of cases the bully was 'a more senior colleague', and the 'midwifery manager' was cited by 41% (Royal College of Midwives 1996). Roberts maintains that this state of oppression will continue to exist until nurses (and, presumably, midwives) reject the negative images of their own culture and replace them with pride in their own abilities to function autonomously (Roberts 1983).

A number of the students did still lack confidence even at this stage of their programme, particularly when sent to an area in which they had not worked for a long period of time:

I went in <to the labour ward> last week and I was absolutely terrified, it was nine months since I'd been there, and I was suddenly a senior. And how can you? You feel so insecure in yourself. And you feel people around you are saying 'God, she's not tuned in at all' but it's not that you're not, it's just that you haven't been there. +Jenny, 5th Nov. 96, 3rd int., C, 100-110

This is one of the many adverse results of the ranking system employed in a hierarchy, and later publications will discuss this aspect of the findings in more detail. Within a hierarchical system, 'senior' students are deemed to be knowledgeable and competent even though they may have assisted at fewer deliveries than has a so-called 'junior' student. Within a true educational system each student can be assessed on his or her own capabilities and experience, and given individually planned assistance to learn. It may, however, be difficult to change to this philosophy as the hierarchy in nursing and midwifery is a secure power structure, because the power wielded by the top-ranking members (e.g. ward sisters) is accepted by those in the lower echelons (e.g. staff nurses and students) without question (Hugman 1991).

Many of the students still professed themselves ignorant of certain procedures. Often they stated that they felt ashamed of their ignorance at this late stage in their education:

... I never thought of assessing how engaged the head was until I saw a senior sister up in the labour ward and...she said: 'oh, yeah, she's two-fifths engaged there, you know from your hands'. I'm thinking, here I am that only happened two months ago that should have been shown to us a year ago (chopping down with hands). +Alice, 6th Dec. 96, 3rd int., E, 147-156

There still appeared to be a shortage of both space and staff in the maternity hospitals:

... I've never seen a hospital to be so understaffed in my life. The birth rate is up at the moment...they've known for months that they were going to have this influx and yet nothing was done about it....there's extra beds pushed everywhere...privacy went out the window because you didn't have even a curtain around each bed. +Gertie, 13th Nov. 96, 3rd int., C, 177-186

... the place is bedlam, there's extra beds up everywhere and everybody's under pressure and you can't even get a cot in beside a mother any more and you're hurting your back because you're leaning in to get a thermometer in the morning... +Andrea, 6th Dec. 96, 3rd int., E, 247-255

Such overload of work has been shown in one small study to lead to job dissatisfaction in nurses (McNeese-Smith 1999) and certainly caused many grumbles among these students. In some ways, the shortage of staff was an artificial one in that staff midwives were reluctant to perform what they considered to be student midwife duties. In her study of nursing, Melia (1981) also showed that students do 'the dirty work' while staff nurses perform less onerous tasks. This artificial divide between staff and student work means that students do not learn to undertake staff midwife roles.

The staffing levels fell so low that in one hospital the students were taken out of class onto the wards, even though there were recently qualified staff from that hospital still looking for work. Although that was a rare occurrence, students were frequently taken from areas where they were allocated for their six-week placement, in order to provide relief work in short-staffed wards.

The emphasis on rushing the work because there was not enough staff to give more relaxed care, meant that the whole point of labour care – to support the woman – became lost in the students' haste to accomplish required tasks:

... pain relief, you'd love them to take something...they make your job more difficult, hanging out of you. +Noelle, 11th Nov. 96, 3rd int., C, 309-311

I never brought such a heap of rubbish up to the labour ward in my life...primagravidae in with shows and not a pain in the world. We had a very busy day anyway with the inductions but out of all the ones that I brought, I would say seventy-five per cent of them were either sent home or sent to the ward, they were rubbish. Waste of time! They'd come in and I'd say to the girl: 'what are you in with?' and she'd say 'I had a show' and I'd say: 'is it your first baby?' 'yes, it is' Oh God! (casting eyes up). +Heather, 6th Nov. 96, 3rd int., B, 3-18

This does not demonstrate the expected 'professional/friend approach' or the 'individualised approach' described by Fraser et al. (1998) as desirable in all qualified midwives, but more of a process-centred approach which does not value women as they go through one of the most significant experiences in their lives. The meaning of the word 'midwife' is 'with woman', indicating that the midwife's role is to be with a woman, encouraging and supporting her. This support and care of a known midwife results in more women looking back on their labour experience as 'wonderful' or 'enjoyable', and in more women feeling in control of their labours (Flint 1989). With increasing numbers of women presenting at maternity hospitals in Ireland and with no increase in the number of staff, the care given to these women will be of a lower standard. This lowering of the quality of care may go unrecognised, as it is unlikely that the classic indicators of perinatal and maternal mortality rates will change.

One of the students described her view of the way in which maternity care was provided in her hospital:

It's like this rotary belt you know, get her labour going, get the baby out, get her down stairs, get the other woman in, get this thing going (gesturing on each phrase). *It's losing the personal touch and it's not allowing the woman to be herself and to labour in her own way.* +Olive, 2nd Nov 96, 3rd int., D, 841-849

This 'depersonalisation' of birth (Kitzinger 1992) has reduced what used to be a significant phase in human life to a mere physiological process under the command and direction of medical 'experts'. The majority of students thought that there was too much intervention, principally by obstetricians, in normal childbirth and it is not surprising that, within this system, some midwives take on the obstetric rhetoric and make it their own (Murphy-Lawless 1991). Kirkham (1996) writes of how the dichotomy between technology on the one hand and the needs of the women on the other cause tensions for midwives, whose first loyalty is to the women in their care.

Staff and students working in this type of situation are also socialised into the use of such insulting language as that demonstrated above by Heather and become desensitized to it, ceasing to realise how offensive it sounds (Greenwood 1993). Hewison (1993) believes that 'the significance of the language used [in obstetrics] extends beyond semantics and style' and that our writings and speech have social and political implications that may have far-reaching effects.

Most of the students appeared to be ambivalent about whether they would like to stay in midwifery or go back to general nursing. For many it was a matter of going where there was a job of any sort, rather than choosing a career path and the majority were determined that they would not stay in their host hospital because the working hours were punitive for temporary staff. A number of the students, however, expressed the pleasure they derived from giving midwifery care and intimated that they would like to continue in this field:

It's nice to deliver a normal delivery by yourself, check the baby, do all those things...I feel it's a great sense of achievement. To bring a life into the world...it's very satisfying...+Pam, 27th Nov. 96, 3rd int., A, 221-233

Summary

The overwhelming sense that one gathers from these students is that they were, indeed, 'thrown in the deep end'. They were released into the clinical areas after one or two weeks of theoretical teaching, had an initial brief introduction to the work and were then expected to 'get on with it' and function as part of the workforce. The majority spent their first weeks or months of midwifery education frightened and unsure, afraid of putting a foot wrong in an environment that did not appear to be conducive to learning and support. The students suffered from role conflict and loss of status, which was all the more severe because it was unexpected. Their general nursing knowledge and skills, so hard-won, appeared to be of little use to them. The work itself seemed to consist mainly of basic nursing tasks, which were seen as boring and repetitive, and more complex midwifery tasks, which they were unsure of attempting on their own.

Because there was not enough staff to give more relaxed care, the students felt that they had to rush through their assigned work. The result of this was that the whole point of labour care – to support the woman – became lost in the students' haste to 'finish the work'. The shortage of staff was exacerbated by the fact that in some hospitals there was a set time by which certain tasks had to be performed, many of the tasks were unnecessary and staff midwives were loath to perform 'student midwife duties'.

Limitations

Students in two hospitals kept diaries only and were not interviewed. Students in one hospital were interviewed only and did not keep diaries. However, every hospital had between 21% (3) and 80% (16) of their student population involved in the qualitative part of the study, which gave a reasonable chance for those students' views to be aired. Also, in the two hospitals where no single interviews were done, a longer group interview was undertaken in order to give them an opportunity to express any views not shared by students in the remainder of the hospitals in Ireland. The questions forming the main part of the final questionnaire were derived from the qualitative data, so that the findings of this section of the study served to confirm the qualitative findings.

Conclusions and recommendations

It appears that midwifery care in Ireland, as described by these students, is governed not by a midwifery model, or even by a medical one, but by an economic model (Martin 1989) which emphasises swift through-put of clients. Maternity care in Ireland needs to be re-examined systematically and pilot schemes introduced that offer women more choice and control in childbirth, and midwives more autonomy of practice (Keenan 1999). Staffing levels must be examined and the use of routines and non-research based care should be phased out. Individualised care for women is essential with, if possible, a move toward more continuity of care. All these recommendations have been made and many have been acted upon in the UK over the last decade, principally in response to the 'Changing Childbirth' document (Department of Health 1993), but similar advances in the standard of care are only recently coming into maternity services in Southern Ireland.

To introduce such major changes in roles and socialisation of practitioners, the education of students needs to focus on the development of autonomous practice through the facilitation of knowledge development, understanding and the gaining of clinical decision-making skills (Holland 1999). This may be achieved not only through the usual two-year post-registration programme for qualified nurses, but also through a 'direct-entry' approach to midwifery education which has not been available in Southern Ireland for over a quarter of a century. A pilot 'direct entry' midwifery education programme has now commenced, in June 2000, in Trinity College, Dublin and its two linked maternity hospitals, which aims to address many of the issues raised in this paper in its pursuit of the optimal education experience for students.

Overall, in this study the setting appeared to be one of work, rather than learning, and the students' status that of junior employee rather than 'learner'. Ways of improving this situation could be to provide an increased amount of theoretical time and a longer period of classroom teaching prior to their first allocation to the clinical area. The 13 weeks previously allocated for theoretical input in the post-registration midwifery education programme in Southern Ireland was far too short (Begley 1999b) and has, from April 2000, been extended to 26 weeks (Department of Health and Children 1999, personal communication). Part of this extra time could be used to give students a period of supernumerary allocation in all clinical areas during which they should actually give care, not just observe care being given, as active participation is better from both the educational and job satisfaction points of view (Baillie 1993). These developments would counteract, to some extent, the effects of the industrial model on students of midwifery.

Students may now be assisted, with support from educated mentors, to plan care in a holistic way that will enable them to develop their midwifery skills in the future. This will result in increased autonomy for midwives and in more enhanced, empowering care for the women of Ireland.

Acknowledgements

This study could never have taken place without the active participation of all the students involved and I thank them for their whole-hearted enthusiasm and interest. Thanks are also due to the matrons and principal tutors in the seven midwifery education hospitals who granted permission for the study to be conducted. Financial support for part of this study was gratefully received from The Royal College of Surgeons in Ireland, An Bord Altranais and Gillespie Ltd.

REFERENCES

Baillie L 1993 Factors affecting student nurses' learning in community placements: a phenomenological study. Journal of Advanced Nursing 18: 1043-1053

Ball J 1989 Postnatal care and adjustment to motherhood. In: Robinson S, Thomson A (eds) Midwives, research and childbirth, vol. 1. Chapman and Hall, London

Begley CM 1996 Using triangulation in nursing research. Journal of Advanced Nursing 24 (1): 122-128

Begley CM 1997 Midwives in the making: a longitudinal study of the experiences of student midwives during their two-year training in Ireland. Unpublished PhD thesis. Trinity College, University of Dublin

Begley CM 1999a A study of student midwives' experiences during their two-year education programme. Midwifery 15: 194-202

Begley CM 1999b Student midwives' views of 'learning to be a midwife' in Ireland. Midwifery 15: 264-273

Benner P, Tanner C 1987 Clinical judgement: how expert nurses use intuition. American Journal of Nursing January: 23-31

Bradby M 1990 Status passage into nursing: another view of the process of socialization into nursing. Journal of Advanced Nursing 15: 1220-1225

Byrne U 1989 Family planning information: the contribution of the midwife. Unpublished BNS thesis. University College Dublin

Chamberlain M 1997 Challenges of clinical learning for student midwives. Midwifery 13: 85-91

Clarke M 1978 Getting through the work In: Dingwall R, McIntosh J (eds). Readings in the sociology of nursing. Churchill Livingstone, Edinburgh

Coates VE, Gormley E 1997 Learning the practice of nursing: views about preceptorship. Nurse Education Today 17: 91-98

Coleman H 1989 Transition to motherhood: a study of the experience of primiparous mothers in the six weeks following discharge from maternity hospital. Unpublished BNS thesis. University College Dublin

Council of the European Communities 1980 Council Directive 80/155/EEC, No. L33/8. EC, Brussels

Coxon T 1990 Ritualised repression. Nursing Times 86: 35-37

Davies E 1993 Clinical role modelling: uncovering hidden knowledge. Journal of Advanced Nursing 18: 627-636

Davies R, Atkinson P 1991 Students of midwifery: 'doing the obs.' and other coping strategies. Midwifery 7: 113-121

Department of Health 1993 Changing Childbirth HMSO, London

Donnison J 1988 Midwives and medical men: A history of the struggle for the control of childbirth. Historical Publications, London

Earnshaw GJ 1995 Mentorship: the students' views. Nurse Education Today 15: 274-279

Field PA, Morse J 1985 Nursing research: The application of qualitative approaches. Croom Helm, London

Flint C 1989 Continuity of care provided by a team of midwives the Know Your Midwife scheme In: Robinson S, Thomson AM (eds). Midwives, research and childbirth, vol. 2. Chapman and Hall, London

Fraser D, Murphy R, Worth-Butler M 1998 Preparing effective midwives: an outcome evaluation of the effectiveness of pre-registration midwifery pro grammes of education. The English National Board for Nursing, Midwifery and Health Visiting, London

Golden J 1980 Midwifery training: The views of newly qualified midwives. Midwives Chronicle and Nursing Notes 93 (1109): 190-194

Gray M, Smith L 1999 The professional socialization of diploma of higher education in nursing students (Project 2000): a longitudinal qualitative study. Journal of Advanced Nursing 29 (3): 639-647

Greenwood J 1993 The apparent desensitization of student nurses during their professional socialization: a cognitive perspective. Journal of Advanced Nursing 18: 1471-1479

Hewison A 1993 The language of labour: an examination of the discourses of childbirth. Midwifery 9: 225-234

Holland G 1999 Professional nurse autonomy: concept analysis and application to nursing education. Journal of Advanced Nursing 30 (2): 310-318

Holloway I, Wheeler S 1996 Qualitative research for nurses. Blackwell Science Ltd., Oxford

Hugman R 1991 Power in caring professions. Macmillan, London

Keenan J 1999 A concept analysis of autonomy. Journal of Advanced Nursing 29 (3): 556-562

Kirkham M 1996 Professionalization past and present: with women or with the powers that be? In: Kroll D (ed.) Midwifery care for the future. Bailliere Tindall, London

Kitzinger S 1992 Ourselves as mothers. Doubleday, London

Martin E 1989 The woman in the body: a cultural analysis of reproduction, 2nd edn. Open University Press, Milton Keynes

McNeese-Smith DK 1999 A content analysis of staff nurse descriptions of job satisfaction and dissatisfaction. Journal of Advanced Nursing 29 (6): 1332-1341

Melia KM 1981 Student nurses' accounts of their work and training: a qualitative analysis. Unpublished PhD thesis. University of Edinburgh

Murphy-Lawless J 1991 Piggy in the middle: the midwife's role in achieving woman-controlled childbirth. The Irish Journal of Psychology 12: 198-215

Murphy-Lawless J 1998 Reading birth and death: A history of obstetric thinking. Cork University Press, Cork

O'Neill ES 1999 Strengthening clinical reasoning in graduate nursing students. Nurse Educator 24 (2): 11-15

Pollert A 1981 Girls, wives and factory lives. Macmillan Press Ltd., London

Proctor S 1989 The functioning of nursing routines in the management of a transient workforce. Journal of Advanced Nursing 14: 184-185

Roberts SJ 1983 Oppressed behaviour: implications for nursing. Advances in Nursing Science 5: 21-30

Quinn FM 1995 The principles and practice of nurse education, 3rd edn. Chapman and Hall, London

Royal College Of Midwives 1996 In place of fear. Royal College Of Midwives, London

Seed A 1991 Becoming a registered nurse: the student's perspective. Unpublished PhD thesis. Leeds Polytechnic, Leeds

Seymour E, Buscherhof JR 1991 Sources and consequences of satisfaction and dissatisfaction in nursing: findings from a national sample. International Journal of Nursing Studies 28 (2): 109-124

Shead H 1991 Role conflict in student nurses: towards a positive approach for the 1990s. Journal of Advanced Nursing 16: 736-740

Treacy MM 1987 'In the pipeline': a qualitative study of general nurse training with special reference to nurses' role in health education. Unpublished PhD thesis, University of London

Wagner M 1994 Pursuing the birth machine: the search for appropriate birth technology. ACE Graphics, Camperdown

Walsh M, Ford P 1989 Nursing rituals: research and rational actions. Butterworth Heinemann, Oxford

Mind... the gap!

Maternal mental illness

Shona Hamilton

As midwives we have managed to cross cultural boundaries and meet some of society's more difficult problems head on. We have come to recognise post-partum mental health problems under the umbrella of postnatal depression. However, we have not fully embraced the deeper issues in the mental health arena, such as suicide. Suicide remains humanly shocking and one of the last bastions of social stigma. Combine suicide with discussions on mental health and maternal death and we have a minefield of emotions, prejudices and fears.

Midwives have continually embraced social and professional trends and explored these within the broad context of midwifery. We have analysed society's shift from normality to technology, homebirth to hospital and now once again we have embraced afresh the concept of normal childbirth. We have empirically investigated drug abuse, teenage pregnancy, and domestic violence. We have become open to scrutiny through risk management and critical incidents, yet we seem unable to fully examine the problem of maternal death through suicide and discuss the contributory mental health problems. In order to embrace normal midwifery and empower women we talk of being 'with women', of guiding, of counselling, acting as advocates, yet this type of relationship is impossible if we do not fully understand or appreciate the mental health problems experienced by the women in our care.

Midwives and obstetricians have made huge advances during the last century in reducing maternal and infant mortality. Clinical governance and risk management have ensured (albeit controversial) changes in the way we execute our professional duties. The Confidential Enquiries into Maternal Deaths (CEMD) findings have altered maternal care and ensured a reduction in maternal mortality.[1] However, the emphasis has been on physical illness and physical complications rather than on the psychological problems that lead to suicide. This, of course, is in keeping with the medical model of care, which most women continue to receive during pregnancy. The medical model accentuates the technological to the detriment of the interpersonal.

The medical model remains the most dominant and antiquated model of care within midwifery and still exerts powerful influence over the care midwives provide.[2] Such emphasis on technology, medicolegal issues and medical care has been detrimental to the psychological and preventative issues that must be addressed in the arena of mental health. This ethos results in women's mental health issues being neglected and inadequately assessed. High visibility needs such as infant feeding, safe delivery and overt physical problems are given priority within a fractionalised system, thus leaving women's psychological needs forgotten. This is far removed from the high quality women-centred care to which each midwife aspires.

Ill health or health problems conjure up a picture of physical complaints. These perceptions are probably due to our foundations in the medical model. Yet the World Health Organization describes health as 'not merely the absence of disease, but a state of complete physical, mental and social well-being'.[3] This definition highlights the need to include psychological ill health in our concept of health and well-being. Health promotion issues have become more pertinent in midwifery over the last decade and midwives make huge contributions to health issues such as nutrition and smoking. Dunkley[4] explains how physical, social and mental facets of health are interlinked. Thus initiatives that aim to promote physical wellbeing to the exclusion of mental and social facets may prove to be ineffective. In order to advance it is essential that the profession embraces health education issues and empowers women to take command of their own destiny.

So are mental health difficulties an issue of some magnitude or merely a factor relevant to only a small group in our communities? Puri et al[5] report that one in five people suffer from unwanted psychological symptoms such as anxiety, despondency and insomnia. GPs treat approximately one in six of their client group for primarily psychiatric disorders, and in a further sixth of the population, psychological factors are important contributors to illness. In terms of pregnancy, Goldberg et al [6] assert that ten per cent of women suffer from minor affective disorders in the first trimester and this number increases during the third trimester of pregnancy. It is estimated that somewhere in the region of 10 -15 per cent of women suffer from postnatal depression.[7] The number of women suffering from postpartum psychosis is lower, at two in 1000, but significant. What is also notable is the fact that the incidence of puerperal psychosis has remained constant for over a century.[8]

Health professionals often evaluate their treatment and interventions in terms of outcomes, a rather unemotional and statistically based indicator of quality care. Clinical outcomes rarely incorporate quality of life issues or the psychological factors that define health. One of the most traumatic outcomes of mental health problems is suicide. It is hard to equate this act to statistical references, risk avoidance and risk reduction. However, in order to highlight the severity of this problem one must look at the number of individuals who chose to end their life by their own hand. Bongar et al [9] state that 12 per 100,000 people commit suicide each year. It appears that the suicide rates among men are considerably higher than in women. National statistics estimate the rate for women around 4 per 100,000 population. The CEMD report highlighted that 42 women died as a result of psychiatric illness and 28 of those women committed suicide during a triennium.[1] Death from mental illness has now become the leading cause of maternal death.

So why are we so reluctant to discuss this matter? Suicide is usually a result of what Shneidman[10] calls 'psychache': the anguish, pain or ache that takes hold of the mind and causes distorted thinking and deep distress. Emotional pain does not fit within the confines of our daily work. It cannot be alleviated through physical means; there is no 'sticking plaster' we can apply. Physical pain can be relieved through touch, massage, support and medication. Physical problems are inherently much easier to address and a scientific model is simply applied. Emotional pain requires a much deeper level of therapeutic commitment from midwives, a commitment energised only through the creation of trust and safety. This type of relationship remains almost impossible to achieve within the confines of a fractionalised maternity system. This is not meant to be disparaging as midwives provide excellent emotional care to pregnant women. Nevertheless, in the context of mental health this emotional care has to be at a more profound level.

Hunt and Symonds[11] highlighted the communication patterns within midwifery care, stating the main goal was to 'get through the work'. This once again has been reflected by Kirkham et al,[12] who reported on women's perceptions of midwives in the clinical environment, showing that midwives focused on clinical tasks rather than listening and facilitative skills. An over-adherence to the medical model is one of the major causes of communication deficits between health professionals and clients.[13] Those at the forefront of care provision must embrace the appropriate communication and counselling skills needed to deal with these vulnerable women.

Whilst discussing maternal death, mental health issues and suicide, many authors have focused on the concept of 'taboos', society's and individuals' inability to discuss openly such painful subjects. Taboo does not fully explain our attitudes and preconceptions; rather it depicts a forbidden topic. Goffman's theory of stigma more aptly illustrates the negative feelings evoked by mental health issues.[14] Goffman asserts that those labelled as different come across sanctions due to societal conceptualisations about what constitutes difference. Mental health patients through out history have been portrayed as 'possessed', 'mad', 'crazy', 'lunatics'. They have been burned at the stake for being witches, locked up as sexual deviants and rehabilitated in asylums. In recent times the media's portrayal of mental health has reinforced society's view of violent psychiatric patients – thus instilling fear. Yet the relationship between mental disorder and violence has been empirically contested.[15] These stereotypes and associated negative characteristics create barriers that lead to discrimination and prejudice. Mental health problems evoke silence, embarrassment and fear thus leading to social exclusion and isolation. This isolation will exacerbate those feelings of 'being different' and may even compound psychological symptoms. Schreiber and Hartrick's [16] study revealed women's negative perceptions of depression. The women within the study regarded themselves as deviant and they enacted stigma.

Mental health problems in the community are widespread, yet societies continue to hold deep-rooted, culturally sensitive, negative beliefs about mental illness.[17] Religious, personal and professional values and beliefs are challenged in the face of suicide, an act that defies the notion that all life is sacred. Maybe this is more relevant in the context of midwifery where new life is our 'business'. Within the context of nursing and medicine the discourse surrounding euthanasia and assisted death has opened the debate publicly. It is not surprising, however, that the terminology is somewhat softer. Euthanasia evokes images of a peaceful, dignified death. Suicide evokes images of execution, hanging, drowning and violent acts, and fills us with horror. Suicide and attempted suicide have only been decriminalised in Ireland since 1993 and in the UK since 1961. Previously, individuals who took their own lives could not be buried on sanctified ground. In Ireland, suicide would have been regarded as the most deadly of mortal sins. These religious and moral beliefs are still deeply embedded in our culture and still influence the way we perceive suicide in the 21st century.

Client-midwife relationships are the fulcrum of effective efficient midwifery care. Each midwife is responsible for the psychological, social and physical wellbeing of childbearing women. It is essential that we initiate open discussions regardless of taboos and stigmas about suicide and maternal death. One of the few studies involving perinatal mental health issues explored midwives' knowledge of mental health problems and their experiences in dealing with these issues.[18] The study showed midwives had some knowledge of the subject but further education was required in order to deliver effective care. There is a plethora of empirical evidence and remarkable initiatives in the field of postnatal depression. However the CEMD report expressed concerns about defining all mental health problems under this diagnosis.[1] Society has come to recognise postnatal depression as a common illness among women and it is, therefore, an acceptable and palatable diagnosis.

It is clear that suicide is a pertinent concern for society today. In recognising a problem one realises a solution must be sought. That may be as complex as suicide itself. It certainly means that risk assessment must take place in the antenatal period and the appropriate systems of support must be implemented. Of course, in a stretched and overworked organisation, this may appear unattainable. It will certainly require input from our psychiatric colleagues and liaison service. Yet, as Morgan and Killoughery[19] state, liaison psychiatry is not a funding priority and its viability is tethered to the attitudes of hospital doctors. As psychological disorders remain within the realms of non-emergency, low visibility diagnoses, then there is little chance of acquiring the necessary funding. Psychiatry has always been regarded as the Cinderella service of primary care as postnatal care is the Cinderella service in maternity. It is now time that psychological care is given the priority it deserves and that vulnerable women receive the support needed to improve their quality of life.

Suicide is not only a tragedy in terms of loss of life but also leaves an indelible mark on families, friends, colleagues and acquaintances. It causes all concerned to question their acts and omissions under the cloud of immense guilt. It unfortunately defines people by the nature of their death rather than the achievements of their life. Midwives must investigate further suicide as a cause of maternal death and identify strategies to address this problem.

It would be easy to conclude with rhetoric and endorse research, one-to-one midwifery care, advanced communication skills and risk assessment. This would, however, be a vain attempt at promoting best practice. What is required is a strategy that goes some way towards generating more positive perceptions of people with mental health problems, a strategy that tackles the stigma within society and enables us to promote mental health in the same manner as we promote physical health. As Alverez[20] so aptly states, no single theory will untangle an act as ambiguous and with such complex motives as suicide, but we can untangle some of the emotional turmoil experienced by women, in the hope that these women do not seek a permanent solution to a temporary problem.

REFERENCES

1 Department of Health. The Confidential Enquiries into Maternal Deaths in the United Kingdom. London: HMSO; 2001

2 Bryar RN Theory for midwifery practice 1st ed. London: Macmillan Press Limited; 1995

3 World Health Organization. Preamble of the constitution of the World Health Organization Geneva: WHO; 1948

4 Dunkley J. Health promotion in midwifery practice: a resource for health professionals. London: Bailliere Tindall; 2000

5 Puri BK, Laking PJ, Treasden IH. Textbook of Psychiatry. 1st ed. London: Churchill Livingstone; 1996

6 Goldberg D, Benjamin S, Creed F. Psychiatry in Medical Practice. 2nd ed London: Routledge; 1994

7 Ugarriza D. Screening for postpartum depression. Journal of Psychosocial Nursing 2000;38:44-51

8 Gaskell C. A review of puerperal psychosis. British Journal of Midwifery 1999;7:172-174

9 Bonger B. Suicide. Oxford: Oxford University Press; 1992

10 Shneidman ES. Understanding suicide. USA: American Psychological Association; 2001

11 Hunt WS, Symonds A. The social meaning of midwifery. London: Macmillan Press Ltd; 1995

12 Kirkham M, Stapleton H, Thomas G, Curtis P. Checking not listening: how midwives cope. British Journal of Midwifery 2002;10:447-450

13 Dickson D, Hargie O, Morrow N. Communication skills training for health professionals. 2nd ed. London: Chapman and Hall; 1997

14 Goffman E. Notes on the management of spoiled identity. New Jersey: Prentice-Hall; 1963

15 Pilgrim P, Rogers A. Mental disorder and violence: an empirical picture in context. Journal of Mental Health 2003;12:7-18

16 Schreiber R, Hartrick G. Keeping it together: how women use biomedical explanatory model to manage the stigma of depression. Issues in Mental Health Nursing 2002;23:91-105

17 Crisp AH, Gelder MG, Rix S. Stigmatisation of people with mental illnesses. British Journal of Psychiatry 2002; 177: 4-7

18 Stewart C, Henshaw C. Midwives and perinatal mental health. British Journal of Midwifery 2002;10:117-121

19 Morgan JF, Killoughery M. Hospital doctors' management of psychological problems – Mayou and Smith Revisited. British Journal of Psychiatry 2003;182:153-157

20 Alvarez, A. The savage God: a study of suicide. 3rd ed. 2002; London: Bloomsbury Publishing plc

Reflecting on being with women

- How are you 'with' women in your area of practice? Increasingly, I hear midwives say it is difficult to be with women because of all kinds of constraints on their practice. Are there things that could be done to increase your ability to be with women? If so, how can you act to change those things?

- Have you been in a situation where a woman wants to make a choice that you feel is 'wrong'? What did you do? In retrospect, would you take the same action, or would you do things differently? Could you find ways to share what you learned from this experience with other midwives who may face similar situations one day?

- A question that builds upon this is in asking whether there is a line between needing to be a source of unbiased information and offering a personal opinion, and if so, where it is. Some women report frustration that, when they ask their midwives what they would do if they were in the woman's place, the midwives may decline to tell them. Is there sometimes a place for sharing a personal feeling or opinion, alongside making clear that this is only a personal opinion? Or is this a misuse of professional 'power'?

- What resources do you have locally for women who want more information about an issue? Do you have 'informed choice' leaflets which you can lend out? Can you direct women who do not have access to the Internet at home to local facilities that offer free access? Do you have a handout of websites, references or sources of information on the most commonly asked-for topics? What can you offer women who are unable to read, or who don't speak English?

Labour and birth

It has been frequently noted that the kind of environment that 'gets the baby in' (i.e. is conducive for lovemaking) is also the kind of environment that most effectively 'gets the baby out'. By comparing labour and sex, Judith Ockenden looks at how we might be able to help women get 'in the mood' for labour and, in doing so, highlights the impropriety of imposing standardised labour 'templates' on women. These templates have, for the past few decades, included routine interventions such as vaginal examination and electronic fetal monitoring, and Beverly Beech adds her voice to the growing body of literature, which is positioned against the idea of using such interventions habitually.

Mary Nolan revisits the subject of birth plans, some ten years after they began to be used in the UK, looking at what women's desires are, how birth plans can best be used as a tool to help women explore their desires, and how this all sits alongside the concept of woman-centred care.

Not that woman-centred care was a feature of the woman whose story is told in Joanna Berry's case study. This is one of the all-too-frequent examples of a situation where a woman was not allowed to eat in labour and was 'denied ... the choice of the type of care she wanted'. Apart from the psychosocial implications of denying women their fundamental right to eat and drink, one of my concerns about this kind of situation is that, by refusing women hospital-sanctioned food in labour, we are encouraging them to eat surreptitiously, out of sight of their midwives. In at least one situation that I know of, a woman who had brought food into a hospital and eaten secretly during her labour ended up needing a general anaesthetic, but didn't feel able to tell the anaesthetist that she had recently eaten because she knew this was 'against the rules'.

There are, of course, many areas where women's experiences are dictated by local culture rather than what is 'natural', 'normal' or informed by evidence. In her summary of the research relating to the third stage of labour, Lois Wattis notes that, 'obstetric practices and preferences largely dictate hospital policies, both of which are slow to change.' I find it remarkable that many hospitals are still basing policies on 'evidence' that is far less than sound. Yet even where evidence exists which shows that something can be truly beneficial (such as the use of water for labour and birth), this has still not become a realistically available option for a large proportion of childbearing women. Judith Ockenden asks some very pertinent questions around why the benefits of water in labour and birth are not being used more by women in hospitals. Despite the mostly positive coverage in the press about this issue a few years ago, a woman's choices (along with so many other things) appear to be dependent on her post-code, and the nature of professional beliefs about birth in the area in which she lives.

Finally, and on a more positive note, Marion Heres and colleagues compared the differences between the hour of birth in women whose spontaneous labours and births were attended by midwives or obstetricians. Given that the 'hour of birth' is determined by the length of labour as well as its time of onset, it is perhaps not completely surprising that there is a difference between labour attended by midwives and obstetricians. However, midwives may be surprised by the degree of difference – the presence of an obstetrician during spontaneous labour can delay birth. Yet another reason to choose a midwife!

The hormonal dance of labour

Can we teach women how to get 'in the mood' for labour?

Judith Ockenden

We have noted remarkable similarities between the changes and behaviour of the birthing woman and those of other sexual responses.[1]

In a sexual relationship, we sometimes talk about the 'right chemistry' between partners. People dance around each other, actually and metaphorically, until the conditions are right for sex. During this courtship, many biochemical and physiological events are leading to sexual arousal. In labour, too, our body chemistry must be correctly choreographed so that the movements of labour and birth can be accomplished successfully.

The right chemistry

The full elucidation of the biology and physiology of labour is still in progress, but a detailed outline of the interactions is now known. Here are a few essential points.[1-6]

- During pregnancy, the stretch-contract reflex of the smooth muscle of the myometrium is inhibited by progesterone and beta-endorphins.
- Before labour starts, the amount of oestrogen in the body increases relative to progesterone.
- The increased oestrogen levels cause the number of oxytocin receptors in the uterus to increase fivefold. The concentration of oxytocin does not change significantly, but the proliferation of receptors means that any oxytocin present can have a much greater effect.
- Oxytocin frees prostaglandins, mainly from the decidua. They promote the change in structure of the collagen 'superglue' of the cervix which softens the cervix.
- Oxytocin also initiates the release of calcium ions stored in the myometrial cells. Together with prostaglandins, they promote the formation of

electrical connections (gap junctions) between the muscle cells, so that the contraction can spread over the entire uterus.
- The damping down of contractions by beta-endorphins may be a modulating effect in labour, aiding the coordination of contractions. They also modulate the perception of pain and may provide a reward for coping with stress, in the same way that runners may get a 'high' from overcoming muscular fatigue.

With good direction and freedom of movement, the combination of all these steps leads to synchronised contractions that are strong and effective.

Orchestration

If hormones choreograph the dance of labour, the brain and nervous system orchestrate the music for the dance.

Oxytocin is made in the hypothalamus and transported along nerve cells to the posterior pituitary gland, where it is stored. It is released into the bloodstream in response to nerve stimulation of the reproductive tissues – the Ferguson reflex for example. The hypothalamus is under the control of the limbic cortex, the most primitive part of the cerebral cortex. This part of the brain coordinates physiological responses and instinctive human behaviour.[1,2]

Labour and birth, like sex, is instinctive, innate, primeval. Or, to have the best chance of working properly, it should be! But these primitive rhythms can be overridden by the higher, thinking parts of the cerebral cortex.

Response to stress

Labour is hard work. It hurts. And you can do it.[7]

In the first stage of labour, beta-endorphins can help

Figure 5.1.1 The booking visit

GP	And what can I do for you, Mrs Smith?
Woman	Well, Doctor, my husband and I have been married for a while now and we were thinking of having sex.
GP	Yes, fine, I'll arrange for you to go to the hospital.
Woman	Well, actually we rather hoped to do it at home?
GP	Sex at home? And is this your first time?
Woman	Yes....
GP	Well, I know it might all go fine... but first time in particular there can be unexpected problems. You'd be better off in hospital with experts to keep a careful eye on you.
Woman	That all sounds a bit off-putting. Surely it's a natural event?
GP	Yes, but things do go wrong and you don't want to take any chances. In hospital there's all the emergency equipment on hand – just in case it's needed.
Woman	It all sounds so clinical, and the hospital beds look so high and narrow, not like our comfy bed at home. We won't have much room for movement.
GP	Well, you don't have to use the bed in the early stages, but in the end, although people have these exotic ideas about different positions, most of them end up choosing the conventional position on the bed. It does give the medical staff the best possible view of what's happening.
Woman	It sounds so different from what we'd hoped for. We rather fancied being at home with soft background music, candles, a nice meal and a bottle of wine – you know, to help us relax.
GP	Well, you can enjoy those at home to start with if you like; keep the meal light and go easy on the wine – too much alcohol can cause problems. You needn't go into hospital until things are well underway, after all, it's only a short drive for you. In hospital, of course, you may not be allowed to eat and drink, but then you won't want to at that stage. As for the candles, they would probably set off the fire sprinklers!
Woman	Won't transferring to hospital upset the flow of things?
GP	Maybe, but it'll soon pick up again once you are settled in. The staff are very good at helping people to settle.
Woman	Won't having all those people around be rather inhibiting?
GP	Oh, you won't be showing them anything new. They won't be embarrassed.
Woman	But I would be!
GP	No, not really. Once you get going you'll be totally engrossed in what you are doing.
Woman	Oh, I don't know. I really imagined somewhere familiar and private for the first time; we redecorated the bedroom especially, bought some lovely new sheets...
GP	Well, you wouldn't want to spoil them would you? It can be a rather messy business. Look, why don't you talk this over with your husband and come back together next week?
Woman	All right, I think that's a good idea. Goodbye, Doctor.

Adapted with permission from an original 'playlet' by Jill Alderton and Jill Oliver.

women to enter their own 'world'. For her physiochemistry to function optimally at this time, she must feel safe. Birth is inherently stressful, and stress initiates the body's alarm response. Once this is triggered, the sensory information about the woman's situation is then analysed by the higher centres of the cerebral cortex. With good support and knowledge of what is happening, the brain does not verify the alarm response and the limbic cortex returns the physiological activity of labour to normal. The woman has adapted to the stress – a condition known as *eustress*.[1]

If, however, the woman encounters the unknown, becomes embarrassed or frightened, the alarm response is verified. The activities of the more primitive limbic cortex are interrupted and the body prepares for 'fight or flight' by producing a surge of adrenaline. There is failure of adaptation to the situation and *distress* ensues.[1]

The music has become discordant, and the dance becomes clumsy and uncoordinated. And there is an unwelcome addition to the repertoire of chemical dancers: adrenaline.

Adrenaline inhibits the production of endorphins, clearing them from the body while its surge lasts. In the first stage of labour it causes the circular muscles in the lower part of the uterus to contract strongly. This inhibits the baby's presenting part from pressing as effectively on the cervix, so reducing the oxytocin surges and slowing labour. These muscles are then acting in direct opposition to the other two sets of uterine muscles – the longitudinal and figure-of-eight muscles. The uterine contractions may become uncoordinated at the same time as natural pain relief is diminished. Redirection of blood to the limbs and panic breathing may lead to hypoxia in the uterine muscles, causing more pain and heightened alarm. The vicious circle is complete. With a clash of cymbals, the hormones no longer dance but are tossed about in the cascade of intervention. Contractions and pain may suddenly increase in intensity if syntocinon is administered or if membranes are ruptured. An epidural might restore calm, but interfere with the Ferguson reflex and pelvic floor activity in the second stage, so increasing the likelihood of an assisted birth. Once out of step, it is difficult to get back in time.

When the baby is born safely, 'that's all that matters'. Until the next pregnancy – when the seeds of fear and anxiety planted by past distress begin to grow, and too much background noise obscures the dance music.

Facing the music

It's all very well to wax lyrical about dancing and sex, but how far can we really take these analogies? Although it can be devastating for a couple if sex goes wrong, the situation is not potentially life-threatening.

We assume that sex is a normal human activity. If there are physical or psychological problems, then we may seek help. And, thankfully, help is available if it is needed.

The medical model of birth assumes that there will be problems. Labour has to be managed. This does not mean promoting *eustress* and preventing *distress* by truly being 'with woman'. It means trying to make the labour of every woman conform to a template. These attitudes, ingrained over decades, are reinforced by the media and by those health professionals who are entrenched in the current system. As a result, the people who seem to know least about how to birth 'normally' are those it most affects – new parents.

There are many who have accepted and understand the psychophysiological model of birthing.[1,2] Unfortunately recent research shows that those who have the knowledge and skills required

... have not only been marginalised, they are barely visible... Midwives' efforts are thwarted at every turn when they are forced to work in ways that do not appear to meet the needs of women or indeed themselves.[8]

Denis Walsh[9] has shown how barriers to change in midwifery are subtle and deep-seated, but that they can be overcome when evidence and audit are effectively combined. The growing strength and organisation of the Birth Centre Network (which can be found at www.egroups.com/group/birthcentres) is also a positive force for restoring the natural rhythm of labour and birth. Jane Walker,[10] in a recent article about the Edgeware Birth Centre, discusses how this model of care has not only 'broken the mould' but conforms to current strategic planning for health and the NHS.

Not many of us would say that sex is only about the organs that participate in intercourse, and whether they are healthy and working properly. Neither are we expected to conform to a set timetable or pattern of behaviour. There are well-rehearsed steps in the dance, but their combination and expression is individual.

And so it is with birthing. To paraphrase Irving Berlin: *There may be trouble ahead, but... let's face the music and dance!*

REFERENCES

1 Ginesi L, Niescierowicz R. Neuroendocrinology and birth 1: stress. BJM 1998; 6(10): 659-63.

2 Ginesi L, Niescierowicz R. Neuroendocrinology and birth 2: the role of oxytocin. BJM 1998; 6(12): 791-6.

3 Robertson A. Empowering Women: Teaching active birth in the 90s. Camperdown, Australia: Ace Graphics, 1994.

4 Morrison JJ. Physiology and pharmacology of uterine contractility. In: Studd J (ed.) The Yearbook of the Royal College of Obstetricians and Gynaecologists 1996. London: RCOG, 1996.

5 Jowitt M. The Reactive Uterus or the Birth Day Balloon. Midwifery Matters 1997; 74: 14-8.

6 McNabb M. Hormonal interactions in labour. In: Sweet BR (ed.) Mayes Midwifery. 12th edition. Balliere Tindall: 1997.

7 England P, Horowitz R. Birthing from Within: An extraordinary guide to childbirth preparation. Albuquerque, New Mexico: Partera Press, 1998.

8 Shallow H. Teams and the marginalization of midwifery knowledge. BJM 2001; 9(3): 167-71.

9 Walsh D. And finally... how do we put all the evidence into practice? BJM 2001; 9(2): 74-80.

10 Walker J. Edgeware Birth Centre. What is the significance of this model of care? MIDIRS Midwifery Digest 2001; 11(1): 8-12.

Birth plans

A relic of the past or still a useful tool?

Mary Nolan

Sheila Kitzinger claims to have introduced birth plans in the UK after discussions with Penny Simkin who pioneered them in the United States.[1] Like Kitzinger, Simkin is well known as a childbirth educator and campaigner for maternity rights, and has written almost as many books as her English colleague on the subject of woman-centred care. The aggressive medicalisation of birth in the USA, where 'gynaecologists' are the primary caregivers and caesarean section rates have always outstripped rates on this side of the Atlantic, made any strategy for assisting women to reinstate themselves in the birth of their children welcome. In 1989, Simkin[2] described the function of the birth plan as informing 'everyone involved in (the mother's) care what options are important to her, what her priorities are, and how she would like to be cared for'. Aids to communication were vital in a birth environment where:

> the mother... hardly ever knows her nurses... and if her own doctor is not on call when she goes into labour, she will be assisted by a substitute doctor who may be a complete stranger.

After crossing from America to the UK, birth plans enjoyed a period of great popularity in the 1980s when approximately 33% of obstetric units encouraged their use as a matter of policy.[3] They fell out of fashion in the 1990s when the promises of *Changing Childbirth*[4] led women and midwives to believe that a written plan was obsolete in the brave new world of continuity of care and carer, where 50% of women would be delivered by a midwife known to them. If maternity services were now to be truly flexible and responsive to women's individual needs, so that mothers were 'at ease in the environment of childbirth',[4] there would clearly no longer be a need for birth plans.

By the end of the '90s, when the structures of care described in *Changing Childbirth* had been tried and found difficult to realise, birth plans began to enjoy a resurgence of popularity. At the beginning of the twenty-first century, women continue to be invited by their hospitals to complete tick-box birth plans, or draw up their own.

Research into birth plans

In 1985, Ekeocha and Jackson[5] analysed the first 100 plans completed by women booked for hospital confinement in Huddersfield. The birth plan employed in the study was a forced-choice questionnaire in which the phrasing of some of the questions definitely 'forced' the responses. So women were asked whether during labour, they would favour:

- Continuous monitoring of baby's heart rate by electronic machine
- Correcting an unduly slow labour by rupture of the membranes (breaking the waters)
- Correcting an unduly slow labour by an intravenous infusion (drip).

What woman would not wish to 'correct' a labour that was 'unduly' slow? Notice as well the supremacy of the medical terminology: 'continuous monitoring, 'rupture of the membranes' and 'intravenous drip'. This is a birth plan that quite clearly presupposes a medical model of birth.

In 1998, Jones et al[6] described a small study of 42 women who presented at the Northern General Hospital in Sheffield with a birth plan. The results were striking – only 40% of these women achieved a spontaneous vaginal delivery compared with 60% of those without a birth plan. Every kind of intervention, except epidural, was experienced more frequently by the birth plan women than by the control group. Speculating as to the reasons for this, the authors concluded that, far from improving relationships between mothers and obstetric and midwifery staff, birth plans often caused 'irritation' which 'adversely affected the obstetric outcome'. The study was, of course, a very small one, and it is interesting that none of the first three named authors was a midwife. The article describes midwifery as a 'medical speciality' and although midwives were interviewed for the study, the midwife's own voice is not heard in the report of the findings.

The hijacking of birth plans by the medical profession has been very much evident in articles on the subject. Writing about birth plans and informed choice in the national newsletter of the National Childbirth Trust, Peattie[7] describes how mothers should discuss their plan with a midwife, and then quotes a consultant obstetrician as saying:

Around 20% of first-time mothers receive some form of medical intervention during labour, so it is very important for midwives and doctors to discuss these issues with women so that they are well informed in advance.

This sounds as if discussion should centre on ensuring that women understand the circumstances in which their birth plans must be put to one side, rather than on how to facilitate the choices that they would like to make. Kitzinger[8] felt that many hospitals 'were using birth plans to reassure pregnant women and to achieve patient compliance' while Jean Robinson[9] commented wryly:

Future researchers might... study why requests for more intervention like induction, epidurals or elective caesarean do not seem to cause hostile response even though they are more expensive... It's when women ask for 'hands off' care that they become unpopular.

Midwives' attitudes

Too[10] interviewed ten midwives to ascertain their views on whether birth plans helped women achieve choice and control during childbirth. One of her respondents felt that women were 'incapable of making rational decisions' in labour, and four commented that 'because of the time constraints and lack of staff, it was often quicker to decide for the women than to go through the lengthy process of dialogue and negotiation to find a way for action which respected the women's wishes' .

Jones et al[6] speculated whether birth plans led to more intervention because of the attitudes of health professionals towards them:

On questioning a complete shift of midwives, it was apparent that patients' birth plans usually provoked some degree of annoyance. This was mainly because the requests were sometimes felt to be inappropriate.

Anecdotal evidence would certainly suggest that midwives sometimes feel a woman is questioning their commitment to acting in her best interests when she arrives on the delivery suite with a detailed birth plan. 'We do that here anyway', I heard a midwife say recently in response to a woman's written request to be allowed to choose her own positions for labour and delivery. Why

then did this woman feel the need to write a birth plan? Perhaps because her experience and that of women she had talked to suggested to her the need to highlight this choice.

What do women ask for?

Price's analysis[11] of 20 birth plans found that women regularly mentioned:

* Choice of pain relief
* Birth companions
* Remaining mobile
* Having a managed third stage
* Avoiding an episiotomy.

However, they also asked for less predictable things, such as wanting a sibling to come into the delivery room immediately after the birth of the baby, and preferring to have the baby cleaned and wrapped before being handed to them. Price comments:

These issues may have little impact on professional practice, but were clearly important to the individuals concerned.

Advantages of birth plans

In many parts of the country, it is likely that a woman will meet a large number of caregivers during her pregnancy, and perhaps even in labour. Midwives would like to provide individually tailored care to meet the woman's needs, but this is difficult when there haven't been sufficient opportunities to get to know her properly. A birth plan provides a speedy way of helping the midwife understand what kind of birth would leave the woman feeling most satisfied and whether there are any particular cultural or religious issues that are important for her.

For the woman, drawing up a birth plan is an opportunity for her to reflect, in the midst of a probably busy life, on the forthcoming birth of her baby. Two thirds of the women in Brown's and Lumley's study[12] found it helpful to have thought about and written down their preferences beforehand. It is ideal if this opportunity for reflection is shared with a midwife who has time to explain to what extent the hospital is likely to be able to accommodate her wishes. In this ideal situation, the birth plan becomes 'a negotiated management plan of labour and delivery'.[7]

Disadvantages of birth plans

Birth plans have been criticised for:

* inflexibility
* creating unrealistic expectations about the choices

that can be made when resources are very limited
- causing difficulties if women's wishes conflict with hospital protocols.

None of these is likely to apply if the woman has had the opportunity to discuss her birth plan with a midwife. Women are not often totally unreasonable, and can be helped to understand the need for flexibility. If many of the birth plans written by women conflict with hospital protocols, either the protocols need reconsidering, or we need to find better ways of helping women understand why they are in place.

What kind of birth plan?

Tick-box birth plans do little to empower women or to make them feel that they are at the centre of their own care. The choices offered are not necessarily the ones that are of interest to them. They are easy to explain to women and easy to complete, but they do not help women think through what they want, nor do they provide midwives with insights into individual needs. They are a lazy way of being seen to involve the woman in her care, without really involving her at all.

If there is no time at antenatal clinics for women to discuss and write down their ideas for birth, childbirth education classes provide an alternative setting. Towards the end of a series of classes, women can be invited to use the information they have gained to identify what they feel are the most important aspects of care for them. If there are women in the group who find it hard to express themselves on paper, or who need help in reflecting on the material that has been covered during classes, the educator could suggest that people group together to draw up their birth plans. This worked very well at one

of my classes when one mother helped another who could neither read nor write to draw up her birth plan. The mother who assisted was probably far more able than any health professional to help the other woman, simply because she used lay people's language, and talked about the issues from the point of view of a pregnant woman.

Try offering simply a blank page with an invitation at the top:

Please write down your ideas for labour and birth – what you would like to happen and what you would not like to happen. If you have special needs because you have a disability, or there are cultural or religious ceremonies that are important to you, please write about these, too.

The women write their ideas in their own words. The words they choose, and the order in which they write things will give lots of clues as to their aspirations.

Woman-centred care

Many women in Whitford's and Hillan's study[13] felt that not enough attention had been paid to what they had written on their birth plans. If what women want is impossible to provide within the hospital setting, should the women be blamed for their inflexibility or should the birthing environment be reassessed? If a large number of women write that they want to labour without pain-relieving drugs, should this be dismissed as 'unrealistic' because 70% of primips at this particular hospital have epidurals, or is it a challenge to provide better labour support?

If birth plans are considered by some staff a waste of time because women always ask for what the hospital provides anyway, why do women go on asking for those things?

REFERENCES

1 Kitzinger S. Sheila Kitzinger's Letter from England: Birth Plans. Birth 1992; 19: 36-7.
2 Simkin P. The Birth Partner. Massachusetts: The Harvard Common Press, 1989.
3 Garcia J, Garforth S. Midwifery, policies and policy making. Midwives, research and Childbirth, Vol. II. London: Chapman and Hall, 1991.
4 Department of Health. Changing Childbirth: Part 1 – Report of the Expert Maternity Group. London: HMSO, 1993.
5 Ekeocha CEO, Jackson P. The 'birth plan' experience. British Journal of Obstetrics and Gynaecology 1985; 92: 97-101.
6 Jones MH, Barik S, Mangune HH, Jones P, Gregory SJ, Spring JE. Do birth plans adversely affect the outcome of labour? BJM 1998; 6(1): 38-41.

7 Peattie S. Is informed choice a legal right? New Generation 1998; 17(2): 18-9.
8 Kitzinger S. Birth plans: how are they being used? BJM 1999; 7(5): 300-3.
9 Robinson J. The birth plan game. BJM 1999; 7(10): 642.
10 Too SK. Do birth plans empower women: a study of midwives' views. Nursing Standard 1996; 10(32): 44-8.
11 Price S. Birth plans and their impact on midwifery care. MIDIRS Midwifery Digest 1998; 8(2): 189-91.
12 Brown SJ, Lumley J. Communication and decision-making in labour: do birth plans make a difference? Health Expectations 1998; 1(2): 106-16.
13 Whitford HM, Hillan EM. Women's perceptions of birth plans. Midwifery 1998; 14(4): 248-53.

Electronic fetal monitoring
Inherited clinical guidelines

Beverley A Lawrence Beech

In April 1999 the Department of Health commissioned the Royal College of Obstetricians and Gynaecologists (RCOG) to develop guidelines for Electronic Fetal Monitoring (EFM). When the National Institute for Clinical Excellence was established by the Government, on 1st April 1999, to provide patients, health professionals and the public with authoritative, robust and reliable guidance on current 'best practice' they inherited the EFM Guidelines from the RCOG and have now published the Guideline Development Group's recommendations.

The types of evidence under consideration were divided into categories based on guidelines which originated from the US Agency for Health Care Policy and Research (Table 1) and the Group's recommendations were graded into categories (Table 2).

Six recommendations were graded A

- For a woman who is healthy and has had an otherwise uncomplicated pregnancy, intermittent auscultation should be offered and recommended in labour to monitor fetal wellbeing.
- In the active stages of labour, intermittent auscultation should occur after a contraction, for a minimum of 60 seconds, and at least:
  - Every 15 minutes in the first stage
  - Every 5 minutes in the second stage.
- Continuous EFM should be offered and recommended in pregnancies previously monitored with intermittent auscultation:
  - If there is evidence on auscultation of a baseline <110 or >160 bpm
  - If there is evidence on auscultation of any decelerations
  - If any intrapartum risk factors develop.
- Units employing EFM should have ready access to fetal blood sampling facilities.
- Where delivery is contemplated because of an abnormal fetal heart-rate pattern, in cases of suspected fetal acidosis, fetal blood sampling should be undertaken in the absence of technical difficulties or contraindications.

Table 5.3.1 Levels of evidence

Level	Types of evidence
Ia	Evidence obtained from systematic review of meta-analysis of randomised controlled trials.
Ib	Evidence obtained from at least one randomised controlled trial
IIa	Evidence obtained from at least one well-designed controlled study without randomisation
IIb	Evidence obtained from at least one other type of well-designed quasi-experimental study
III	Evidence obtained from well-designed non-experimenatal descriptive studies, such as comparative studies, correlation studies and case studies
IV	Evidence obtained from expert committee reports or opinions and/or clinical experience of respected authorities.

Table 5.3.2 Grading of recommendations

A	Requires at least one randomised controlled trial as part of a body of literature of overall good quality and consistency addressing the specific recommendation (evidence levels Ia, Ib)
B	Requires the availability of well-conducted clinical studies but no randomised clinical trials on the topic of the recommendation (evidence levels IIa, IIb, III)
C	Requires evidence obtained from expert committee reports or opinions and/or clinical experience of respected authorities. Indicates an absence of directly applicable clinic studies of good quality (evidence level IV)
✔	Good practice points: recommended good practice was based on the clinical experience of the Guideline Development Group

- In the presence of abnormal FHR patterns and uterine hypercontractility not secondary to oxytocin infusion, tocolysis should be considered. A suggested regime is subcutaneous terbutaline 0.25 milligrams.

Ten recommendations were graded B

- Continuous EFM should be offered and recommended for high-risk pregnancies where there is an increased risk of perinatal death, cerebral palsy or neonatal encephalopathy.
- Current evidence does not support the use of the admission cardiotocography (CTG) in low-risk pregnancy and it is therefore not recommended.
- Fetal blood sampling should be undertaken with the mother in the left-lateral position.
- Contraindications to fetal blood sampling include:
  - Maternal infection (e.g. HIV, hepatitis viruses and herpes simplex virus)
  - Fetal bleeding disorders (e.g. haemophilia)
  - Prematurity (<34 weeks).
- During episodes of abnormal FHR patterns when the mother is lying supine, the mother should adopt the left-lateral position.
- In cases of uterine hypercontractility in association with oxytocin infusion and with a suspicious or pathological CTG, the oxytocin infusion should be decreased or discontinued.
- In cases of suspected or confirmed acute fetal compromise, delivery should be accomplished as soon as possible, accounting for the severity of the FHR abnormality and relevant maternal factors. Ideally this should be accomplished within 30 minutes.
- Absolute outcome measures of fetal/neonatal hypoxia to be collected at a local and regional level should be:
  - Perinatal death
  - Cerebral palsy
  - Neurodevelopmental disability.
  Collection and interpretation at a national level would then be possible.
- Intermediate fetal/neonatal measures of fetal hypoxia to be collected should be:
  - Umbilical artery acid-base status
  - Apgar score at five minutes
  - Neonatal encephalopathy.
  These should be collected on a local (hospital/Trust) level.
- Umbilical artery acid-base status should be assessed by collection of paired samples from the umbilical artery and umbilical vein.

Sixteen recommendations were graded C

- Continuous EFM should be used where oxytocin is being used for induction or augmentation of labour.
- Women must be able to make informed choices regarding their care or treatment via access to evidence-based information. These choices should be recognised as an integral part of the decision-making process.
- Women should have the same level of care and support regardless of the mode of intrapartum fetal monitoring.
- Trusts should ensure that there are clear lines of communication between carers and consistent terminology is used to convey urgency or concern regarding fetal wellbeing.
- Prior to any form of fetal monitoring, the maternal pulse should be palpated simultaneously with fetal heart-rate auscultation in order to differentiate between maternal and fetal heart rates.
- If fetal death is suspected despite the presence of an apparently recorded fetal heart-rate (FHR), then fetal viability should be confirmed with real-time ultrasound assessment.
- With regard to the use of intermittent auscultation:
  - The FHR should be auscultated at specified intervals
  - Any intrapartum events that may affect the FHR should be noted contemporaneously in the maternal notes, signed and the time noted.
- With regard to the use of EFM:
  - The date and time clocks on the EFM machine should be correctly set
  - Traces should be labelled with the mother's name, date and hospital number
  - Any intrapartum events that may affect the FHR should be noted contemporaneously on the EFM trace, signed and the date and time noted (e.g. vaginal examination, fetal blood sample, siting of an epidural)
  - Any member of staff who is asked to provide an opinion on a trace should note their findings on both the trace and maternal case notes along with the date, time and signature
  - Following birth, the care-giver should sign and note the date, time and mode of birth on the EFM trace
  - The EFM trace should be stored securely with the maternal notes at the end of the monitoring process.
- Prolonged use of maternal facial oxygen therapy may be harmful to the fetus and should be avoided. There is no research evidence evaluating the benefits or risks associated with the short-term use of maternal facial oxygen therapy in cases of suspected fetal compromise.

- Classification of fetal blood sample (FBS) results:

Fetal blood sample results (pH)*	Subsequent action
≥7.25	FBS should be repeated if the FHR abnormality persists
7.21-7.24	Repeat FBS within 30 minutes or consider delivery if rapid fall since last sample
≥7.20	Delivery indicated

All scalp pH estimations should be interpreted taking into account the previous pH measurement, the rate of progress in labour and the clinical features of the mother and baby.

- Continuous EFM only provides a printed recording of the FHR pattern. The interpretation of the FHR record is subject to human error. Education and training improve standards of evaluating the FHR.
- Trusts should ensure that staff with responsibility for performing and interpreting the results of EFM should receive annual training with assessment to assure that their skills are kept up-to-date. Details of key elements of training are in the full guideline.
- EFM traces should be kept for a minimum of 25 years.
- Tracer systems should be developed to ensure that CTGs removed for any purpose (e.g. risk management, teaching purposes) can always be located.
- Maternal outcome measures that should be collected include:
  - Operative delivery rates (Caesarean section and instrumental vaginal delivery).
- Umbilical artery acid-base status should be performed as a minimum after:
  - Emergency Caesarean section
  - Instrumental vaginal delivery.

Three recommendations were graded ✔

- A grading system for FHR patterns is recommended. This incorporates both the proposed definitions of FHR patterns and categorisation schemes.
- Settings on CTG machines should be standardised, so that:
  - Paper speed is set to 1cm per minute
  - Sensitivity displays are set to 20 beats per minute (bpm)/cm
  - FHR range displays of 50-210 bpm are used.
- Where there is clear evidence of acute fetal compromise (e.g. prolonged deceleration greater than three minutes), fetal blood sampling should not be undertaken and the baby should be delivered urgently.

The Guideline Development Group

The Group consisted of a multi-professional team of 13 doctors (of whom seven were obstetricians), one midwife, two consumers and a health economist who gathered together to consider the evidence of clinical and cost effectiveness. It is yet another example of a medically-dominated group producing guidelines which will be required to be used by another professional group, whose views could not possibly be given equal weight when there was just one, token, practitioner present.

There is a huge philosophical divide between the medical and woman-centred approach to birth. The medical model sees birth as a dangerous, risky event where one must deliver the baby as quickly as possible, and, in the meantime, find out as much as possible about what is going on inside the woman's uterus. The woman-centred approach sees the birth as a physical, spiritual, and potentially empowering event, where the majority of women will, with support and encouragement, birth their babies successfully. The former view perceives that death can be avoided or prevented by the appropriate technology and the latter sees death as an event which occasionally occurs and will sometimes occur with no possible explanation. Neither approach will eliminate death at birth: the tragedy is that enthusiasts for the medical model believe that they can.

RCTs and meta-analysis

As early as 1976 a randomised controlled trial of EFM revealed that it did not improve outcomes but almost doubled the Caesarean section rates in the process.[1] An almost endless stream of studies since then have come to similar conclusions. As Macintosh has suggested in a critique of EFM[2] a trial of 85,000 women would be required to reveal a reduction in the fetal hypoxia death rate from 2 in 1500 to 1 in 1500. Meta-analysis, where data from individual studies are combined, can provide sufficient numbers to answer some of the questions. By combining studies from different clinical settings, which measure different outcomes, the conclusions may depend upon what the reviewers sought to include or exclude. Furthermore, epidemiologists have expressed concern at the unknown number of studies which never see the light of day because they came to conclusions which were not positive, this further skews any analysis no matter how rigorous the reviewers have been.

The limitations of RCTs are perhaps best demonstrated by the recommendation that:

In the active stages of labour, intermittent auscultation should occur after a contraction, for a minimum of 60 seconds, and at least:

- Every 15 minutes in the first stage
- Every 5 minutes in the second stage.

The RCTs used this regime as a comparison, what is not available is a trial that compares this regime with a supportive, observant, and 'hands off' midwifery approach.

Auscultating a woman in line with these guidelines could become another rod for the midwife's back. Certainly, there is justification for this if the midwife is concerned, but for those women who wish to have a normal birth, having their labours constantly interrupted by a midwife with a pinard or doppler could be as disruptive as pinning them to the bed with a monitor strapped across their abdomens. Are we going further down the road where the midwife ends up paying more attention to the protocols than to the wellbeing of the mother?

What do the consumers think?

Electronic fetal monitoring was developed in the 1960s, but it was not until the 1970s that childbirth groups began gently to question its use and an early article ended with a quote from a perceptive mother:

I ... wonder whether too much reliance on mechanical measuring devices may eventually undermine the ability of midwives and obstetricians to 'sense' what is going on without them[3]

The questions about its value have increased in intensity over the years but despite one's reservations about a medically dominated Group these Guidelines are to be welcomed. They represent a significant step towards assessing the value or otherwise of electronic fetal monitoring. One of the most welcome recommendations in the Guidelines is the acknowledgement that

Current evidence does not support the use of the admission cardiotocography (CTG) in low-risk pregnancy and it is therefore not recommended

One advantage of this procedure, for the staff who persist in using it, is that it is a ritual which turns the active woman into a passive patient. She learns, right from the beginning that she is now under medical control. The labour is no longer hers, and she is required to comply with the hospital protocols that many staff wrongly consider over-rule the woman's wishes. It will be interesting to see what is developed in its place, and how long it takes for this unnecessary procedure to sink into oblivion.

As enthusiasm for electronic fetal monitoring developed, the majority of women were subjected to this intrusive and painful intervention. Even though many consumers are critical of its widespread use, it nonetheless comes as a shock to understand that only six

out of 34 recommendations are based on the highest standard of analysis – at least one randomised controlled trial. It is a shocking indictment of obstetric care that after forty years of enthusiasm for this technology the bulk of the recommendations are based on 'evidence obtained from expert committee reports or opinions and/or clinical experience of respected authorities'. Clinical opinion and respected authorities killed thousands of babies by recommending that women put their babies face down to sleep. Respected authorities recommended that every first time mother should have an episiotomy. These recommendations need to be considered carefully.

The 'high risk' woman and baby

An early paragraph in the Guidelines states:

EFM was introduced with an aim of reducing perinatal mortality and cerebral palsy. This reduction has not been demonstrated in the systematic reviews of randomised controlled trials (RCTs). However an increase in maternal intervention rates has been shown.

Yet, despite EFM's acknowledged failure to reduce perinatal mortality and cerebral palsy the Clinical Practice Algorithm suggests that women who are in the following categories – previous Caesarean section, multiple pregnancy, breech presentation – will automatically be offered continuous electronic fetal monitoring. This 'offer' will immediately increase the risk to them of the very thing that many women in these groups wish to avoid – Caesarean sections.

Some of the other categories recommended for continuous EFM are pre-eclampsia, meconium-stained liquor, fetal growth restriction and oligohydramnios, all of which are notoriously misdiagnosed, and in each case the severity of the condition, if it exists in each individual woman's case, should influence any recommendation.

The Clinical Practice Algorithm is headed by the statement: 'Consideration should be given to maternal preference and priorities'. Those who do the 'considering' also do the over-ruling, and too often 'offering' is interpreted as 'must have'. Those women who refuse the offer often find themselves under intense pressure to comply and if that fails they can find themselves accused of irresponsibility and putting their baby at risk.

The final section of the Guidelines lists future research recommendations:

- Evaluate the performance of EFM compared to intermittent auscultation in a low risk pregnancy setting with regard to perinatal mortality
- Evaluate the performance of different forms of intermittent auscultation, and how the performance of these modalities is affected by different frequencies

of monitoring in comparison to EFM
- Evaluate the performance of admission CTG.

For the last forty years thousands of women and babies have been subjected to unproven and poorly evaluated technology. Consider how the suggestion that a rise in the water temperature could cause brain damage in a baby born into a pool resulted in huge numbers of hospitals withdrawing their water birth service immediately, yet forty years of EFM research, which repeatedly demonstrated no benefit and higher rates of damage, results in yet more calls for more research because of these unanswered questions.

These Guidelines, by exposing the lack of good quality research, show how far the medical model has been imposed on normal birth, changing it from an intimate, physiological, event to a technological exercise in controlling, monitoring and recording, while ignoring the emotional and psychological impact on the women, babies and their families.

What kind of Guidelines would have been issued had the group consisted of equal numbers of midwives to obstetricians, and a substantial number of consumers? For too long maternity care has been dominated by the medical approach. One hopes that when these guidelines are reviewed the new Group will be more balanced, and by then there will be research which answers the questions the consumers want answered.

REFERENCES

1 Havercamp AD, Thompson HE, McFee JG et al. The evaluation of continuous fetal heart rate monitoring in high risk pregnancy. Am J Obstet Gynecol 1976; 125: 310-7.

2 Macintosh MCM. Continuous fetal heart rate monitoring. Journal of the Royal Society of Medicine 2001; 94(1): 14-6.

3 Hill J and Taylor A. Fetal Monitoring: A consumer viewpoint. Journal of Maternal and Child Health 1997; December: 472-4.

Eating and drinking in labour
A case study

Joanna Berry

This incident occurred following the admission of a 28-year-old primigravid woman (Judy) with a spontaneous onset of labour at 9am. Judy's labour was progressing well with no complications. Judy had declined breakfast when at home and when she first came into hospital. By 12.00 Judy was hungry, and was offered a sandwich by the catering staff, but according to the protocol Judy was informed that she was only permitted to sip water.

Judy was considered to be in early labour as she was not contracting regularly and was mobile. Although she was not in confirmed established labour at this time she was in the delivery suite. It is difficult to understand why she was not able to have a sandwich considering that she was hungry but as she was in the delivery suite it was indicated that the policy should be followed.

Later in the afternoon Judy's labour was established. By 5pm she was found to have ketones in her urine and Hartmanns solution was commenced. Once the intravenous infusion was set up, Judy was more or less immobile on her bed. Although Judy had wanted a normal delivery, her baby was born by forceps at midnight, by which time Judy was very tired.

Commentary

There still appears to be controversy on the issue of eating and drinking in labour. This is reflected by the disparity between hospital policies.[1-3] Since the late 1940s withholding food and water for all labouring women has been a standard practice. Mendelson[4] proposed this after having conducted a retrospective study of 44016 women undergoing obstetric anaesthesia. Of these, 66 women aspirated stomach contents into their lungs. Mendelson concluded that the aspiration of gastric fluid containing hydrochloric acid was responsible for the syndrome which now bears his name. The policy he recommended was designed to reduce stomach volume, thereby decreasing morbidity and mortality from gastric aspiration. Importantly Ludka and Roberts[5] point out that at the time of Mendelson's study general anaesthesia was administered with greater frequency for deliveries, combined with the use of an opaque face mask that obstructed the view of the airway, and the application of cricoid pressure was not always used.

In this instance the policy for fasting was instigated too early as Judy was not in established labour – she was not contracting regularly and she was fully mobile. This emphasises the importance of a midwife using her autonomy and not imposing polices without assessing each woman individually. The failure to provide Judy and her partner with a rationale for fasting so early in labour consequently caused unnecessary stress and a subsequent cascade of interventions. Midwives are in a position of power, which can be insidious,[6] and when women are compliant it is easier to follow policies than to think through their individual needs.

The Department of Health emphasises the value of research-based practice and states that practice should be based on sound evidence.[7] Withholding of food is not evidence-based. It is important that as midwives we should practise autonomously and be able to differentiate women's needs. Reflecting on this incident has given me a better understanding of protocols for eating and drinking in labour, but the outcome for Judy was a cascade of interventions that denied her the choice of the type of care that she wanted. This might have been avoided and this outcome of labour could affect her attitudes to subsequent pregnancies.

REFERENCES

1   Garcia J and Garforth S. Labour and delivery routines in English consultant maternity units. Midwifery 1989; 5: 155-62.
2   Michael S, Reilly C, Caunt J. Policies for oral intake during labour. Anaesthesia 1991; 46: 1071-3.
3   Berry H. Feast or famine? Oral intake during labour: Current evidence and practice. British Journal of Midwifery; 5(7).
4   Mendleson CL. The aspiration of stomach contents into the lungs during obstetric anaesthesia. American Journal of Obstetrics and Gynaecology 1946; 52: 191-205.
5   Ludka LM and Roberts CC. Eating and drinking in labour: A literature review. Journal of Nurse-Midwifery; 38: 199-207.
6   Kirkham. A feminist perspective in midwifery: Midwifery role and status. MIDIRS information pack.
7   Department of Health. Changing Childbirth: Report of the Expert Maternity Group. London: HMSO, 1993.

The third stage maze
Which practice pathway for optimum outcomes?

Lois Wattis

As a midwifery student negotiating the steep learning curve of clinical experience in several settings with numerous instructors, the birth of the placenta proved to be a bewildering maze of 'dos and don'ts'. Which oxytocic was ordered, and what dose? Whether to clamp the cord immediately or await cessation of pulsation, and which direction to 'milk the cord' when placing the clamps? Whether to 'guard the uterus' directly or through a folded sterile sheet? Whether to await 'signs of separation' or initiate controlled cord traction (CCT) immediately? Whether to release the clamp on the cord to 'drain the placenta' to assist separation or leave the cord clamped? And what about informed maternal consent regarding available choices? How much understanding do mothers really have regarding which oxytocic will be used and the likely side-effects? How often are mothers consulted regarding their preferred method and position for placental expulsion, and given the opportunity to examine the mysterious organ which has sustained their newborn throughout their pregnancy?

A heightened awareness of the hazards of third stage developed after witnessing two incidents where the umbilical cord was snapped due to an obstetrician's impatient application of CCT, and an inverted uterus caused by an ashen-faced GP/obstetrician resulting in emergency surgery. After seeing numerous new mothers' births marred by nausea and vomiting following syntometrine administration and several 'trapped' placentae requiring manual removal, I consulted peers, mentors, tutors, texts and databases in an effort to navigate the 'third-stage maze' to find a personal pathway of evidence-based best practice. This paper focuses on the choice of oxytocic, and umbilical cord clamping and traction in third stage care.

Active or expectant management

The third stage of labour extends from the birth of the baby to the expulsion of the placenta and membranes.[1]

Modern midwifery and obstetric management of the third stage varies significantly between countries, states, domains and practitioners. Care given to the birthing woman and neonate has evolved from an eclectic combination of historical, anecdotal, philosophical and research-based factors. This stage of the birth is identified as a time of great potential hazard and caregivers must make choices about whether to take an active approach, an expectant (physiological) approach, or a 'piecemeal' combination of both approaches.[2]

The third stage of labour may be managed 'actively' which involves administration of a prophylactic oxytocic after birth of the baby, early cord clamping and cutting, and application of controlled cord traction (CCT – originally called the Brandt-Andrews method) to deliver the placenta. Alternatively, 'expectant' management involves allowing the placenta to deliver spontaneously, or aided by gravity or nipple stimulation.[3] Procedures of pushing down on the uterus (Dublin or Traditional method) or its vigorous squeezing (Crede method) have largely been abandoned.[4]

In Australian hospitals the third stage is usually managed actively and is dictated by hospital policies. Prophylactic use of an oxytocic, cord clamping and delivery of the placenta by CCT are the norm.[5] Most practitioners await 'the signs of separation' which are a trickle or flow of blood, followed by signs of descent of the placenta into the uterine lower segment as the uterus becomes smaller, harder, and narrower as it rises in the abdomen, and cord lengthening, before clamping and applying CCT. The latter 'signs' are actually components of the expectant method hence a 'piecemeal' approach is often adopted.[2] Some caregivers also await cessation of cord pulsation prior to clamping the umbilical cord. True physiological management is more likely to be available for women birthing at home in the care of an independent registered midwife who is unrestricted by hospital policies.[5]

Management of third stage seems to be a 'pot-pourri of practices' with a kind of 'russian-roulette' of associated risks. Complications in third stage of labour are minimised if the woman has achieved maximum health in pregnancy and is not anaemic prior to labour. Prolonged labour causing exhaustion or dehydration, or having a full bladder at the beginning of third stage can all contribute to poor uterine action and increased risk of problems.[6]

In very general terms it would appear those birthing at major tertiary institutions may be less likely to experience potentially dangerous interventions due to the structured (some would say rigid) guidelines and protocols in place, which are updated in response to research findings. Women birthing at smaller hospitals implicitly trust practitioners to provide optimum care in limited environs but could be at increased risk for several reasons. General practitioners and obstetricians working in areas other than tertiary settings may be slow updating their practice in line with research findings, or worse, may disregard evidence-based recommendations in favour of their own experiences. Likewise, midwives may continue with familiar practices without questioning the evidence-base underpinning routine actions.

What is 'normal'?

As the baby is born, separation of the placenta usually begins with the uterine contraction which expels the baby's trunk, and is completed with the next one or two contractions.[5] Because the baby's body is no longer taking up space in the uterus, its size (and therefore the placental site) is decreased by about half. The placenta is tightly compressed by the contracted uterus and some fetal blood is pumped back into the baby's circulation. Simultaneously maternal blood is forced back into the veins of the decidua basalis, but is unable to return to the maternal circulation due to the contracted and retracted state of the myometrium. This causes the congested veins to rupture, the villi to shear off the spongy decidua basalis, and the inelastic placenta to become wrinkled and peel away from the uterine wall.[6] Bleeding is controlled physiologically by three processes: The action of the 'living ligatures' which are interlacing spiral fibres which contract around the maternal vessels to prevent further blood loss; the pressure exerted on the placental site through apposition of the firmly contracted walls of the uterus; and blood clots at the placental site, in the sinuses and torn blood vessels.[6] The umbilical arteries constrict at birth so blood does not flow from the infant to the placenta, however the umbilical vein remains dilated allowing blood flow from the placenta to the infant via gravity during the first three minutes after birth.[7] When the baby starts breathing pulsations

cease in the umbilical cord.[4] Nature has provided wonderously for both mother and baby from conception to first breath, and to the breast.

Historical overview of interventions

So how did intervening in the natural process of third stage become 'normal practice'? Cutting the cord as soon as the baby was born was first carried out in the seventeenth century, around the same time as women started lying down in bed to give birth, rather than using a birthing stool. The extra blood loss from the cut cord and consequent soiling of bed linen also led to clamping (by knot or tie) of the severed cord ends.[8] Cutting the cord deprives the baby of the blood remaining in the placenta but does not affect the (natural) way by which the placenta separates from the uterus. Clamping the placental blood flow sets up a counter-resistance, causing formation of a blood clot behind the placenta. Experts cannot agree whether clamping the cord aids or slows the separation process, however the formation of a retroplacental clot is not believed to be a (natural) physiological event.[7] With the cord clamped the placenta remains plump and bulky rather than compressed and compact during uterine contractions, tending to make placental expulsion difficult and more prone to retention.[8] Pulling on the cord was advocated by doctors to facilitate separation and expulsion of the placenta before the cervix closed in response to uterine involution, however inversion of the uterus was sometimes a life-threatening consequence of this action. These factors all led to an increased incidence of post-partum haemorrhage, manual removal of the placenta and infection. The cascade of intervention continued as the need for anaesthetics and surgery to remove various retained products of conception also increased.[8]

During the 1920s postpartum haemorrhage (PPH) accounted for 22 per cent of maternal deaths in the UK. In the 1930s the discovery of the oxytocic drug ergometrine was hailed as a major breakthrough for controlling PPH when used immediately after childbirth. The maternal death rate fell steadily when ergometrine became readily available, however improved nutritional and health status of mothers is also believed to have influenced morbidity and mortality rates.[8] During the 1940s several uncontrolled studies claimed beneficial effects of ergometrine's routine use during third stage. Unfortunately ergometrine's side-effects were also profound, and the incidence of retained placenta due to the drug's tonic effect on the uterus, plus hypertension, nausea, vomiting and severe afterbirth pains detracted from its lifesaving benefits.[2]

In the 1960s the availability of syntometrine (a combination of syntocinon and ergometrine) offered an alternative prophylactic oxytocic drug with similar but less severe side-effects. Its value was claimed to lie in the rapid effect of oxytocin and the sustained effect of ergometrine.[2] Studies showed that administration of oxytocics results in an important reduction in the risk of postpartum haemorrhage, and when combined with use of CCT accelerates the third stage of labour significantly.[6] Active management of the third stage of labour became routine, and was officially recommended by the WHO in 1994, especially in the developing world where PPH is the commonest cause of maternal death.

Choice of oxytocic agent

The routine use of oxytocics to reduce the risk of PPH has been the subject of debate and clinical trials over recent years. Initially research revolved around oxytocic choice and timing of administration, but few questioned the wisdom of third stage interventions and their impact on women's childbirth experience. Syntometrine has been shown to be superior to oxytocin alone in reducing PPH in some controlled trials.[3,6] Others found no significant difference between intramuscular syntometrine 1ml and oxytocin 10iu in rates of PPH and this view is further substantiated by a recent meta-analysis of trials.[9-11] Side-effects of the ergometrine (contained in syntometrine) such as nausea, vomiting and headache, its vasopressor action resulting in hypertension, and its association with reduced prolactin levels must be weighed against its marginal superiority over oxytocin alone in reducing the risk of PPH.[12]

The experience of vomiting is not a common reaction after the stress of giving birth, rather a common side-effect of syntometrine.[13] Recommendations for the use of syntocinon alone have prevailed in recent times, including the findings of the most comprehensive study of the management of third stage to date – the Hinchingbrooke randomised controlled trial.[14]

The value and place of naturally-occurring oxytocin in response to nipple stimulation should not be overlooked when considering safe management of the third stage of labour. The nipples are very sensitive immediately following birth and any touch of the baby's mouth or tongue can stimulate oxytocin release in the mother's body. A powerful surge of oxytocin probably greater than at any other time during the labour occurs with suckling, assisting expulsion of the placenta and avoidance of haemorrhage. It also raises the mother's skin temperature, warming the baby, and floods her with nurturing feelings which are key elements in the initial attachment process between mother and baby.[15]

Nevertheless, the 'trade off' effect between the two drugs continues to confound decision-making on choice of oxytocic in many settings. Practitioners develop an allegiance to trusted oxytocics and changes to policies and practices can challenge long established belief systems. Interventions to reduce the risk of PPH such as choice of oxytocic drug, and how or when it is given may be irrelevant when other contributing factors to PPH are considered. Mismanagement of the third stage by massaging, squeezing or otherwise 'fiddling' with the uterus can disrupt the rhythm of myometrial activity causing only partial separation of the placenta and subsequent excessive bleeding. Induced, augmented, prolonged or rapid labours can increase risks of PPH, while genital tract lacerations and coagulopathies may also be responsible for haemorrhages.[6]

Practice pathway – oxytocics

Midwifery and obstetric care is increasingly directed by the findings of well-formulated research, and a critical and analytical approach to the development of evidence-based practice is actively promoted. The provision of a safe, satisfying third stage of labour not only demands examination of routine practices in a clinical sense, but also in light of the childbearing woman's expectations and perceptions of their childbirth experience, and neonatal outcomes.

Meta-analysis of research provides practitioners with clarified results, but if the experts cannot agree how can a fledgling midwife be expected to decide, and safely guide women in their choices? The direction to take through the third stage maze demands careful consideration as well as flexibility. For the majority of women birthing in Australian hospitals a choice between active and expectant management of third stage is not an available option. Active management is advocated in the name of safety and women wanting truly physiological management of third stage may only achieve this through birthing at home or some birth centres. Enkin describes the combination of active and expectant techniques as a 'piecemeal' approach.[2] This terminology seems unnecessarily derogatory – philosophical purity is irrelevant. Amalgamation of the two methods providing the benefits of both while minimising risks seems a reasonable approach for evidence-based practice – perhaps 'complimentary' would better describe this mode of care.

Recent research indicates syntocinon is preferable to syntometrine due to the adverse maternal side-effects of the latter. Practitioners who continue to order syntometrine as their first choice in prophylactic oxytocic need to 'revisit their guidelines'.[13] The benefits of utilising endogenous oxytocin through early breastfeeding stimuli must feature as a preferred natural adjunct to prophylactic oxytocic administration.[15]

Cord clamping and traction

During the 1930s and 1940s Brandt and Andrews modified Aristotle's method of delivering the placenta by cord traction, replacing the traditional or Dublin method of fundal pressure. The Brandt-Andrews method involved application of tension (but not traction) to the umbilical cord with one hand, with the other hand placed on the abdomen pushing the uterus upwards off the placenta.[16] Controlled cord traction is a refinement of this method, and its routine use coincided with the introduction of oxytocic drugs. The use of oxytocics hastened and intensified uterine involution following birth of the baby necessitating active intervention to remove the placenta before closure of the cervical os. When administered intramuscularly syntocinon acts within 2.5 minutes, and ergometrine within 6-7 minutes creating a climate of relative urgency in third stage. When syntometrine is used the placenta should be delivered with the first uterine contraction after the birth of the baby, usually between 2-4 minutes, otherwise placental entrapment may occur.[16]

Active management of third stage usually entails clamping and dividing the umbilical cord relatively early, before beginning controlled cord traction. Pre-empting physiological equilibration of the blood volume within the fetoplacental unit in this way may predispose to retained placenta, postpartum haemorrhage, fetomaternal transfusion and impact on neonatal wellbeing, particularly relating to respiratory distress.[2] CCT is associated with a lower mean blood loss and shorter third stage, however trials provide insufficient data to warrant firm conclusions about its effects on either postpartum haemorrhage or manual removal of the placenta.[2] Manual removal of the placenta is an unpleasant procedure with its own serious complications of haemorrhage, infection or genital tract trauma. Recent research indicates umbilical vein injection of saline solution plus oxytocin appears to be effective in the management of retained placenta, and provides a far less invasive treatment option.[17]

Consensus of opinion on the timing of clamping is not easy to achieve. Delayed cord clamping results in a placental transfusion to the baby between 20% and 50% of neonatal blood volume depending on the timing of clamping, positioning of the baby in relation to gravitational flow from the placenta, and whether an oxytocic is used. Delay in clamping of as little as 30 seconds may have important clinical benefits for the baby, particularly if it is preterm.[2] In support of this, other authors propose the cord of the preterm baby born by caesarean section should not be clamped nor an oxytocic given until the cord has stopped pulsating because early clamping deprives the baby of vital blood volume, and giving an oxytocic before clamping risks overloading the baby's circulation.[18] Opposing views are also held regarding preterm infants, stating delayed cord clamping is associated with hyperbilirubinaemia due to the increased volume of RBCs, and respiratory distress resulting from movement of excess plasma volume that cannot be accommodated in the lungs leading to decreased lung compliance and functional residual capacity.[7]

Early cord clamping results in lower haemoglobin values, haematocrits and bilirubin levels in the newborn, and should be avoided in rhesus negative women because it increases the risk of fetomaternal transfusion. Allowing free bleeding from the placental end of the cord reduces the risk of fetomaternal transfusion which may be important with regard to blood group isoimmunisation.[2] Non-clamping of the maternal end of the severed cord to allow free bleeding from the undelivered placenta is practised routinely in Pithiviers, France, and is believed to aid placental detachment in the absence of oxytocic use.[19] Nevertheless, rapid cord clamping and cutting, and retention of the clamp at the maternal end (often to facilitate application of CCT) is commonly practised by midwives instructing midwifery students. Is it any wonder students become confused?

Neonatal wellbeing is believed to be enhanced by the provision of additional red cells which maintain a higher haemoglobin level and extra iron stores in the infant.[20] A study conducted in 1997 reviewed the haematologic status of infants after two months and found those who had been managed with delayed cord clamping had significantly higher haematocrit values and haemoglobin concentrations than those who had early cord clamping. The result suggests waiting until the cord stops pulsating before clamping is a feasible low-cost intervention that can reduce anaemia in infants, especially in developing countries.[21] The World Health Organization recommends late cord clamping in normal birth.[22]

Practice pathway – cord clamping

Early or late cord clamping remains a debatable issue. There appears to be clear benefits for fetomaternal physiological equilibrium when interventions such as cord clamping and traction are minimised. Much of the urgency commonly attached to third stage is unnecessary. Awaiting cessation of cord pulsation before clamping and cutting, allowing free drainage of the maternal end of the severed cord, and patiently observing for the signs of separation and descent of the placenta can be readily incorporated into the management of the uncomplicated birth without compromising safety. Adoption of an upright maternal position to facilitate expulsion of the placenta with the aid of gravity can reduce the likelihood of application of excessive traction and its potentially dangerous sequelae.[14] Allowing the parents the opportunity to examine the products of conception if they wish (and to keep them if that is part of their plan) can physically and emotionally complete their total birth experience.

Informed consent

Obstetric practices and preferences largely dictate hospital policies, both of which are often slow to change. The woman's experience of birth may be neglected by professionals whose focus is on physical care and monitoring progress to detect deviation from the normal. Safety is of paramount importance, but women also have high emotional expectations of this momentous event in their lives. When expectations are fulfilled women can review their unique experience with pride and a sense of achievement. With confidence and self-esteem enhanced women are less likely to experience problems bonding to their baby, or to suffer from postnatal depression.[6]

The basic principle of a woman's right to know all the risks and benefits of proposed treatments is accepted as the foundation of equitable and effective maternity care. A number of factors influence a woman's ability to exercise her right to make informed choices. Access to accurate valid information, the limitation of information reflecting personal bias of the advisor, or the woman's inability to understand or evaluate information due to her physical or emotional state of health may affect decisions. Women may feel pressured, coerced or rushed into agreeing with a mode of care, denied the right to change their mind, or lack support for their chosen plan. Women need a strong sense of identity, plus skills in negotiation and the ability to be assertive to find their way through the healthcare maze. Throughout pregnancy and birth the midwife can be 'a lighthouse guiding the way through a sea of confusion and inequality'.[15]

Consideration of women's preferred method of third stage management is demonstrated in the important paper published in *The Lancet* known as the Hinchingbrooke randomised controlled trial.[14] The trial was carried out in a setting where the philosophy of care emphasised helping women to give birth with minimal intervention, including during the third stage of labour. The midwives were confident with both active and expectant management for women at low risk of PPH. Apart from a slightly higher mean birthweight of babies

in the expectant-management than in the active-management group, there was no evidence of any other differential effects of the two policies on maternal or neonatal outcomes either in the short term or at 6 weeks after the birth. Maternal posture (upright or supine) during placental expulsion was found to have no influence on the risk of PPH.[14]

When the Hinchingbrooke trial sought women's perceptions of their birthing experience, feedback indicated feelings of satisfaction with the management of the third stage were similar in both groups (94.2% expectant; 96.8% active). However women in the expectant group felt more 'in control' during third stage (87.5%), compared to 83.4% in the actively managed. The pleasing aspect of this study is that women were consulted. The level of understanding among childbearing women of their options reflects a comprehensive and unbiased antenatal education process, in that part of Britain at least. The conclusions of this study may be used to enable individual women, together with their caregivers, to weigh up the relative importance of the various outcomes.

The final recommendation of the trial advocated the use of active management with oxytocin (not syntometrine) in hospital settings. The challenge for practitioners centers on the need to give balanced information to women during the antenatal period supporting informed choice, and to develop and maintain competence in both expectant and active management of third stage.[14]

Caring for the woman's psychological wellbeing during the intrapartum period is intrinsic to the delivery of holistic midwifery care. Knowing, respecting and endeavouring to assist the woman to fulfil her personal birth plan whenever possible is integral to achieving a satisfying outcome for many women.

The frightening and dangerous experiences of retained placenta, uterine inversion, or PPH with likely sequelae of anaesthesia, separation from the newborn and extended postpartal recovery are potential negative outcomes of a poorly managed third stage of labour. Some of the more disturbing memories parents carry away from the experience of an at-risk birth are those created by unthinking application of 'stormtrooper obstetrics'.[23] The dramatic intrapartum period can leave lasting impressions, and may enhance or inhibit the family's ability to integrate the birth experience into their lives and move on to productive parenthood.[23]

REFERENCES

1 Llewellyn-Jones D. Fundamentals of Obstetrics and Gynaecology. 6th Edn. London: Mosby, 1994.

2 Enkin M, Keirse MJNC, Renfrew MJ & Neilson JP. A guide to effective care in pregnancy and childbirth. 2nd Edn. Oxford: Oxford University Press, 1995.

3 Prendiville WJ, Elbourne D & McDonald S. Active versus expectant management of the third stage of labour (Abstract) 1998. http://www.update-software.com/ccweb/cochrane/revavstr/ab000007.htm

4 Beischer NA & Mackay EV. Obstetrics and the newborn. 2nd Edn. Sydney: Holt Saunders P/L, 1986.

5 Bennett A, Etherington W & Hewson D. Childbirth Choices. Melbourne: Penguin Books Australia Ltd, 1993.

6 Sweet B. Mayes Midwifery: A textbook for midwives. 12th Edn. London: Balliere Tindall, 1997.

7 Tucker A, Blackburn S & Loper DL. Section placental development in maternal, fetal and neonatal physiology. Philadelphia: WB Saunders Co, 1992.

8 Priya JV. Birth traditions and modern pregnancy care. Dorset: Element Books Ltd, 1992.

9 Jouppila P. Postpartum haemorrhage. Current Opinions in Obstetrics and Gynaecology 1995; 7: 446-50.

10 McDonald S, Prendiville WJ & Elbourne D. Prophylactic syntometrine versus oxytocin for delivery of the placenta (Abstract) 1999. http://www.updatesoftware.com/ccweb/cochrane/revabstr/ab000201.htm

11 Drife J. Management of primary postpartum haemorrhage. British Journal of Obstetrics and Gynaecology 1997; 104(3): 275-7.

12 Soriano D, Dulitzki M, Schiff E. A prospective cohort study of oxytocin plus ergometrine compared with oxytocin alone for prevention of postpartum haemorrhage. British Journal of Obstetrics and Gynaecology 1996; 103(11): 1068-73.

13 Anderson T. MIDIRS comments: A prospective cohort study of oxytocin plus ergometrine compared with oxytocin alone for prevention of postpartum haemorrhage. MIDRS Digest 1997; 7(2): 193.

14 Rogers J, Wood J, McCandlish R, Ayers S, Truesdale A, Elbourne D. Active versus expectant management of third stage of labour: The Hinchingbrooke randomised controlled trial. The Lancet 1998; 351: 693-9.

15 Robertson A. Empowering women: Teaching active birth in the 90s. Camperdown, NSW: Ace Graphics, 1994.

16 Myles MF. Textbook for midwives. 10th Edn. London: Churchill Livingstone, 1995.

17 Carroli G & Bergel E. Umbilical vein injection for management of retained placenta (Abstract) 1999. http://www.updatesoftware .com/ccweb/cochrane/revabstr/ab001337.htm

18 Rosevear SK & Stirrat GM. Handbook of obstetric management. London: Blackwell Science, 1996.

19 Odent M. Birth Reborn: What childbirth should be. 2nd Edn. New York: Random House, 1984.

20 Johnston PGB. The newborn child. 8th Edn. London: Churchill Livingstone, 1998.

21 Grajeda R, Perez-Escamilla R, Dewey KG. Delayed clamping of the umbilical cord improves haematologic status of Guatemalan infants at 2 months of age. American Journal of Clinical Nutrition 1997;65(2): 425-31.

22 World Health Organization. Care in normal birth: A practical guide. Geneva, WHO 1996.

23 May K. Psychosocial implications of high-risk intrapartum care. In: Foundations of Practice, Curtin University of Technology Article 9, 42-5.

Water labour and birth
Time to let it flow

Judith Ockenden

One midwifery manager simply tells women: 'We do not allow water births. My midwives are not trained for it.' She said the same thing last year. And the year before. Meanwhile no training has been arranged. Just what is so difficult about water labour and birth training? We are not talking rocket science for heaven's sake. (Robinson, 2001)

This is an anecdote. I could add several more of my own, from comments received from parents at my antenatal classes. It's not that our units do not have pools (they are very good units), but parents on a tour of them are sometimes subtly discouraged from using them. The benefits listed in the leaflets given out are not always reinforced by those midwives who are not trained in management of water labour and birth. The pools are greatly underused.

Yet, when I speak to women about their experience of using birthing pools, the vast majority are very positive about them. One woman employed a private midwife recently to ensure she could use a birthing pool. She had been told that due to staff shortages she could not otherwise be guaranteed use of the pool.

If I was beginning my childbearing career again, I would certainly be keen to use a birthing pool. My opinion has not been formed only as a result of listening to the experience of others, although I do consider these reports to be valuable. It has also comes from evaluating the evidence.

Is water beneficial in labour and birth?

A recent study (Burns, 2001) of over 1300 women, with comparative controls, found that:

- water immersion is rated very highly by both women and midwives
- it was equally attractive to primigravidae and multigravidae
- women who used the pool for a period of their labour were significantly less likely to have an epidural
- perineal outcomes were improved in waterbirth
- there was no increased admission to the special care baby unit
- there was no increase in postpartum haemorrhage, despite almost half the women having a spontaneous third stage.

These findings reinforce other studies with regard to women and babies. For example:

- In 1996, Johnson (1996) showed that babies were more likely to swallow than breathe because of the so-called 'diving reflex'.
- In 1998, the British Journal of Midwifery published an audit report (Brown, 1998) which concluded that waterbirth is no more dangerous than land birth, and that women liked water as it made them feel in control of their labour.
- In August 1999 a study was published (Gilbert & Tookey, 1999) which showed that the perinatal mortality rate among 4032 births in water was similar to that for low risk land births: 1.2 per thousand. Furthermore, none of the five deaths that occurred were attributable to birth in water.
- In December 1999, Beake published a literature review (Beake, 1999) of water labour and birth which concluded that there is 'no research evidence not to support its use'.

Some studies (Garland & Jones, 1994; Otigbah, Dhanjal & Harmsworth, 2000) have shown a decrease in the duration of labour in water, particularly in first stage. but this has not been confirmed by several other reports. Overall, midwifery research (Burns, 2001; Brown, 1998; Gilbert & Tookey, 1999; Beake, 1999; Otigbah, Dhanjal & Harmsworth, 2000; Garland & Jones, 2000) has found:

- no difference in length of labour, apgar scores, or blood loss

Box 1 Why does being in water help?

Perhaps we should begin using the term hydrotherapy (Harris, 1999) rather than waterbirth. As Michel Odent (2000) points out

...the reason for the birthing pool is not to have the baby born in water but to facilitate the birth process and to reduce the need for drugs and other intervention.

- A woman's body in water seems to weigh less because of the buoyancy effect of water. It is easier for her to support her body, which decreases muscular tension. With a decrease in tension there may be a decrease in catecholamines, and an increase in oxytocin and endorphins. This leads to a more coordinated pattern of labour (Ockendon, 2001).
- Equal pressure is exerted on all parts of the body beneath the water. Pressure is not felt on one part more than another, so helping to diffuse the discomfort of labour.
- There is suppression of the renin-aldosterone system and vasopressin hormones, leading to reduced blood pressure through vasodilation. It also increases diuresis, so it is important to maintain hydration.
- Water is a good conductor of heat. In warm water, there is an increase in local tissue metabolism, temperature at the surface and muscle relaxation. Heat and pain are thought to travel along the same nerve, so the conduction of the heat sensation limits the pain sensation.
- Peripheral vascular pressure and therefore pulse rate is decreased by heat and hydrostatic pressure. Central blood flow increases, which may increase uterine blood flow.

In addition to these physiological effects, a woman in a birthing pool is:
- upright and mobile
- in a private environment and more in control of her actions and less accessible to interventions.

- more 1st and 2nd degree tears in primips in water; more 3rd and 4th degree tears on land
- more intact perineums in water, including few episiotomies
- less analgesia in water
- no increase in infections to mothers or babies
- no water-related complications for mothers or babies.

In addition, these and a single entirely qualitative article (Hall & Holloway, 1998) showed high rates of satisfaction with labour in water.

What hasn't been addressed in much of the research, and what I found most interesting about the Burns study (Burns, 2001) was the high effectiveness rating that midwives gave to labour in water. A similar number of midwives and mothers found the birthing pool more helpful rather than less helpful. Perhaps this is not surprising. Karlene Davis, President of the Royal College of Midwives, said at a recent conference (NCT, 2001) that what makes women happy is usually what makes midwives happy too – because they derive much of their job satisfaction from giving women a satisfying

experience of becoming a mother.

So, if midwives and mothers like waterbirth, why is its use still so limited?

What is damming the flow?

A possible clue to the reasons for continued resistance to water labour and birth can be found in the latest edition of A Guide to Effective Care in Pregnancy and Childbirth (Enkin, Kierse, Neilson et al, 2000), where the following comments can be found on p.317:

Critics maintain that there may be an increased risk of infection for both mother and baby, possible inhibition of effective contractions, increased risk of perineal trauma, postpartum haemorrhage, water embolus, and trauma to the baby....

Caregivers, too, may be at risk from infection and back injury.

No clear benefits to mothers and babies were identified....

Four randomised controlled trials were discussed (possibly those discussed in Beake (1999)?), which had shown neither benefits or complications, although it was conceded that a recent Canadian study found that women reported less pain after immersion, and 80% said they would like to use water again. No mention was made of the research published in midwifery journals, but a paragraph was devoted to individual cases where babies had died, despite almost all these deaths having been found not to be attributable to birth in water (Gilbert & Tookey, 1999; Kitzinger, 2000).

Garland & Jones (2000) explored the reasons for the medical profession ignoring the evidence published by midwife researchers. The key is that the medics prefer a clinical research approach: essentially randomised controlled trials, whereas many of the reports in midwifery journals have adopted the audit approach: mainly retrospective, non-randomised studies, often with matched controls. They acknowledge that audit cannot predict for any individual mother and baby whether her outcome would be better in water, but can only work in probabilities. They also, however highlight the practical and moral drawbacks of trying to apply randomised controlled trials in this context.

Their reasoning is supported by examining the findings of a randomised controlled trial published this year (Eckert, Turnbull & MacLenan, 2001). The authors concluded that 'Bathing in labour confers no clear benefits for the labouring woman and may contribute to adverse effects in the neonate'. Results were recorded according to 'intention to treat', but only 71% of those in the 'bath group' used it, and 26% of the 'non-bath group' had access to a bath, although it is not stated how many used it. Midwives simply did not feel that it was ethical to deny women access to the bath if they wanted to use it. Seventy-one protocol violations occurred in all. The authors state that the provision of 'baths' was new at the hospital at the time the study began, and 'water immersion was not a routine option of care...and no protocol had been established for the use of the bath'. No mention was made of staff training. A woman 'could partake of a bath for as little or long as she wished during labour'. This is clearly against recommendations (Odent, 2000) that women should be encouraged to use the pool after 5cm dilatation. I could go on.

It should be pointed out that all proponents of waterbirth seem to agree that it is essential that questions are asked and research conducted, so that guidelines can emerge and evolve. In this context, Enkin et al (2000) give us a further clue about the causes of resistance:

There is no consistency in the criteria used to guide practice.

This issue has now been addressed by the Midwifery guidelines for the use of water in labour (Burns & Kitzinger, 2000), and by the ongoing collection of data with which to review and update these guidelines. (To take part in this exercise or get further information, visit www.sheilakitzinger.com/Waterbirth.htm.)

Another clue might come from the work of Otigbah et al (2000) who suggested that the decreased need for analgesia may result from continuous midwifery care. Whether or not this is true, it highlights the need for continuous care during water labour, a difficult thing to achieve in understaffed maternity units.

The lack or underuse of pools stems partly from the lack of midwife-led units in some areas, and from the strict criteria applied to whether women are low risk and therefore eligible. If water lowers blood pressure, for example, why not use it for women with pregnancy-induced hypertension or pre-eclampsia? After all, it is perfectly possible to monitor mothers and babies in water, and it is well established that continuous monitoring has no benefit in outcomes over intermittent auscultation (Enkin, Kierse, Neilson et al, 2000, p.273).

If a hospital in Switzerland can offer waterbirth to all of its labouring women, without any detrimental effects to mother and baby (Geissbuhler & Eberhard, 2000), why can't all other hospitals do the same? It is careful management that is important, of any birth.

Is the real reason for resistance to freer access to waterpools suggested by a quotation from Samuel Johnson in 1755?

Change is not made without inconvenience, even from worse to better.

The cost of provision of equipment and training staff, and having to have continuous midwife presence during water immersion – these things may be very inconvenient in over-stretched hospitals.

What midwives can do

Managers need to be convinced of the efficacy and safety of any procedures in hospitals. As well as the evidence I have presented here about how much women and midwives value labour and birth in water, there are well established physiological effects of immersion in water that account for many of the benefits (Box 1). The weight of evidence now clearly shows that childbirth in water is as safe as that on land if guidelines are followed.

If you are convinced:

• Promote the benefits to women, including encouraging them to go to antenatal aquanatal sessions so that they can appreciate the water environment (Garland, 2000). In the chapter on antenatal education, Enkin et al (2000) suggest:

Once a critical mass of mothers becomes aware of the fact that options are available to them, major changes in obstetrical practice may ensue.

• Attend training sessions for managing water labour and birth. The Midwives' Code of Practice says each midwife should acquire competence in new skills through adequate preparation (UKCC, 1988). This training will also include the safeguarding of the midwife's health and safety.
• Promote the benefits to colleagues and, where possible, present evidence to support the relaxation of conditions under which women can use the pools (Geissbuhler & Eberhard, 2000).

The underuse of pools is a multiple misfortune. It is a waste of resources, a lost opportunity for many women to improve their experience of giving birth, and also for many midwives to improve their job satisfaction.

REFERENCES

Beake S. 1999. Water birth: A literature review. MIDIRS Midwifery Digest, 9(4), 473-7
Brown L. 1998. The tide has turned: Audit of waterbirth. British Journal of Midwifery, 6(4), 236-43
Burns E, Kitzinger S. 2000. Midwifery guidelines for the use of water in labour. Oxford: Oxford Centre for Health Care Research and Development, Oxford Brookes University
Burns E. 2001. Waterbirth. MIDIRS Midwifery Digest, 11(suppl. 2), S10-S13.
Eckert K, Turnbull D, MacLenan A. 2001. Immersion in water in the first stage of labour: A randomised controlled trial. Birth, 28(2), 84-93
Enkin M, Kierse MJN, Neilson J et al. 2000. A Guide to Effective Care in Pregnancy and Childbirth. Oxford: Oxford University Press

Garland D, Jones K. 1994. Waterbirth: 'First stage' immersion or non-immersion. British Journal of Midwifery, 2(3), 113-20

Garland D, Jones K. 2000. Waterbirth: Supporting practice with clinical audit. MIDIRS Midwifery Digest, 10(3), 333-6

Garland D. 2000. The uses of hydrotherapy in today's midwifery practice. In Complementary therapies for pregnancy and childbirth, 2nd edn, ed D Tiran & S Mack, pp 225-37. Edinburgh: Bailliere Tindall

Geissbuhler V, Eberhard J. 2000. Waterbirths: A Comparative Study. A prospective study on more than 2000 waterbirths. Fetal Diagnosis and Therapy, 15, 291-300

Gilbert RE, Tookey PA. 1999. Perinatal mortality and morbidity among babies delivered in water: Surveillance study and postal survey. British Medical Journal, 319(7208), 483-7

Hall SM, Holloway IM. 1998. Staying in control: Women's experiences of labour in water. Midwifery, 14(1), 30-6

Harris KT. 1999. Hydrotherapy: An alternative method for relieving labour pain. Mother Baby Journal, 4(5), 15-20

Johnson P. 1996. To breathe or not to breathe. British Journal of Obstetrics and Gynaecology, 103, 202-3

Kitzinger S. 2000. Sheila Kitzinger's letter from Europe: The waterbirth debate updated. Birth, 27(3), 214-6

NCT. A National Service Framework for Maternity Care. NCT Conference, London, 15th June 2001

Ockenden J. 2001. The hormonal dance of labour. The Practising Midwife, 4(6), 16-8

Odent M. 2000. Abstract, comments and updated recommendations. MIDIRS Midwifery Digest, 10(1), 63-4

Otigbah CM, Dhanjal MK, Harmsworth G et al. 2000. A retrospective comparison of water births and conventional vaginal deliveries. European Journal of Obstetrics and Gynecology and Reproductive Biology, 91(1), 15-20

Robinson J. 2001. Demand and supply in maternity care. British Journal of Midwifery, 9(8), 510

UKCC. 1988. Midwives' Rules and Code of Practice. London: UKCC

The hour of birth

Comparisons of circadian pattern between women cared for by midwives and obstetricians

Marion H B Heres, Maria Pel, Marion Borkent-Polet, Pieter E Treffer, Majid Mirmiran

Objective: to examine the difference, if any, between midwives' care and obstetricians' care in the circadian pattern of the hour of birth in spontaneous labour and delivery.

Design: a descriptive study comparing the circadian pattern of the hour of birth between women cared for by a midwife or an obstetrician.

Setting: data were derived from the Perinatal Database of the Netherlands (LVR), comprising 83% of all births under midwives' care and 75% of all births under obstetricians' care.

Subjects: 57 871 women receiving midwives' care and 31999 women receiving obstetricians' care with spontaneous labour and spontaneous delivery.

Main outcome measures: differences in the circadian rhythms between women receiving midwives' care and obstetricians' care.

Findings: there was a difference in the circadian pattern of the hour of birth between midwives' and obstetricians' care. Peak times differed 5.43 hours (CI 4.23-7.03) for primiparous and 3.34 hours (CI 3.00-4.08) for multiparous women between the midwives' group and the obstetricians' group.

Conclusion: this study demonstrates a remarkable difference in circadian pattern of the hour of birth between midwives' care and obstetricians' care. In obstetricians' care the duration of normal labour appears to be prolonged, presumably by an increased level of stress. In normal birth the care of midwives is preferable.

The hour of birth is the result of the time of onset and the duration of labour. Onset of labour and hour of birth show a circadian rhythm, a fact relatively unknown among obstetricians, which has been rediscovered many times, only to be forgotten again (Yerushalmy 1938, Malek 1952, Simpson 1952, Charles 1953, King 1956, Kaiser & Halberg 1962, Smolensky et al. 1972, Glattre & Bjerkedal 1983, Panduro-Baron et al. 1994).

Obstetric care in the Netherlands makes a clear distinction between primary and secondary care, founded on a selection-based approach. Low-risk pregnant women receive prenatal care and are attended during labour by independent midwives or general pracitioners (Treffers et al. 1990, Oppenheimer 1993). Midwives only deliver term singleton babies in the vertex presentation and are not authorised to administer oxytocics before the birth of the baby. Of these births 55% take place at home. Fetal surveillance during labour under the care of midwives is by intermittent auscultation. If medical or obstetric problems arise either during pregnancy or labour (such as preterm labour or post-term dates) pregnant women are referred to secondary care (obstetricians). During labour pregnant women at increased risk are attended by obstetricians. Fetal surveillance during labour, supervised by obstetricians, is generally by electronic monitoring.

The purpose of our study was to use this Dutch system of obstetric care as a model to study whether there is a difference between primary and secondary care in the circadian patterns of birth, under conditions excluding all obstetric interventions which could influence the hour of birth, such as induction or augmentation of labour, caesarean section or vaginal operative delivery. Naturally obstetric interventions have a great influence on the hour of birth, thus we were only interested in the circadian pattern of birth after spontaneous labour and spontaneous delivery.

Methods

In 1985 the voluntary registration of primary perinatal care (LVR 1) was started in the Netherlands. The participation rate has increased over the years so that in 1990 77% of the midwives' practices registered 83% of all babies born under midwives' care. Data are compiled anonymously. The LVR 1 form includes 38 items on prenatal care, delivery and postnatal care. The voluntary registration of secondary care (LVR 2) started in 1982; in 1990 75% of all babies born under secondary care were registered. These data are also compiled anonymously. The LVR 2 form includes 34 items on prenatal care, delivery and postnatal care. Data management is compiled by the SIG, the Information Centre for Health Care.

We used the 1990 data of this National Perinatal Database, with the permission of the LVR privacy committee. Two reference groups were created: the LVR 1 reference group consists of the total LVR 1 population (all births under the care of midwives), and the LVR 2 reference group comprises term vertex singletons, with spontaneous onset of labour and spontaneous delivery, under the care of obstetricians.

The data set on midwives' care encompasses 57 871 women, delivering term vertex singleton babies; the onset of labour was spontaneous, and during labour no oxytocic drugs were given. In the Netherlands midwives are not authorised to administer oxytocics before the birth of the baby. All deliveries were spontaneous. The data set on obstetricians' care encompassed 81 451 women. In this data set a selection was made: only term vertex singletons with a spontaneous onset of labour and a spontaneous delivery, without use of oxytocic drugs before the birth of the baby were considered, in total 31 399 women. Both the data set on midwives' care and the selected group of women from the data set on obstetricians' care only comprise women who delivered spontaneously at term, without any intervention influencing the hour of birth. The circadian patterns of the hour of birth of these two groups were compared. As parity has a distinct influence on the duration of labour, primiparous and multiparous women were analysed separately.

To compare circadian rhythms between groups cosinor analysis was applied (Halberg et al. 1977). Differences between the hour of birth in the subgroups were analysed with the use of x^2 test.

Findings

There was a clear difference between the circadian rhythm of the hour of birth of the midwives' and the selected obstetricians' groups of women in both parity

Figure 5.7.1 (a) Primary care group, primiparous women; (b) Primary care group, multiparous women; (c) Secondary care group, primiparous women; (d) Secondary care group, multiparous women.

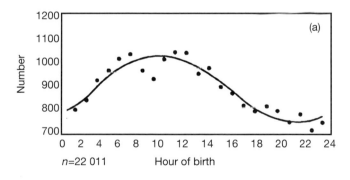

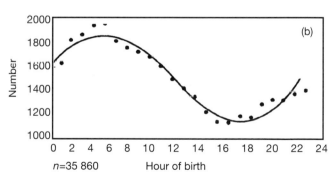

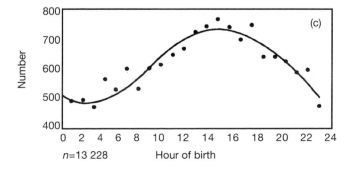

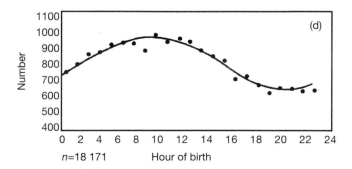

Table 5.7.1 Association of circadian rhythm of hour of birth with level of care

Population	n	P	r²	P
Primiparous				
primary care	22011	8.42	0.89	0.005
seondary care	13228	14.25	0.89	0.005
Multiparous				
primary care	35860	5.00	0.95	0.005
secondary care	18171	8.34	0.94	0.005

n = number of births; P = peak time (Acrophase), in hours and minutes; r^2 = percentage of the variance accounted for by the curve-fitting model; P = P-value of curve-fitting model.

groups (Table 5.7.1 and Figure 5.7.1 a-d). Both parity groups show a great difference in peak times between the midwives' and obstetricians' groups. In the women under the care of midwives peak times of delivery were around 08.42 hours (primiparous women) and 05.00 hours (multiparous women) were found. In the obstetricians' group the peak delivery times occurred later, at 14.25 hours (primiparous women) and 08.34 hours (multiparous women). The difference between both groups was 5.43 hours (CI 4.23-7.03) for primiparous women and 3.34 hours (CI 3.00-4.08) for multiparous women.

Discussion

This study clearly demonstrates for the first time, that compared with the women under care of the midwives, the women cared for by obstetricians show a delayed time of birth. We were not interested in the total group of women under the care of obstetricians, but only in the selected group who, although they were at increased risk, were allowed to go into spontaneous labour and in whom no indication for augmentation with oxytocics or assisted delivery occurred.

The moment of birth is determined by the time of onset of labour and by the duration of labour. The literature is unanimous about a circadian pattern of the onset of labour with a fixed peak around midnight (Malek 1952, Charles 1953, King 1956, Shettles 1960, Cooperstock et al. 1987, Honnebier 1993, Backe 1991), similar for both parity groups (Malek 1952, Charles 1953, Cooperstock et al. 1987, Oppenheimer 1993, Honnebier 1993). Due to the longer duration of labour in primiparous women the circadian rhythm of the hour of birth shows a later peak time than in multiparous women. The LVR database does not provide data on the peak of onset of labour, but we have no reason to assume that it would be different compared with the data of all the previous studies or that there would be a difference

between both care groups. The LVR 2 reference group of women was in the care of obstetricians because they were considered to be at increased risk of complications. However, in this particular group of women the obstetrician found neither indication to induce or augment labour, nor to apply instrumental or operative delivery. Therefore, the risk status itself could not be the cause of the delayed time of birth.

The only explanation for the delayed peak time in secondary care deliveries is a longer duration of labour in these women. It is known that in all mammalian species the course of labour is influenced by environmental disturbances: anxiety and fright prolonging the duration of labour (Yerushalmy 1938, Naaktgeboren1989). In humans it has been demonstrated that stress extends the duration of labour (Malek1952, Lederman et al. 1978). The length of labour is shortened considerably in association with the presence of a supportive companion during labour (Klaus et al. 1986, Flint et al. 1989). Possibly a less continuous and comforting support of obstetricians and residents combined with electronic fetal monitoring and the less comforting atmosphere in hospitals leads to higher stress hormone levels and thereby to a delayed course of labour.

Another factor could possibly be the awareness of the woman that her pregnancy and labour are not regarded as low risk, which may increase her stress levels, and thereby could inhibit contractility and uterine placental blood flow (Myers 1975, Backe 1991). Within the group of women under the care of midwives we compared the women delivering at home with those giving birth in a hospital, but we did not find a difference in the peak times between these two groups. A reassuring influence of midwives' care is in agreement with the results of randomised trials of midwife managed care compared to shared care or care supervised by obstetricians. These studies show that women express greater satisfaction with midwives' care (Flint et al. 1989, MacVicar et al 1993, Waldenström & Nilsson 1994, Turnbull et al. 1996).

In conclusion in spontaneous labour, obstetricians' care delayed the moment of birth by prolonging the duration of labour, probably by an elevated level of stress. Therefore, the care of midwives appears to be the most appropriate care in normal birth as also recommended by the World Health Organization (1996).

Acknowledgement

We would like to thank Patty Elferink-Stinkens and Matheé Swenne-van Ingen for supplying the data, Guus Hart and Eus van Someren for their statistical advice, and Fulco van der Veen for his critical appraisal of the manuscript.

REFERENCES

Backe B 1991 A circadian variation in the observed duration of labor. Possible causes and implications. Obstetrics & Gynecologica Scandanavia 70: 645-648

Charles E 1953 The hour of birth. A study of the distribution of times of onset of labour and delivery throughout the 24-hour period. British Journal of Preventative Social Medicine 7: 743-759.

Cooperstock M, England JE, Wolfe RA 1987. Circadian incidence of labor onset hour in preterm birth and chorioamnionitis. Obstetrics and Gynecology 70:852-855

Flint C, Poulengeris P, Grant A 1989 The 'Know YourMidwife' scheme – a randomised trial of continuity of care by a team of midwives. Midwifery 5: 11-16

Glattre E, Bjerkedal T 1983 The 24-hour rhythmicity of birth. Obstetrics & Gynecologica Scandanavia 62:31-36

Halberg F, Carandente F, Cornelissen G et al. 1977 Glossary of chronobiology. Chronobiologica 4(suppl 1): 1-189

Honnebier MBOM 1993 The role of the circadian system during pregnancy and labor in monkey and man. Unpublished thesis, University of Amsterdam

Kaiser IH, Halberg F 1962 Circadian periodic aspects of birth. Annals of the New York Academy of Science 98:1056-1068

King PD 1956 Increased frequency of births in the morning hours. Science 123: 985-986

Klaus MH, Kennell JH, Robertson SS et al. 1986 Effects of social support during parturition on maternal and infant morbidity. British Medical Journal 293:585-587

Lederman RP, Lederman E, Work BA, 1978 The relationship of maternal anxiety, plasma cathecholamines and plasma cortisol to progress in labor. American Journal of Obstetrics & Gynecology 132:495-500

Malek J 1952 The manifestation of biological rhythms indelivery. Gynaecologica 133: 365-372

MacVicar J, Dobbie G, Owen-Johnstone L et al. 1994 Simulated home delivery in hospital: a randomized controlled trial. British Journal of Obstetrics and Gynaecology 100:316-323

Myers RE 1975 Maternal physiological stress and fetal asphyxia: a study in the monkey. American Journal of Obstetrics and Gynaecology 122: 4759

Naaktgeboren C 1989 The biology of childbirth. In: Chalmers I, Enkin M, Keirse MJCN (eds). Effective care in pregnancy and childbirth. Oxford University Press, Oxford

Oppenheimer O 1993 Organising midwifery led carein the Netherlands. British Medical Journal 307:1400-1402

Panduro-Baron G, Gonzalez-Moreno J, Hernandez-Figueroa E 1994 The biorhythm of birth. International Journal of Gynaecology and Obstetrics 45:283-284

Shettles LB 1960 Hourly variation in onset of labor and rupture of membranes. American Journal of Obstetrics and Gynaecology 79:177-179

Simpson AS 1952 Are more babies born at night? British Medical Journal 2: 831

Smolensky M, Halberg F, Sargent F 1972 Chronobiologyof the life sequence. In: Itoh S, Ogata K, Yoskimura H (eds) Advances in climate physiology. Igaku Shoin Ltd, Tokyo

Treffers PE, Eskes M, Kleiverda G et al. 1990 Home birth and minimal medical interventions. Journal of the American Medical Association 264: 2203-2208

Turnbull D, Holmes A, Shields N et al. 1996 Randomised, controlled trial of efficacy of midwife-managed care. Lancet 348: 213-218

Waldenström U, Nilsson CA 1994 Experience of childbirth in birth center care. A randomized controlled study. Acta Obstet Gynecol Scand 73:547-554

World Health Organization 1996 Care in normal birth: a practical guide. WHO, Geneva (WHO/FRH/MSM/96. 24)

Yerushalmy J 1938 Hour of birth and stillbirth and neonatal mortality rates. Child Development 9:373-378

Reflecting on labour and birth

- If you were going to design an ideal environment for birth, how would it look? What would women see, hear, smell, touch? Is this a reality for the women you work with? Are there even small ways in which we can alter or adapt existing birth rooms to make them any nearer to this ideal?

- Do you think the word 'allow' is ever appropriate in midwifery? (As in, "we do/don't allow you to do/choose this"?) Do you use it? Under what circumstances? Is this an aspect of your practice with which you are happy, or which you might want to consider changing?

- Along the same lines, how can we explain policies and obstetric preferences to women in ways where they understand that this is a preference but that they have an absolute right to make a different choice? In what ways can we manage the need to offer choice to women without prejudicing our own position and relationship with colleagues and employers?

- Under what circumstances (if any) is it acceptable to 'do good by stealth'? (For instance, by advising a woman that, if she eats while you are out of the room, then you will not know about it, or by extending the time a woman can spend in second stage by delaying vaginal examination or diagnosing a stubborn anterior lip?) How can we remove the need to 'do good by stealth'?

- Is there anything we can do as midwives to even out the geographical and cultural discrepancies, which mean that women's choices and experiences are dependent on where they live? Is it appropriate to inform women about these differences, in order to enable them to realise that there are very few hard and fast rules about birth, and that the choices they are offered may be context-dependent?

- Are there audits and research studies being carried out in your area such as the one by Heres et al, which may not require large amounts of funding, but can add to the body of midwifery knowledge? Could you become involved in this? What questions would you explore if you could, and who might be able to help you with this?

Focus on:

Elements of risk

SECTION CONTENTS

When birth goes wrong

Rosalind Weston

Eclamptic fits, major post-partum haemorrhage, shoulder dystocia, cord prolapse – these are words that send shivers down midwives' spines. The realities of life and death can draw close at birth, whether we find ourselves in a busy tertiary obstetric unit, or at a home birth up a farm track in the middle of winter miles from the nearest DGH. The challenge of birth in the twenty-first century is to blend and combine the art and science of midwifery – especially when birth 'goes wrong!' How can we empower ourselves as midwives and the women that we care for in labour? Firstly by developing our intuitive skills of 'watching, waiting, listening, holding, touching, trusting, knowing,' along with emergency procedures to deal with unexpected and serious complications.

For the past decade I have worked as an independent midwife as well as in a rural maternity unit, 35 miles away from a DGH. This has taught me some principles in recognising and dealing with abnormalities in labour. Several case scenarios stand out, which I will use to illustrate these lessons.

The first principle is to remember that extreme and life-threatening emergencies occur rarely. Before situations get to this stage, there are often warning signs that give you time to take appropriate action. In this 'new age' of clinical governance, quality and risk management, we must be careful not to stifle the normal physiology of birth by over-managing all potentially 'risky' situations. One intervention often leads to a cascade of others – which in turn can contribute to complications and birth emergencies. There are, of course, other times when labour 'goes wrong' without any prior warning. This is where attending the excellent ALSO course, or some other intensive emergency training, can help to ensure that when problems do occur, they are recognised and dealt with immediately and appropriately.

Most Trusts and midwifery teams now recognise the value of planned and regular 'emergency drills' on the labour ward. These undoubtedly contribute to good risk management strategies and, as the CESDI (1998, 2000) reports highlight, to reducing maternal and perinatal morbidity and mortality.

When I am stuck at a red traffic light or waiting for my child to come out of school, I regularly replay in my mind 'what if' emergency scenarios. I do not do this out of anxiety, but so that when I attend a labour I am mentally alert and ready. This helps me to bring little or no fear into the birthing environment – something which makes an enormous difference for a labouring woman. If emergencies arise, the appropriate manoeuvres and procedures are at the forefront of my mind, and can be quickly activated.

Fear is a powerful emotion, both for a woman in labour and for midwives dealing with emergencies. This is not the time to be checking equipment or to discover that something is not working! If clear methods of communication are established beforehand, records are kept accurate and contemporaneous, (CESDI 1998, CESDI 2000, UKCC 1998) and appropriate action is taken by all personnel, the likelihood of errors occurring that would contribute to a poor birth outcome is greatly reduced.

Cord prolapse

I was caring for a woman who had had two previous normal births in the community unit. She was in spontaneous labour, but there was a delay in the first stage. The membranes were intact. She was getting tired, and the contractions were waning in strength and frequency. The vertex was mid-cavity on vaginal examination with a bulging bag of forewaters. I discussed the situation with her, and explained that performing an artificial rupture of membranes might encourage more regular, effective contractions and prevent a transfer to a DGH. There was copious clear liquor as I performed a controlled ARM with an amnihook and my fingers – and then I felt something which I had never felt before: a pulsating cord to the side of the presenting part – and we were 50 minutes from a DGH! I quickly explained to my midwife colleague and the woman what had happened and what we needed to do. 'Call the ambulance, turn into a knee chest position, give oxygen, do not remove my fingers from her vagina, and transfer fast!'

Forty minutes of flashing blue lights, winding roads and one very queasy midwife later we arrived at the previously alerted DGH. The Registrar met us and asked to check the vaginal examination. 'No!' I said firmly. 'There's a prolapsed cord and I can feel a cord pulse: we need to get into theatre straight away!' I have never been so glad to hear a newborn babe's cry from my position under the green drapes in the theatre!

The woman met me again several times in the unit during the early weeks and months after this experience because she was having disturbing dreams and memories. Our accessibility as a team in her community ensured an immediate response to her needs, and a familiar person with whom to talk, which greatly facilitated her return to emotional health.

Calm, clear communication

The next principle I set myself is to develop a relationship of understanding and information-sharing with the woman and, if possible, with her partner too. Ideally, this should be developing antenatally. The challenge in a busy labour ward is for a midwife to achieve this level of trust and communication in a few short and intense hours. (Kirkham, 1994: 1-19)

Women often approach their pregnancies and labours with high expectations. Realistically, these will not always be met. The expectations of a live and healthy mother and baby have never been greater than at the start of the 21st century in the UK. The DoH Report 'Why Mothers Die' (1999) however, makes sober reading. The reality is that a number of women still do die in childbirth, the main killers being thrombosis, haemorrhage and eclampsia, although, poignantly, domestic violence has for the first time made an entry into the statistics. In preparing women and their partners antenatally, we tread a fine line. Our main concern is to build confidence in their abilities to give birth without intervention whilst at the same time we are fully aware that The Good Birth Guide (www.drfoster.co.uk, 2001) reminds us that in some hospitals 20% of women will have a Caesarean, 10% will require an instrumental delivery and 10-15% may need induction or augmentation of labour. It does not require a mathematician to work out that almost 50% of all women in labour may therefore require some degree of obstetric assistance at their births. Some of these may be entirely justified – but others lead to inappropriate use of technology and to births 'going wrong,' as Wagner (1994) so brilliantly argues. The provisional results from the National Sentinel Study of Caesarean Sections seem to be showing similarly worrying trends, with no significant reduction in either morbidity or mortality.

In leading workshops on setting up midwifery-led units, Dimond (1994) writes that one of the main concerns midwives had was whether a woman would refuse to transfer in the event of complications. The principle that I have applied in my practice to help overcome this possibility is broadly along the same lines: maintaining openness, honesty and clear communication with the couple throughout. As Young (1999) suggests, the best person to be concerned about the wellbeing of the unborn child is usually the woman herself.

Women and their partners need clear, unbiased information on which to base their decisions. So long as they understand the rationale for these decisions, the vast majority of women will not refuse advice, treatment or transfer. When women feel in control and involved in decision-making, even when complications do ensue, they become 'empowered.' It is when women feel out of control and left out of the decision-making process that they are more likely to look back on their labour as an unhappy event or even to sue (Berg & Dahlberg, 1998: 23-9).

Even when emergencies do occur there is still much we can do to create an environment which respects the woman as a person with feelings and emotions rather than an object to be rushed to theatre.

Coping with hospital transfer

Another example from my practice illustrates this principle of showing respect for a woman's feelings. A woman who had had a previous Caesarean for delay in the first stage of labour contacted me for a home birth. As she would normally be considered 'high risk' for a home birth, I involved both my supervisor and her consultant in the decision-making process. She had thought the issues through and made an informed choice to stay at home.

She called me in the early hours of a spring morning when she was at term. She was in early labour and picking daffodils in the garden! By the time I arrived she was having regular contractions and was coping very well. Later in the morning she filled her birthing pool to assist her in dealing with more painful contractions. Her cervix was 5 cms dilated, thin and well applied to the presenting part. All was going well, but by lunchtime she was becoming very tired, and not feeling that she was dealing well with the contractions. Another vaginal examination revealed no change. It seemed as if this labour was now following the same course as her last one. She drank some energy-rich nourishment, tried to rest and lie down on her side between contractions. I assessed her again two hours later, and since there was still no change, we needed to transfer to hospital. She was disappointed but resigned.

Labour is often about 'what goes on in a woman's head,' as much as the physiological birth process. I encouraged her not to give up, especially since there was no fetal distress and no signs of obstruction. Wainer Cohen (1991) suggests that women who have had a Caesarean section often need more help and support around the same time in her labour when she had her previous operation. The way this delivery developed demonstrates this point.

The senior registrar fully recognised her great desire to avoid having another Caesarean, so we started a small amount of syntocinon to augment the labour, and set up an epidural. This enabled her to get some much-needed rest and regain her energy levels. Four hours later she was fully dilated! Now that the epidural was wearing off, she had some urges to push, but could not do so effectively in her semi-recumbent position. With the support of the registrar and my midwifery colleagues, she got out of bed and used my birth stool to bring the baby down onto the perineum. Since she still could not push the baby out, however, she returned to her bed and gave birth to her baby with the gentle help of the registrar and a Ventouse. An empowered woman and midwife, working in close cooperation with a multi-professional team, achieved this outcome at a time when labour appeared to have gone wrong. Even though her initial plans for a home birth did not work out, she still had much to celebrate!

Breech at home

Another woman had had two previous vaginal births, one of which was a breech delivery. She booked with me for a home birth at nearly 38 weeks but this baby too was presenting in an extended breech position. As in the previous scenario, I discussed the situation with both my supervisor and the consultant as well as the woman herself concerning her desire to deliver a breech birth at home.

At 39 weeks, the woman phoned me, reporting ruptured membranes. I went immediately to her home. There was clear liquor and I refrained from performing a vaginal examination in order to reduce the likelihood of infection. The breech was engaged and the regular fetal heart at 140-160 bpm reassured me that there was unlikely to be a cord presenting. Over the following hours she began to contract irregularly and mildly. Her husband was working a long way away but was returning home as quickly as possible. She wanted to know what progress she was making, so in view of her parity, I performed a vaginal examination. Her cervix was thick, partially effaced and 3-4 cms dilated. I also found a presenting part that felt unlike anything I had ever come across before. There were ridges and small 'knobbly bits' alongside a breech presentation. There was a compound presentation of a hand!

It was not possible to remain at home. I made arrangements to transfer to hospital, but because she was not in established labour, and there was no sign of fetal distress, I felt justified in heeding her desire to wait until her husband was with her. We were warmly greeted on arrival at the labour ward, and the hospital team worked together with me well to facilitate a birth outcome that the woman had not been anticipating. As I was helping her to prepare for a spinal anaesthetic prior to the Caesarean section, she leant over my shoulder and whispered, 'This isn't what I wanted, but I know it has to happen.'

Women are amazingly philosophical when it comes to birth, and are more than aware of the need to ensure the wellbeing of their babies. Once again we can see how having the continuity of a known carer during the labour can reduce the amount of fear and pain a woman experiences at that time – all of which contributes to reducing the number of births that go wrong (Enkin, Keirse & Neilson 1991). It also leads to more satisfying birth memories, even if complications do occur.

There is a delightful PS to this complicated birth. When I visited postnatally, her baby was lying on her chest with her left arm and hand curled around her bottom, just as she had been in the womb! This visit helped both me and the mother to make sense of her birth, and justified the reason for the Caesarean. It 'completed the circle.'

Emotional recharge

When labour goes wrong, women and their families need as much love and support, and appropriate evidence-based care as possible. Midwives equally need that support – and the opportunity to express their feelings after a traumatic birth. I am fortunate to work in a small team of highly supportive colleagues. We constantly peer review our practice, both formally and informally. This provides a great opportunity for 'caring and sharing', as the Association of Radical Midwives call some of their workshops.

The challenge is to translate these practices into large and busier labour wards, when midwives may finish a late shift having cared for a woman giving birth to a stillborn baby and find themselves the next morning dealing with several emergency Caesarean sections with little or no time to 'debrief'. Unless specific time is woven in and dedicated to reflecting on practice and to recharging the emotional batteries, many midwives will continue to burn out.

When a midwife has been through a traumatic time, her supervisor needs to be there to listen and care for her. As a supervisor, I cannot stress too highly how important it is to be proactive in creating essential time and space for non-judgmental support. This may go some considerable way towards ensuring that midwives do not become 'hard' in their attitudes to emergency situations and complications of birth as Wray (2001) intimates.

Last week, I reviewed a critical incident with a midwife who had to transfer a multigravid woman in the second stage of labour from a community unit to a DGH. This unusual situation caused her to reflect deeply with me on the scenario. She had asked the woman how she had felt about her labour and birth. She said that she felt 'cherished' by the care she had received from the midwife throughout the day, despite a complication occurring. If we can cherish women, and be cherished ourselves by our colleagues, then we will indeed be developing our intuitive skills of 'watching, waiting, listening, holding, touching, trusting and knowing' – and the likelihood of achieving healthy and satisfying outcomes for both mother and baby will be greatly increased.

Taken together, the principles outlined in this article point the way forward for the profession. They will make a continuing impact on reducing perinatal and maternal morbidity and mortality – and midwives will gain an increased sense of satisfaction in making an all-important contribution to the health of future generations of childbearing women and their offspring.

REFERENCES

Berg M, Dahlberg K. 1998. A phenomenological study of women's experience of complicated childbirth. Midwifery, 14, 23-9

CESDI. 1998. 5th Annual Report, Maternal and Child Health Research Consortium

CESDI. 2000. 7th Annual Report, Maternal and Child Health Research Consortium

Dimond B. 1994. The Legal Aspects of Midwifery. Oxford: Books for Midwives

DoH. 1999. Why Mothers Die: Confidential Enquiry into Maternal Mortality

Enkin M, Keirse M, Neilson J et al. Support in Labour. 2000. In A Guide to Effective Care in Pregnancy and Childbirth, 12th edn. Oxford: OUP

Kirkham M. Communication in Midwifery. 1994. In Midwifery Practice: A Research-Based Approach, ed J Alexander, V Levy, S Roch, pp 1-19. London: Macmillan

UKCC. 1998. Guidelines for Records and Record Keeping.

Wagner M. 1994. Pursuing the Birth Machine: The Search for Appropriate Birth Technology. Ace Graphics

Wainer Cohen N. 1991. Open Season: Survival Guide for Natural Childbirth and VBAC in the 90s. New York: Bergin and Garvey

Wray J. 2001. Being Hard: Reflections on making it to be a Midwife. Practising Midwife, 4(7), 23

www.drfoster.co.uk. 2001. The Good Birth Guide

Young G. The Case for Community-based Maternity Care. 1999. In Community-Based Maternity Care, ed G Marsh & M Renfrew. Oxford: Oxford Medical Publications

Home birth

A paediatrician's story

Frances Wedgwood

'So you're OK intubating your baby within seconds of giving birth, then?' she said, spluttering on her soup. 'Though I imagine it's probably quite hard checking the laryngoscope while you're trying to push a baby out of your vagina.'

My friend and colleague was a paediatrician like me and the most tactful and polite person I know. But giving birth at home? This was clearly a personal affront. I had to be mad.

'Are you going to personally check the midwives' equipment between your contractions then?' another paediatrician friend at the party commented. 'You know what they're like. You can guarantee the suction will be broken or they'll have run out of oxygen.'

My first birth had been a disaster. A long pre-labour. Arrival at hospital much too early. A badly timed epidural, leading to complete stopping of contractions for several hours. Amniotomy. Syntocinon. Fetal distress. Ventouse. Very bad tear. I believed this time I would be safer at home. But I hadn't reckoned on my colleagues' ire. Or their determination to slag off midwives.

'Anyway, I'm not going to stay at home if there's meconium, am I? I'm not an idiot', I remonstrated. 'Besides, there's not going to suddenly be vast quantities of meconium without some previous indications of distress', I added sulkily.

Meconium fears

All my colleagues had said the same thing. The mere mention of home birth really, really pissed them off.

Throughout my paediatric training we were encouraged to view women who had home births as selfish, foolhardy women prepared to stake their babies' lives against some romantic whim.

If someone wanting to deliver at home had to change plans, we rejoiced at the triumph of common sense over New Age nonsense. There was nothing we liked better than when a home birth went wrong and the woman and baby had to be brought back to the safety of the paediatric fold, with a good telling-off. Indeed, you really couldn't trust midwives and obstetricians to look after the baby's interests at all, and if it wasn't for paediatricians most babies would probably be dead.

'I once saw a midwife trying to get a cyanosed baby to breastfeed, for goodness sake', said my friend, determined to convince me.

Times may have changed, the data may not support their views, but they still felt what I wanted to do was really, really risky.

But there was one thing that really irked them, that they kept coming back to. Meconium. Meconium was a dreadful thing that happened to full-term babies when you least expected. Without a paediatrician the baby could die, they said. And for that reason alone I should not have a home birth.

Even I started to doubt my resolution. Perhaps they were right?

Reading up

It prompted me to research the subject. Meconium is surprisingly common. About 13% of live born babies are born through meconium-stained amniotic fluid. Of these, about 5-12% develop the meconium aspiration syndrome (MAS), and of these, about 4% die (Cleary & Wiswell, 1998). Although suctioning the trachea was proposed in 1960, it was not until the mid-1970s that anecdotal reports found it to be effective in preventing MAS (Ting & Brady, 1975). It was widely adopted and in the subsequent decade the incidence of MAS significantly declined (Wiswell, Tuggle & Turner, 1990).

But is it appropriate for all meconium babies? About 75% of babies born through meconium are vigorous within 10-15 seconds of birth. A large, multicentre, randomised, controlled trial of over 2000 full term babies looked at this (Wiswell, Gannon, Jacobs et al, 2000). They found that the routine suctioning of the vigorous meconium-stained infant was no better than expectant management, no matter how thick the meconium was.

But what I couldn't find out, and I'm pretty sure no one else knows either, was how to predict which babies will be vigorous at birth.

Nor could I find out what exactly causes the baby to pass meconium. It clearly isn't just related to labour, as a large percentage of stillbirths have meconium present. But intervention, such as induction, epidurals and syntocinon, does seem to make it more likely, as does post maturity and bigger babies.

Well, I wouldn't be having any of the former at home, though there wasn't anything I could do about the last two. But one thing was sure: if there was meconium there would be no home delivery.

The reality

And so, what happened? Well, nine days past my due date I went into labour. The obstetric registrar had given me a sweep the day before and had dutifully given me the same meconium/post-dates speech, though with considerably more tact. My midwives Linda and Julie arrived at 8am.

Unlike last time, the contractions started with a vengeance, but I was excited. This time things were moving. And I loved being at home. I felt safe. The birthing pool was helping and I dozed off between contractions. (The only downside was the fact that the gas and air mouthpiece didn't fit onto the cylinder – well, you know what midwives are like.) It was going well.

And then my waters went. Meconium. What a surprise.

'Well, it is only Grade 1, but I think we should go to hospital', said Julie. The paramedics arrived within minutes. I was so desperate for that gas and air by this point I walked into the street without a stitch on, fighting off Linda's desperate attempts to get some clothes on me. The neighbours loved it.

But we took the home birth atmosphere into hospital with us. An hour and a half after we got there I gave birth to my daughter on all fours.

But there was one final twist in store. As Imogen's head crowned there was a fountain of thick, tarry meconium. She looked like a squashed greyish gargoyle with green slime spewing from her mouth. But Julie was totally calm. She delivered the head slowly, and with careful grace. She gently suctioned her mouth, taking care not to overstimulate her. Oh, and she called the paediatrician.

When the paediatrician arrived, seconds later, tutting at my enormous foolishness, Imogen was already shrieking and turning a delicious shade of beetroot.

Of course, once she'd got my baby in her clutches, the paed couldn't help herself and thrust the laryngoscope down her throat. I guess she felt she was proving a point. Imogen promptly dropped her Apgar to 2. But the bradycardia was short-lived and a few hours later (having pulled paediatric rank) we were home.

I still don't quite know why there was suddenly so much meconium, but my instincts weren't wrong. There's not going to be vast unexpected quantities of meconium without some previous indication.

My paediatrician friends smile archly when they hear the story, all their fears vindicated. But, with the exception of the unwanted laryngoscope, I got what I wanted. A safe, beautiful, perfectly managed home birth. In hospital.

REFERENCES

Cleary GM, Wiswell TE. 1998. Meconium staining and the meconium aspiration syndrome: An update. Pediatr Clin North Am, 45, 511-29

Ting P, Brady JP. 1975. Tracheal suction in meconium aspiration. Am J Obstet Gynecol, 122, 767-71

Wiswell TE, Gannon CM, Jacobs J et al. 2000. Delivery room management of the apparently vigorous meconium stained neonate: Results of the multicentre, international collaborative trial. Pediatrics, 105, 1-7

Wiswell TE, Tuggle JM, Turner BS. 1990. Meconium aspiration syndrome: Have we made a difference? Pediatrics, 85, 715-21

Media representation of women's health

Maria Barrell

The effects of mass communication on health and health related issues are in general under-estimated. It can inform, educate and entertain but perhaps its influence has not been fully realised.

The media have done a great deal to influence the population and enhance general knowledge.[1] Information is transmitted to the general public via television, newspapers and magazines and the whole spectrum of the population from children to adults can be influenced. It is therefore essential that accurate information on health issues be transmitted to the population via media communication.

The media have achieved much in recent years to present accurate unbiased information, but there remains a specific area where the media may create undue stress and anxiety, and this is women's health.

Women's issues

Women's health and women's issues in general attract a great deal of interest from the press; women are a captured audience. The development of media interest in women has evolved over a number of years. Women were targeted with television and radio programmes and advertising specifically developed to appeal to housewives. With the increasing numbers of women now in paid employment again women are targeted specifically for their increased spending power.

How do the media represent women's health? There is now a plethora of women's issues which are highlighted through the medium of television, advertising, newspapers and magazines which include:

'Breast cancer. Unintended pregnancies. Birth control. Access to abortion. Female HIV infection and AIDS. Heart disease and high blood pressure. Lung cancer and cigarette advertising. Maternal drug and alcohol abuse and fetal effects. Date rape and domestic violence. Infant mortality. Childbirth and caesarean section. Osteoporosis and calcium. Menopause and hormone therapy.' [2]

More than ever before, the risks women face and the care they receive are of increasing interest to members of the medical and public health communities, politicians, insurance companies, consumers and the media.

Women's health topics have jumped from the back of the magazines' women's sections to the news pages, and from daytime television to network primetime. Women's magazines have toughened their coverage to tackle controversial topics like contraception, AIDS, and abortion in addition to more traditional topics such as diet, exercise and cosmetic surgery.[3] There is little doubt: from a media perspective, women are a marketable commodity.

It is suggested the effect of the media on women's health is one risk that has been underestimated. Increased media coverage of women's health does not necessarily mean better coverage, or result in women who are more accurately informed. Many women are motivated to seek advice from health professionals after reading news items or magazines. We know from experience many of the questions women ask can be traced back to a newspaper article or television programme. As midwives we need to know that we can locate accurate information and evidence to present to women either to allay fears or to present potential risk factors in a professional, unbiased, supportive manner.

Demand for information

As midwives, we need to be aware of the effects the media may have, both positive and negative, on women, their families and their lifestyles. The recent *Government Strategy for Health*[4] has highlighted the need for midwives to expand their role into the public health domain, focusing primarily on aspects of women's health and potential risk factors that influence health outcome. With this role expansion and blurring of traditional role boundaries will come increasing demands on midwives.

The traditional midwifery knowledge base will expand as women demand information on a range of subjects ranging from conception to the menopause. The media fuel women's desire for information. As new technologies, drugs and research become news headlines, midwives will have to act swiftly to advise and respond to women's questions and concerns.

Media scares may be unsubstantiated and therefore midwives need to validate information and give women accurate advice. Exposure to media coverage of women's health risks can itself be hazardous to health if those who create the news and those who cover it are not prepared to present a balanced, accurate and informative account of the problem. The aim of media coverage should be to alert those who should be worried and reassure those who should not.[2]

Perceptions of risk

What do women worry about, and what role does the media play in their perception of risk? Research suggests that, in general, there is a gap between the public and experts' views about risks, and which risks are more important.[4]

In the arena of women's health risks, for example, heart disease was long portrayed as a man's disease, despite its long-standing status as the number one killer of women.

Lung cancer, following the revolution in smoking amongst women, has overtaken breast cancer as the top female cancer killer in the United States, but breast cancer still appears to be perceived by women as a far greater risk. Why do women perceive that breast cancer is a greater risk than lung cancer?

Women today are often presented with confusing and conflicting information. The media basing 'facts' on too little information and not presenting all of the evidence may exaggerate potential risks. When media coverage creates public concern and anxiety, it appears that in some instances journalists may do little to explain discrepancies in news reporting. It is suggested that, because of this type of reporting, media coverage may have contributed to health risk uncertainties for women.[2]

No more hype

Research has suggested that there is a need for improvement in current media coverage of women's health. The media, when reporting women's health issues, need to present up-to-date research-based evidence. Potential risk factors need to be presented accurately with the avoidance of media hype and the creation of unnecessary anxiety and stress for women. Information needs to be presented to women with clear advice to seek further information from health care professionals.[2]

Improving media coverage of women's health risks requires better interpretation of research findings for the public. Journalists need to be better equipped to ask the right questions and interpret the answers in a more meaningful way, even when time and space are limited.

In conclusion, it is essential midwives, within their expanding public health role, keep up-to-date with media interest in women's health and ensure that women receive unbiased evidence-based information to enable them to clearly identify personal health risks and reduce fear and uncertainty.

REFERENCES

1 Nobbs J. Sociology. Second edition. London: Macmillan Education, 1980.
2 Russell C. Hype, hysteria, and women's health risks: The role of the media. Women's Health 1993; 3(4): 191-7.
3 Holme R. Mass Media and their Social Effects. Blandford Press, 1975.
4 Department of Health. Making a Difference: Strengthening the nursing, midwifery and health visiting contribution to health and healthcare. London: HMSO, 1999.

Coccydynia: a woman's tail

Isobel Ryder, Jo Alexander

Objective: to review the literature on coccydynia with specific reference to those cases of pregnancy and birth-related onset.

Method: databases (Medline, CINAHL, MIDIRS) were searched using the keywords coccydynia, coccygodynia, coccyx, spine, pelvis, injury, and trauma. The references contained within this review are those which give clear information about clinical cases and are least anecdotal.

Findings: much of the literature is of poor quality when judged by current standards. Where there is no other literature older references remain of interest. There is little information about incidence, prevalence, pathophysiology, methods of differential diagnosis and efficacy of treatment for these women. No qualitative data from women with pregnancy or birth-related coccydynia were identified.

Key conclusions and implications for practice: research into this topic needs to be undertaken if midwives are to be enabled to facilitate early diagnosis and provide care and advice for women with pregnancy and birth-related coccydynia.

Introduction

Coccydynia is the name given to pain in and/or around the coccyx. Churchill's Illustrated Medical Dictionary (Koenigsberg et al. 1989) defined coccydynia as 'persistent pain in the coccyx, whether spontaneous or following a fall on the buttocks' and gave the alternative terms as coccyalgia, coccygalgia, coccygodynia and coccyodynia. The pain is probably caused by musculoneurofascial disruption of the joint (Peyton 1988) and is a symptom (Wray et al. 1991), not a disease in itself. Duncan (1937) suggests that the term coccydynia was used in a generally descriptive way and tended to discourage accurate diagnosis and appropriate management based on the specific nature of the pathology. Coccygeal pain may be of acute or insidious onset and has a multifactorial aetiology. The coccyx is richly innervated thus, once sustained, the pain may be difficult to eradicate (Dandy 1993).

Structure and function

The coccyx lies at the lower end of the spine, on the inferior aspect of the sacrum (Gunn 1992). It is a triangular bone, made up of three to five segments (Gunn 1992) which partially or wholly fuse in adulthood (Martini 1995). The sacrococcygeal joint is articulated by a fibrocartilaginous disc (Williams et al. 1995) which is thicker anteriorly and posteriorly than laterally and is composed of hyaline cartilage. Occasionally the joint is synovial and hence more mobile (Williams et al. 1995). The coccyx is surrounded by sacrococcygeal ligaments that provide support as it undertakes passive movements of extension and flexion.

The coccygeal base is described as the posterior landmark of the anteroposterior diameter of the pelvic obstetric outlet (Williams et al. 1995) and it is the tip of the coccyx which forms the posterior border of the anatomical outlet (Silverton 1993, Verralls 1993). The obstetric outlet is important in relation to the space available to the fetus during birth (Silverton 1993) because the coccyx has the ability to extend during the birth process; it also extends during defaecation. The coccyx forms the site of attachment for the levatores ani muscles, which are important in voluntary control of bladder and bowels and thus are vital in terms of physical, social and sexual health.

An understanding of the anatomy of the pelvis is essential in order that pelvic size and shape can be optimised during labour. Midwives must also be aware of the possibility that pre-existing trauma to the coccyx may affect its ability to flex and extend during birth. Coccydynia may also arise as a result of birth.

The nature of the underlying injury or disease

The nature of the injury, and hence the cause of the pain, may be multifactorial and involve one or more types of tissue. Differential diagnosis is important before effective management can be commenced.

Bone fracture or joint dislocation or disruption have been identified as causes of some cases of coccydynia (Howorth 1959, Borgia 1964, Brunskill and Swan 1987, McRae 1994, Bergkamp and Verhaar 1995). A number of authors suggest that many cases are caused by spasm within the muscle groups surrounding the coccyx or coccygeal joint (Thiele 1937, 1963, Borgia 1964) and Thiele (1937, 1963) specifically mentions the levatores ani and coccygeus groups of muscles. Other suggested causes include degenerative diseases, such as osteoarthritis (Howorth 1959).

Bremer (1896) uses the term 'hysteria', and Hirst and Wachs (1924) allude to a neurotic basis for some cases of coccydynia, but in neither paper is any evidence offered to support this. Wilkinson (1947) comments that the neurosis was more likely to be as a result of the painful condition, rather than the coccydynia a manifestation of hysteria or psychoneurosis, and Duncan (1937) writes that such diagnoses should only be considered when organic disease has been excluded. However, Borgia (1964) reports about a 17-year-old girl he had cared for who, over 12 years had been seen by at least five different doctors. Her mother was about to seek psychiatric referral having been told that this long- standing problem was 'psychologic'. She experienced immediate relief from an injection of local anaesthetic and subsequently underwent coccygectomy with complete success. As recently as 1993 Dandy writes that the pain was more difficult to treat in litigious or neurotic individuals, who seemed more prone to the condition.

Frequency by gender

Some of the literature is very old and appears of poor quality when judged by current standards; in particular, the number and gender of the subjects is not always given. However, the majority of cases appear to be in women (Thiele 1963, Borgia 1964, Hodge 1979, Maigne et al. 1994, Zayer 1996). It has been suggested that the reason for this is the differences in pelvic anatomy between the genders (Duncan 1937). The typical female pelvic bituberous diameter is wider (mean 118 mm) than a man's (mean 85 mm). The anteroposterior diameter (from coccygeal apex to midpoint of the lower edge of the symphysis) is greater in women (mean 125 mm) than in men (mean 80 mm). The greater sciatic notch is wider in women, with a mean width of 53.9 mm, than in men at 40.8 mm, (Caldwell and Moloy 1933). It is suggested that these differences in pelvic outlet mean that the coccyx is more prominent in women and hence potentially more vulnerable to injury (Wray et al. 1991). However, it is important to remember that another key difference is that women have babies and without further evidence it is not possible to say that coccydynia occurs more frequently in women primarily because of differences in pelvic shape.

There has been no analysis of cases in relation to those women who have never taken a pregnancy to term nor given birth. Neither does any of the literature comment about gender differences in diet or lifestyle; for example, posture, participation in exercise and sports or the effect of osteoporosis. These aspects of the condition need further exploration.

Causes of coccydynia

External trauma

The cause of the injury may be acute or chronic trauma to the coccygeal area, but commonly includes direct external trauma, often as the result of a fall into a sitting position, or a direct blow (Bayne et al. 1984, Peyton 1988, Maigne et al. 1994). Bergkamp and Verhaar (1995) describe a case of coccydynia due to a dislocated coccyx. A 26-year-old woman had fallen downstairs with her three-month-old baby in her arms and landed in a sitting position.

Thiele (1963) found external trauma the cause of 50% (162/324) of cases. Of these 35% (56/162) were of acute onset and 65% (106/162) were due to chronic trauma. Peyton (1988) identifies that of the women he studied, 66% (119/180) had a history of trauma (examples given most commonly included falls, but also included road traffic accidents or physical abuse). Cooper (1960) suggests that trauma was the cause of 38% (38/100) of cases studied. In 21/38 the trauma was a fall; three of these cases were pregnant at the time. In 17 of the 38 the trauma was chronic due to prolonged rides or sitting.

Birth

After external trauma, delivery appears to be the second most common cause of coccydynia in women (Thiele 1963, Bayne et al. 1984, Peyton 1988, Wray et al. 1991, Zayer 1996). However, there are no papers on this topic in midwifery journals and only two case reports in recent years, one in an obstetric/gynaecology journal (Brunskill & Swan 1987) and one in a trauma journal (Jones et al. 1997). Both of these papers described women who had sustained a fractured coccyx during delivery.

Petit (1726) provides the earliest recorded case of birth-related coccydynia and this involved anterior displacement of the coccyx during childbirth, subsequently reduced by manipulation; both mother and child survived but there was no information about follow-up. In his texts of 1832 and 1840 Blundell advises fracture of an anteriorly displaced (anchylosed) coccygeal joint for delivery. Artificially fracturing the displaced coccyx during labour so as to facilitate delivery was also described as preferable to the destruction of the fetus (Simpson 1859).

The proportion of all cases of coccydynia which are delivery-related are thought to be in the region of 3-4% (Maigne & Tamalet 1996); however, other studies reported this percentage as higher (Thiele 1963 – 15%; Bayne et al. 1984 – 11%; Peyton 1988 – 6%; Wray et al. 1991 – 14%;). However, to date, no large scale studies have been undertaken and very few of the papers presented this aspect clearly. Thiele (1963) also suggests that there was another group (pregnancy-related) of four women who appeared to develop the condition as a physiological reaction to pregnancy. He is the only author to have identifed this group.

Frazier (1985) describes delivery trauma as a 'common cause of acute coccydynia', but gives no numerical data to support this claim. She added that some women fracture their coccyx during a difficult delivery. The only paper to give an indication of figures in relation to gynaecological cases is that of Peyton (1988) who retrospectively reviewed 180 women with coccydynia (out of 3000 gynaecological patients) over a 10-year period. He found that 6% (10/180) felt that the pain arose following delivery, and when he studied their obstetric records he found that there was an obvious history of difficult second stage of labour.

Brunskill and Swan (1987) report a case where a woman experienced spontaneous fracture of the coccyx during the second stage of labour. The woman had spontaneous onset of labour, epidural analgesia and oxytocic infusion. While pushing she 'felt something crack' and developed 'severe pain in the bottom' so that she was unable to continue pushing and had an epidural top-up followed by instrumental delivery. She had no previous recorded history of injury to the coccyx. Jones et al. (1997) described a similar case where a 'crack' was heard by all in the delivery room which coincided with the onset of acute coccygeal pain. These are the only birth-related case studies reported in some detail.

Surgery

Coccydynia related to surgery to the pelvic region or spine appears to be sub-divided into two groups. The first group developed coccydynia as referred pain following spinal surgery. Bayne et al. (1984) found that seven (including four women) of 48 cases arose following spinal surgery. This group had uniformly poor results following coccygectomy and they suggested that this was due to the referred nature of the pain. The second group had localised surgery (ano-rectal region) and in these cases position during surgery may have influenced onset. Six of 120 cases studied by Wray et al. (1991) arose following surgery, three in lithotomy position (gender not given). Two of the 100 cases treated by Cooper (1960) developed coccydynia after ano-rectal surgery.

Other causes

Bayne et al. (1984) found 12 cases of insidious onset (10 women) and identify that of these 12 cases, three women had a history of pilonidal sinus and four women had participated in anal intercourse prior to developing coccydynia. Origin may also be associated with nearby pathology such as disc prolapses or pelvic disorders including carcinoma (Frazier 1985) and chordoma (Hodge 1979).

Cooper (1960) identifies infection as the cause of coccydynia in 60% (60/100) of cases. Of these, 51 had anal infection, three prostatic, one epidymal and five cervical infections. Thiele (1963) reports that 55% (178/324) patients had anal infections.

Symptoms

The main symptom is localised pain, which may be severe and of long duration (Dandy 1993). The duration of pain for the forty-eight cases that Bayne et al. (1984) studied ranged from three months to 20 years (mean three years). Cases identified by Wray et al. (1991) ranged from six months to 10 years (mean 16 months).

Of the 180 women that Peyton (1988) studied, 36% (n=65) experienced low backache, 20% (n=36) pelvic pressure, 11% (n=20) painful bowel movements or rectal spasm and 7% (*n*=13) dyspareunia. The pain or tenderness may be aggravated by sitting on hard surfaces or with poor posture (Thiele 1963) or sitting for long periods, for example when travelling (Thiele 1963, Frazier 1985) or by prolonged standing, bending or lifting (Peyton 1988). Wray et al. (1991) report that pain is especially severe when sitting or when rising from a sitting position. Other factors which increase the pain include repetitive minor trauma, such as arises from cycling (Peyton 1988, Nakamura et al. 1995), rowing (Wray et al. 1991), or other forms of exercise which put pressure on the coccygeal area. The symptoms may be exacerbated by climbing stairs or be worse during menstruation (Peyton 1988).

Diagnosis

Knowledge of the most common symptoms could provide a basis for careful questioning by the midwife during history taking, thus enabling diagnosis of coccydynia during pregnancy or the postnatal period. It is also possible to observe signs such as obvious discomfort when sitting down or rising from a sitting position (Wray et al. 1991), especially when sufficient time is given to postnatal examination. The nature of the reported pain needs to be explored in order to differentiate between coccydynia and perineal pain.

Where there is anterior displacement of the coccyx it may be possible to feel the exposed sharp edge of sacrum on external palpation, and there will be associated discomfort or pain (McRae 1994). It may be possible to make a diagnosis on rectal examination (Frazier 1985), although midwives do not usually perform this. Radiological examination in a sitting position may confirm diagnosis if the injury involves the bone or joint (Maigne et al. 1994).

The preponderance of female sufferers led Wray et al. (1991) to suggest that when the condition occurred in men there should be a high degree of suspicion of some serious underlying pathology.

Management

If the coccydynia is of traumatic origin (including delivery) it is advised that the acute state be treated by use of non-steroidal anti-inflammatory drugs and non-constipating analgesia, together with local application of ice (Brunskill and Swan 1987) or ice and heat (Peyton 1988). Prevention of further injury and assistance with recovery may be achieved by correcting posture to encourage an upright sitting position so that the body weight is taken on the ischial tuberosities rather than the coccyx (Howorth 1959). In the case of the postnatal woman, specific advice and consideration may need to be given in relation to posture, position and comfort, especially if she is breast feeding. Successful Breastfeeding (RCM 1991) suggests that modern furniture, both in and out of hospital, does not facilitate a good breast-feeding posture while seated. The furniture may be too soft to encourage women to lean forward slightly and any position which results in leaning back will put pressure on the coccyx.

Frazier (1985), Peyton (1988) and Wray et al. (1991) all mention the use of rubber rings to assist the alleviation of pressure on the coccyx for all people with coccydynia. In the postnatal period the use of both ring cushions and valley cushions (UT Care Products Ltd) need to be evaluated (Sleep 1995) in order to exclude complications such as increased oedema, impeded circulation or thrombosis to which it has been suggested they may predispose (Church & Lyne 1994). Peyton (1988) suggested pelvic floor exercises as a method of treatment, however, acute treatment for possible fracture or dislocation would normally involve rest. Since the levator ani muscles are attached to the coccyx any movement involving these muscles will increase the pain.

Brunskill and Swan (1987) used transcutaneous nerve stimulation as a method of pain relief for the woman they describe, starting treatment some six weeks after the birth during which the spontaneous fracture occurred. The pain gradually lessened but the mother was still in some pain three months after birth.

The woman reported by Jones et al. (1997) remained undiagnosed for some six weeks during which time the woman was referred to the physiotherapist and then for osteopathic treatment, which acutely exacerbated the pain. Following radiological identification of a coccygeal fracture, treatment included physiotherapy and ultrasound, and three weeks later the symptoms had improved.

Wray et al. (1991) undertook a five-year prospective study involving 120 patients (101 women) in an attempt to identify which treatments were helpful in cases of coccydynia. Their pilot study (*n*=50, number of women not given) used a step-wise approach from physiotherapy (two weeks of daily ultrasound followed by two weeks of short-wave diathermy) progressing to local injection of steroids and anaesthesia (repeated one month later if required) and then to manipulation and injection (under general anaesthetic). If the patient was still in pain six weeks after this coccygectomy was performed. The pilot study showed physiotherapy to have had a success rate of 16% (8/50) and they suggested that this was not a useful method of treatment.

The randomised trial which followed, (*n*=120, 101 women) compared local injection with manipulation and injection. Unfortunately the paper is rather unclear about both the numbers involved and the findings. Local injection (steroids and anaesthesia) was described as a relatively straightforward outpatient procedure and with a success rate of 60% (17/29), they suggested that it should be used as the first line of management. They found that any improvement was likely to be achieved following the first two injections (Wray et al. 1991). If unsuccessful, they used manipulation of the coccyx under general anaesthesia along with another local injection, which had an 85% success rate (28/33). Coccygectomy was performed on those patients (23) who did not respond to these treatments or who relapsed following repeated treatment.

Bergkamp and Verhaar (1995) undertook surgical reduction for a woman who had dislocated her coccyx in a fall three months postnatally. She had no pain after rehabilitation and at two years post-operatively.

Enemas, acupuncture and chiropractic adjustments were some of the therapies that other practitioners had attempted prior to Peyton (1988) undertaking massage for the cases he discussed. He describes the process that he used, which was based on the technique used by Thiele (1937, 1963), but states that massage should never be used in the acute stage. Of the 180 women that Peyton (1988) studied he managed 96% using massage. It is difficult to interpret how successful this form of management was as the number of women followed up and the duration are not given. However, he indicates that of those who were followed up (for between one and 22 years after massage) 61.5% were 'cured', 27% were improved, and 11.5% were not improved. Howorth (1959) is the only author to specifically mention that there may be a place for postnatal massage of the sacro-coccygeal region and muscles when they are in spasm.

Coccygectomy (excision of the coccyx) as the surgical form of treatment appears to be highly effective for some cases. Peyton (1988) successfully treated three of the 11.5% women who had not responded to the treatments offered previously with this surgery. Wray et al. (1991) managed 23 of 120 cases using this method. These 23 cases had not responded to earlier treatments (injection or manipulation) or had relapsed following these treatments. Of the 23 patients, 21 had complete and sustained relief. Zayer (1996) performed ten coccygectomies on selected cases and found that nine cases were asymptomatic at follow-up. He suggests that it is important to exclude those with symptoms not related to the coccyx and that having tried conservative treatments first, coccygectomy might be of benefit. Borgia (1964) and Bayne et al. (1984) suggested that coccygectomy was contraindicated if the pain was referred from the spine.

Implications for midwifery practice

There is a lack of specific information about pregnancy and birth-related coccydynia and this is important if midwives are to be able to accurately diagnose this symptom. In particular there is a lack of empirical evidence in relation to: .

- incidence of pregnancy and birth-related coccydynia
- pregnancy and birth-related factors which may predispose to coccydynia
- differential diagnosis in the postnatal period
- comparative efficacy of the various methods of treatment
- women's reports of the nature of this pain.

Accurate information about incidence may not become available until there is more awareness about the condition and there is an effective method of diagnosing it. Coccydynia may often be mistaken for perineal pain. Research into coccygeal injuries arising during pregnancy and birth is currently ongoing by the authors.

Midwives are in a position to facilitate early diagnosis and to provide care and advice for women with pregnancy or birth-related coccydynia, but they need more information on which to base their care.

REFERENCES

Bayne O, Bateman J, Cameron H 1984 The influence of etiology on the results of coccygectomy. Clinical Orthopaedics and Related Research 190: 266-272

Bergkamp A, Verhaar J 1995 Dislocation of the coccyx: a case report. Journal of Bone and Joint Surgery 77-B: 831-832

Blundell J 1832 Lectures on midwifery. Field & Bull, London

Blundell J 1840 Principles and practice of obstetric medicine. J Butler, London

Borgia C 1964 Coccydynia: its diagnosis and management. Military Medicine 129: 335-338

Bremer L 1896 The knife for coccygodynia a failure. Medical Record 1: 154-155

Brunskill P, Swan J 1987 Spontaneous fracture of the coccygeal body during the second stage of labour. Journal of Obstetrics and Gynaecology 7 (4): 270-271

Caldwell W, Moloy H 1933 Anatomical variations in the female pelvis and their effect in labor with a suggested classification. American Journal of Obstetrics and Gynecology 26: 479-505

Church S, Lyne P 1994 Research based practice: some problems illustrated by the discussion of evidence concerning the use of a pressure relieving device in nursing and midwifery. Journal of Advanced Nursing 19: 513-518

Cooper W 1960 Coccygodynia: an analysis of 100 cases. Journal of the International College of Surgeons 33: 306-311

Dandy D 1993 Essential orthopaedics and trauma, 2nd edn. Churchill Livingstone, Edinburgh

Duncan G 1937 Painful coccyx. Archives of Surgery 34:1088-1104

Frazier L 1985 Coccydynia: a tail of woe. North Carolina Medical Journal 46 (4): 202-212

Gunn C 1992 Bones and joints: a guide for students, 2nd edn. Churchill Livingstone, Edinburgh

Hirst J, Wachs C 1924 Labor injuries to the coccyx and their treatment.

American Journal of Obstetrics and Gynaecology 7: 199-205

Hodge J 1979 Clinical management of coccydynia. Medical Trial Technique Quarterly 25 (3): 277-284

Howorth B 1959 The painful coccyx. Clinical Orthopaedics 14:145-161

Jones M, Shoaib A, Bircher M 1997 A case of coccygodynia due to coccygeal fracture secondary to parturition. Injury 28 (8): 549-550

Koenigsberg R, Lovell Baker E, Heptinstall R et al. (eds) 1989 Churchill's Illustrated Medical Dictionary. Churchill Livingstone, New York

Maigne J, Guedj S, Straus C 1994 Idiopathic coccygodynia: lateral roentgenograms in the sitting position and coccygeal discography. Spine 19 (8): 930-934

Maigne J, Tamalet B 1996 Standardized radiologic protocol for the study of common coccydynia and characteristics of the lesions observed in the sitting position. Spine 21 (22): 2588-2593

Martini F 1995 Fundamentals of anatomy and physiology, 3rd edn. Prentice Hall. New York

McRae R 1994 Practical fracture treatment, 3rd edn. Churchill Livingstone, Edinburgh

Nakamura A, Inoue Y, Ishihara T et al. 1995 Acquired coccygeal nodule due to repeated stimulation by a bicycle saddle. Journal of Dermatology 22: 365-369

Petit J 1726 A treatise of the diseases of the bones (translated from the French). T Woodward, London

Peyton F 1988 Coccygodynia in women. Indiana Medicine 81 (8): 697-698

Royal College of Midwives 1991 Successful breastfeeding. RCM, London

Silverton L 1993 The art and science of midwifery. Prentice Hall, New York

Simpson J 1859 Coccygodynia and diseases and deformities of the coccyx. Medical Times and Gazette 1: 1-7

Sleep J 1995 Postnatal perineal care revisited. In: Alexander J, Levy V, Roch S (eds) Aspects of midwifery practice. Macmillan, Basingstoke

Thiele G 1937 Coccygodynia and pain in the superior gluteal region. Journal of the American Medical Association 109 (16): 1271-1275

Thiele G 1963 Coccygodynia: cause and treatment. Diseases of the Colon and Rectum 6: 422-436

Verralls S 1993 Anatomy and physiology applied to obstetrics. Churchill Livingstone, Edinburgh

Wilkinson W 1947 Coccygodynia: a review of the literature and presentation of cases. South Surgeon 13: 280-293

Williams P, Bannister L, Berry M et al. (eds) 1995 Gray's Anatomy, 38th edn. Churchill Livingstone, New York

Wray C, Easom S, Hoskinson J 1991 Coccydinia, aetiology and treatment. Journal of Bone and Joint Surgery 73 (2): 335-338

Zayer M 1996 Coccygodynia. Ulster Medical Journal 65 (1): 58-60

The postnatal experience

SECTION CONTENTS

As I sit writing my piece for this section of the book, I am struck that, in the first volume, we separated 'postnatal issues' (which were primarily about the woman's post-birth experience) from the section on breastfeeding. This time, the postnatal experience of the mother and baby are so intertwined in the following articles that it would be impossible to separate them in this way – and this somehow feels more 'right'.

The articles in this section raise some crucial questions, which midwives need to consider in defining where midwifery is moving over the next few years. Lorna Davies' original article on co-sleeping is an example of how, over time, some of the practices that are central to families' lives – such as sharing a family bed – have become re-positioned within the frameworks of Western medicine and modern society to seem deviant, if not positively hazardous. This issue highlights how relative our positions and ideas are, when considered in a context wider than our own belief system.

Another example of an innate practice that our culture has somehow undermined is skin-to-skin contact between families. It seems logical to me that, in pre-industrial societies, particularly those situated in the Northern hemisphere, a mother who did not spend time skin-to-skin with her baby would have had less chance of that baby surviving. Helen Wallace and David Marshall explore some of the literature around the benefits of skin-to-skin contact, considering some of the cultural issues that may have reduced the appeal of this practice for women and the ways in which this might now be addressed.

In examining women's feelings and opinions about their experiences of postnatal care, Debbie Singh and Mary Newburn found that only half of the women in their study felt their emotional, informational and support needs had been met. In this study, the women who were less likely to feel their needs had been met were those who were having their first baby, who had had an operative birth or who were feeding their baby formula milk. Nicky Bean has also considered the views and feelings of formula-feeding mothers in asking whether our reluctance to give out information on artificial feeding is doing more harm than good. Her work certainly begs the question of whether our 'bottom-line' goal as midwives is in preserving what we deem to be natural or normal, or in supporting women's choices, whether we personally agree with them or not.

In an attempt to provide more help for women who have chosen to breastfeed, Alison Blenkinsop discusses her prize-winning 'breast' – a truly useful tool which can aid in demonstrating 'latching on' and other techniques visually (thus potentially reducing problems caused by literacy and language barriers), and without the need for midwives to handle women's breasts in order to explain their suggestions. Linda Mason, Sheila Glenn, Irene Walton and Carol Hughes' research also asked women for their views on the care they received – focusing on the advice given regarding pelvic floor exercises. Their focus on the term 'ad hoc' to describe the differences between the advice and information received by different women is another timely reminder that, where the focus of postnatal care absolutely needs to be on meeting the needs of the individual family rather than on routines, there are a few pieces of information that we might consider vital for all women. And, if this is the case, then our next challenge might be to find more creative ways of sharing information with women, given that the women themselves don't seem to be finding current midwifery services – with all that constrains them – to be meeting their informational needs.

'All through the Night'

Co-sleeping – risky business or survival mechanism?

Lorna Davies

Sleep my child and peace bestow thee,
All through the night
Guardian angels will attend thee,
All through the night
Soft the drowsy hours are creeping,
Hill and dale in slumber sleeping
I my loved ones' watch am keeping,
All through the night

Anon

Eight years ago, I published an article in a British midwifery journal, exploring the concept of mother and infant co-sleeping.[1] While reviewing the literature for the piece, I was unable to unearth one single article that was written specifically for midwives on the subject. The article received a great deal of attention, much of it positive, some less so. I did receive a number of letters from midwives who felt that to even suggest such a practice as bed sharing with a baby was tantamount to professional misconduct.

There is no doubt that eight years on we have moved forward. There is far more information available for both parents who may consider the option of sharing sleeping arrangements with their infants and children, and also for health workers. However, I feel that the dominant rationale for consideration of the issue is still risk, rather than benefit. Although it is imperative that safety issues (including contraindications) around co-sleeping are discussed openly, it is poignant – and perhaps an inevitable reflection of the times in which we live – that the reasons for this discussion are generally centred around the principles of risk management. There are undoubtedly some risks around the practice of bed sharing; these are usually related to other social behaviours that accompany the practice, such as smoking or drinking alcohol. However, is it right that the highlighting of risk factors takes precedence in discussions around what some parents feel instinctively

to be the right choice for them? My feeling is that if we make the practice a positive and enhancing experience for parents, the acceptance of suggested safeguards will become part of the process of following a powerful and instinctive parenting response.

Ninety per cent of the world's mothers carry out some form of co-sleeping arrangement, which would indicate that this is a tried and tested human response that has benefits for both mothers and their infants.[2] In many developing countries, babies are viewed as an extension of the mother until well into toddlerhood. They are carried around on the mother's person, have access to a continuous supply of breastmilk and sleep in the same bed as their mother.[3]

In westernised industrial society we are encouraged to foster social and biological independence in our young as early as possible.[4] Birth is viewed as the moment of separation when the growth of the individual begins. The infant is no longer perceived as being reliant on the mother for physiological wellbeing. The child may be breast fed so still needs the mother to fulfil this function, but otherwise the baby is actively 'trained' to spend a great deal of time being separated physically from the mother for fear of being 'spoiled' or creating too much reliance on the parents.[5]

In fact, solitary infant sleeping is a relatively recent phenomenon, even in western industrialised society. Until 200 years ago, co-sleeping was the norm within all societies.[6] In western industrialised society, this remained to be the case within the lower socio-economic groups until even more recently. Our working class Victorian foremothers could not even consider the luxury of separate sleeping accommodation and whole families would, through necessity, sleep in one bed.[6] It would appear that the practice of infant sleep separation has coincided with an increasingly affluent western lifestyle. The advice proffered by Truby King in his 1934 best selling manual 'Mothercraft',[7] to keep the child in their own room overnight, could not have been achieved by anyone on less than a substantial income. Increasingly, throughout the twentieth century, the ability to provide bigger and better homes with more rooms has encouraged the commercial growth of the baby product industry, and the trend of providing the newborn infant with its own colour coordinated environment.

Ironically, the UNICEF Baby Friendly Initiative, which has proved to be an ally of co-sleeping, with its recognition of the importance of skin-to-skin contact and insistence of rooming in, has spawned the development of a further commercial spectre. Some hospital units are now providing cot attachments that enable mother and baby to be together on the same level in the bed, in an attempt to minimise the criticism levelled by those who propose that babies are unsafe in hospital beds with their mothers.[8] This has offered the opportunity for more commercial enterprise with companies now marketing 'nest arrangements' for parents who choose to sleep with their baby!

Until recently in western culture, sleeping with one's children had not only ceased to be the norm but had become a taboo.[9] This abrupt change in the past few centuries or so seemed to be based on the assumption that infants had adequately altered biologically to adapt to this shift – an assumption that has neither been acknowledged nor tested.[10]

In a paper entitled *The Unknown Human Infant* Michel Odent[11] states: 'One can wonder if the sleep patterns usually considered as physiological are not, in fact, an adaptation to a very special society where the infants are weaned before the age of one year and do not sleep with their mother.'

The integrated infant care system which incorporates co-sleeping with parents is the result of millions of years of evolution; one would therefore imagine that it must provide social, physiological, psychological, and even spiritual benefits for those involved.

It has been suggested that co-sleeping with parents is a contributory factor in SIDS.[12] This suspicion evolved as a result of studies conducted in New Zealand where cot death rates were high among the Maoris who always sleep with their children.[13] However, other contributory factors were not fully taken into consideration. Alcoholism is prevalent among this disadvantaged indigenous group, as is heavy smoking and a history of bronchial problems.[14]

Cot death is rare in many cultures where babies routinely sleep with their mothers. In Hong Kong, for example, where infants co-sleep with parents, the Hong Kong authorities documented only 15 cases of SIDS in a five-year period.[6] Three of these cases were British babies. British and US rates would have suggested 800 to 1200 deaths in that size of population. Epidemiological

observations within co-sleeping Asian communities report the lowest rates of SIDS even when crowded housing and poorer socio-economic status would predict a higher incidence of the syndrome.[15]

Ironically, much of the information pertaining to the benefits of co-sleeping has evolved as a result of research into SIDS. Observation in studies to assess the risk has uncovered physiological benefits, which could have a profound effect on our cultural sleeping habits. A good deal of this information could potentially be used to formulate advice with the aim of decreasing the risk of SIDS.

The discipline of anthropology has cast much light on the physiological attributes of co-sleeping. Medical anthropologist James McKenna believes that this pattern of behaviour provides a more enriched and varied sensory environment that the human infant has evolved to expect. He speculates that: 'Co-sleeping could provide important practice for the neurological and physiological mechanisms which underlie the arousal response.'[16]

Research carried out by McKenna and his team indicates that babies sleeping with their mothers arouse more frequently, and polysonographic traces in controlled experiments suggest that mother and baby wake-sleep patterns synchronise.[16] When sleeping with their mothers, babies feed three times more frequently than those in separated states and their mothers wake between six and 10 times during the night to attend to or check their baby. They frequently have no recollection of this nocturnal activity.

Mosko et al[10] explored infant arousals during mother-infant bed sharing and the implications for infant sleep and SIDS research, and discovered that sleep patterns changed in the pairings resulting in less stage 3-4 sleep (deep sleep) and more 1-2 stage (rapid eye movement) episodes. They concluded that these observed changes might offer protection against SIDS.

Infants are able to process and respond to environmental stimuli during sleep[17] and it is thought that their reactions to external events such as parents changing position or breathing audibly might compensate for a respiratory control defect.

The proximity of a mother to her baby in sleep is another interesting issue. Quite often the mother and her child will lie with their faces only five to eight centimetres apart, which allows intermittent exposure to atmospheric CO_2 concentrations as high as 3%. Haddad et al[18] demonstrated that continuous exposure to 2% CO_2 increased ventilation in infants. It is therefore possible that this intermittent exposure may have significant impact on infant breathing patterns.

Helen Ball, a British social anthropologist, has filmed mother and baby pairings extensively for her research and has identified specific traits of behaviour. For example, she has identified that mothers who are breastfeeding and co-sleeping form a protective 'fetal' position around their infant.[19] Babies who breastfeed as they sleep with their parents are much more likely to lie on their back or on their side.[20] Position of the baby is now recognised to be an important factor in reducing the risk of SIDS.[21]

The impact of the thermal environment is a further factor that may contribute to SIDS. Again it would appear that protective maternal behaviours prevent any compromise to the infant as far as thermal control is concerned. Even during very short arousals, mothers often pat or stroke the head, back or chest of their baby or instinctively move the bedding.[10]

Many parents fear they will suffocate their baby by rolling on them in sleep, a phenomenon known as 'overlay'.[3] The work carried out by Blair and Fleming[22] would suggest that a greater risk in terms of suffocation comes when the parent chooses to sleep on a sofa with the baby who subsequently falls between the cushions and the back of the sofa and suffocates whilst the parent sleeps on, unknowing. This is borne out by several examples of this occurrence in recent years, which were initially cited as bed-sharing tragedies. Ironically, these parents had potentially transferred from the bed because of what they perceived as the risk of overlay in co-sleeping.

Studies carried out in the UK[23] and New Zealand[24] have concluded after multivariate analysis that the increase in risk of SIDS associated with bed sharing is found only to apply to parents who smoke. Blair[22] supports the smoking factor hypothesis and additionally includes alcohol and drugs (including some therapeutic, such as sedatives, as well as recreational drugs) as risk factors. Blair and Fleming[19] also suggested that parents who are ill or exhausted are more at risk of causing overlay and should avoid co-sleeping, and that duvets were probably best avoided during co-sleeping episodes. Jackson[9] states that mechanical suffocation is less likely to occur than cot death by a factor of 200, as long as the above advice regarding smoking, alcohol and medication is followed.

One further interesting factor is the significance of breastfeeding in the co-sleeping debate. There is strong evidence that bed sharing directly promotes breastfeeding.[25] Nocturnal video recordings of mothers and babies demonstrated that bed-sharing infants breastfed for three times longer than babies who were separated at night. McKenna went on to suggest that an increased daily infusion of maternal antibodies may provide bed-sharing, breastfeeding infants with increased protection from infectious diseases, some potentially related to SIDS.

Ball[19] discovered that the protective response of co-sleeping mothers differed from that of their bottle-feeding counterparts, which may indicate that the benefits of co-sleeping are closely linked with feeding practices. This is an area that, in my opinion, requires further consideration and research. If biological synchronicity of child and mother when bed-sharing provides physiological benefit, we might also assume concurrent psychological rewards for both mother and infant in order to drive this behaviour.

It would appear that there has been a backlash in the UK to the emergence of the co-sleeping lobby, in books such as *The Contented Little Baby Book*.[26] In this book, Gina Ford, a 'maternity nurse', cites her own experience of working with babies and small children as the formula for training babies into sleep-wake patterns that ensure the parents get their full quotient of sleep and a much needed rest from their infant. This text is reminiscent of the material produced by Truby King in the 1930s where fathers were advised to lock their babies in the nursery at night and not to allow the mother to have the key, because sentiment may get in the way of logic where the baby was concerned.[7]

Michel Odent[11] believes that a baby needs its mother even more at night because its predominant sense (sight) is at rest. This means that the baby needs to use skin-to-skin touch to gain emotional security. If bed sharing offers the child security, then separation anxiety is minimised.

Bowlby[27] suggested that a baby who was with his or her mother continuously day and night, would evolve into a secure and confident adult. Contrary to making the child more 'clingy', which is another frequently cited reason for not encouraging bed sharing, sleeping with one's children actually makes them more independent by fulfilling their need to feel secure.

Many parents endure sleepless nights while pursuing a series of battles of will with their children over the time and place of going to sleep. However, Jackson[9] suggests that the experiences of a baby who is forced to sleep alone may well develop into sleeping problems in adulthood; the emotional and psychological damage may be self-perpetuating.

The psychological and emotional rewards for the mother when sleeping with her baby must also be considered. Psychologically, a mother who knows that her child is safe and close to her is much more likely to enjoy her new baby, once old wives tales and myths about co-sleeping are put to rest. It is possible that socially enforced separation at night creates ambiguous feelings that could manifest in postnatal depression.

The issues around the benefits for fathers are not as clear-cut and further research is required before these are realised. It is fair to say that in many cultures where co-sleeping is practised, the father does not sleep on the same sleeping surface as the mother and baby, or even in the same room. In discussions about co-sleeping with fathers it has been brought to my attention that many more men than we possibly do realise leave the matrimonial bed during the early days of parenthood, when the baby is waking frequently for feeds. Perhaps this is a design specification of human behaviour to ensure that mother and baby get the opportunity to occupy the eco-niche required to maximise human development. Alternatively, if fathers do remain in the family bed during this period, they too may benefit from the practice. They may experience a less disturbed sleep because the baby's needs are actually met before being made known by crying. Co-sleeping offers the father a chance to be close to his baby and he may feel less left out of the new family arrangement as a result.

Anyone who has spent time sleeping with their baby is aware of what an amazing experience it can be, yet the horror stories in the press of mothers who have 'killed their babies' haunt the parents who have made a choice to co-sleep. Equally, the health professional is faced with frequent criticisms of the practice in healthcare-related publications. The reality of life with a new baby means

that many parents are going to continue to practise co-sleeping with or without the blessing of their midwife, health visitor, GP or other health practitioner. Without their support they are likely to do so covertly, and then maybe they *will* be placing their baby at greater risk. It is therefore essential that we continue to bring the issue out into the open for discussion.

We must stop being solely the harbingers of doom, shroud waving at every given opportunity. Yes, by all means lets advise that smoking, drinking and taking medication may not be appropriate when co-sleeping. Let's inform parents about opting for layers of blankets rather than duvets, and of the potential threat of falling asleep with their babies on a sofa. But let's also consider the potential benefits of a global practice that may lead to improved physical and emotional well being and which may have far reaching effects at a societal level.

'Who sleeps by whom is not merely a personal or private activity. Instead it is social practice, like burying the dead or expressing gratitude for gifts or eating meals with your family or honouring the practice of a monogamous marriage, which (for those engaged in the practice) is invested with moral and social meaning for a person's reputation and good standing in the community.'[28]

REFERENCES

1. Davies L. Babies co-sleeping with parents. Midwives 1995;108(1295) 384-386
2. Young J. Babies and bedsharing...Co-sleeping. MIDIRS Midwifery Digest 1998;8:364-369.
3. Breazeale TI (2001) http://www.visi.com/~jlb/thesis.html
4. Kagan J. The Nature of the Child. New York: Basic Books; 1984
5. Levy TM, Orlans M. Attachment, trauma, and healing: Understanding and treating attachment disorder in children and families. Washington, DC: CWLA Press; 1998
6. Gantley M, Davies DP, Murcott A. (1993) Sudden Infant Death Syndrome; Links with infant care practices. British Medical Journal 1993;306:16-20
7. King T. Mothercraft. Christchurch, New Zealand: Whitcombe and Tombs; 1934
8. UNICEF Baby Friendly Initiative. Sharing a bed with your baby. London: UNICEF; 2001 available at URL http://www.babyfriendly.org.uk/resourcefile/data35.asp
9. Jackson D. Three in a Bed 3rd ed. London: Bloomsbury;1995
10. Mosko S, Richard C, McKenna J. Infant arousals during mother-infant bedsharing: implications for infant's sleep and SIDS research. Pediatrics 1997;100:841-849
11. Odent M. The unknown human infant. Journal of Human Lactation 1990;6: 6-8.
12. Consumer Product Safety Commission (US) http://www.cpsc.gov/cpscpub/pubs/5091.html
13. Scragg R. Bed sharing, smoking and alcohol in the Sudden Infant Death Syndrome. British Medical Journal 1993; 307:1312-18
14. Mitchell E. Ethnic differences in mortality from Sudden Infant Death Syndrome in New Zealand. British Medical Journal 1993;306:13-16
15. Watanabee N, Yotsukura M, Kadoi N, Yashiro K, Sakanoue M, Nishida H. Epidemiology of sudden infant death syndrome in Japan. Acta Paediatrica Japan 1994;36:329-32
16. McKenna J. Experimental studies of infant-parent co sleeping: mutual physiological and behavioural influences and their relevance to SIDS (Sudden Infant Death Syndrome). Early Human Development. 1994;38:187-201
17. Kahn A, Picard E, Blum D. Auditory arousal thresholds of normal and near-miss SIDS infants. Developmental Medicine and Child Neurology.1986;28:299-302
18. Haddad GG, Leistner HL, Epstein RS, Epstein MAF, Grodin WK, Mellins RB. CO_2 induced changes in ventilation and ventilatory patterns in normal sleeping infants. Journal of Applied Physiology 1980;48:684-688
19. Ball HL, Hooker E, Kelly PJ. Where will the Baby Sleep? Attitudes and practices of new and experienced parents regarding co-sleeping with their newborn infants. American Anthropologist 1999;101:143-151.
20. Di Pietro JA, Larson SK, Pores SW. Behavioural and heart rate pattern differences between breastfed and bottle fed neonates, Development Psychology 1987;23:467-474.
21. Department of Health. Sudden Unexpected Deaths in Infancy. London: DoH; 2000
22. Blair PS, Fleming PJ, Smith I. Babies sleeping with parents: case control study of factors influencing the risk of sudden infant death. British Medical Journal 1999;319:1457-62.
23. Blair PS, Fleming PJ, Bensley D, Smith I, Bacon C, Taylor E, Berry J, Golding J, and Tripp J. Smoking and the sudden infant death syndrome: results from 1993-5 case-control study for confidential inquiry into stillbirths and deaths in infancy. British Medical Journal 1996;313:195-198.
24. Mitchell EA, Tuohy PG, Brunt JM et al. Risk Factors for Sudden Infant Death syndrome following the prevention campaign in New Zealand: a prospective Study. Pediatrics 1997;100: 835-840
25. McKenna JJ, Mosko SS, Richard CA. Bed sharing promotes Breastfeeding. Pediatrics 1997;100: 214-19
26. Ford G. The Contented Little Baby Book. London: Vermillion; 1999
27. Bowlby J. Childcare and the Growth of Love. London: Pelican; 1953
28. Goodnow JJ, Miller PJ, Kessel F. Cultural Practices as Contexts for Development. San Francisco: Jossey Bass; 1995

Postnatal care in the month after birth

Debbie Singh, Mary Newburn

Changing Childbirth highlighted the need for woman-centred care throughout pregnancy, birth, and in the postnatal period.[1] In recent years there has been much discussion about the needs of women during pregnancy and childbirth,[2-5] but less emphasis on postnatal care.[6,7] Yet evidence suggests that postnatal care may be the least satisfactory aspect of maternity care for women in the United Kingdom.[8-10] Poor postnatal care can have physical, psychological, and emotional consequences for both the woman and child.[9,11-14]

Compared to evaluations of postnatal services,[15-18] research into women's opinions of postnatal care is sparse.[12,19] However, more research in this area is emerging.[20-24] This study examines a group of women's opinions about postnatal care in the first month after childbirth. The aim was to investigate whether different aspects of postnatal care were meeting women's needs and to motivate more detailed work in this area.

Methodology

After pilot testing, a one page, 20 question survey was published in the members' journal of the National Childbirth Trust and on the Baby World internet site.[25] The survey consisted predominantly of closed-ended questions, with two open-ended questions and an invitation to add further commentary

Women receiving the journal or visiting the website were invited to participate during a month-long data collection period.[26] To guard against memory problems only those who had given birth in 1999 or 2000 were eligible.

Nine hundred and sixty women from throughout the United Kingdom completed questionnaires. The majority had given birth within the last year and for two thirds it was their first baby. Ninety one percent gave birth in hospital, 7% had a home birth and 2% had their baby at a birth centre. Three fifths of the women had a vaginal

birth without major intervention; 17% had an instrumental delivery; 16% had an emergency caesarean and 8% had a planned caesarean.

This non-probability self-selected sampling method was used to allow women from throughout the United Kingdom to participate and to ensure data was collected rapidly. The results can not be generalised to all women in the United Kingdom, but they highlight important issues and themes to be examined by ongoing research. Delivery type and geographic dispersion were relatively representative of the wider population of interest.[27-30]

Findings

Women were asked to rate the information and advice, care, and emotional support that they received from health professionals in the first 3 days after giving birth; 4-10 days after giving birth; and 11-30 days after their baby was born (Table 7.2.1).

Overall, around half said that they had got all of the information, care and emotional support that they needed from health professionals. Yet more than one in ten said that they had received very little or no information and up to a quarter said that they had received no emotional support.

Emotional support

Throughout the three phases of care, women were consistently less satisfied about the extent to which their emotional support needs had been met (Figure 7.2.1). This was especially the case in the period 11-30 days after the birth where more women reported very low levels of care and support, compared with the 4-10 day period (p < 0.05).[31]

'There was no emotional preparation for parenthood or emotional support in tackling the huge change in everyday life which first became apparent after a few weeks. Physical fitness

Table 7.2.1 Levels of postnatal care received

Postnatal Care	% Got All Needed	% Got Some	% Got Little/None
0-3 Days after Giving Birth			
Care	59	26	15
Information / Advice	53	30	16
Emotional Support	49	25	26
4-10 Days after Giving Birth			
Care	64	28	8
Information / Advice	52	37	11
Emotional support	49	32	19
11-30 Days after Giving Birth			
Care	55	29	16
Information / Advice	48	34	18
Emotional support	43	31	26

Note: Percentages are based on responses from 960 women.

Table 7.2.2 Women's perceptions of postnatal care 0-3 days after birth

Postnatal Care Issues	% Always	% Mostly	% Sometimes	% Hardly/Never
Felt fully involved	65	23	7	4
Treated with respect	40	37	18	5
Staff kind and understanding	40	37	20	5
Enough midwives	39	29	20	12

Note: Percentages are based on responses from 960 women.

was taken as proof that everything was OK, but I felt very much left in a black hole.' (First baby, Edinburgh)

Differences in care

First-time mothers and women who had an instrumental delivery or emergency caesarean were less likely to feel positive about the postnatal care they received (p all < 0.05). These trends remained constant throughout the first month after childbirth.

'For a first-time mother I felt I was left to get on and look after my baby even though I had no idea of what I should have been doing. I remember being in tears in hospital and felt that I was being a burden. In the end I felt worse because I felt guilty for disturbing the others.' (First baby, Scotland)

'There was absolutely no recognition by any of the ward midwives that because of the caesarean I needed help to sit up and could not twist and lift my baby out of his crib to feed him over the first two days. My baby was crying, I was crying but they still said I was being 'lazy' and they were 'busy people'.' (First baby, location not provided)

Treatment by staff

Most women thought that they had either 'mostly' or 'always' been fully involved in decisions about their baby's care, and treated with respect by staff who were kind and understanding while they were in hospital (Table 7.2.2). But one in five said that they had only been treated with respect 'some of the time' or 'never' and one in four did not think that staff were kind and understanding. Women who were formula feeding, those having their first child, and those who had an instrumental delivery or caesarean tended to feel less satisfied about the quality of care and level of respect and kindness they received (p each < 0.05).

Continuity of carer

In open-ended questions, many women highlighted continuity of carer as an especially important issue.

'I had a one-to-one midwife from the outset. She was brilliant throughout my pregnancy, during my pregnancy,

Figure 7.2.1 Women who got little or non of the postnatal care they needed

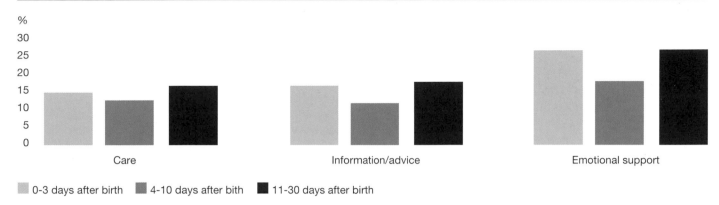

0-3 days after birth   4-10 days after bith   11-30 days after birth

Note: Percentages are based on the responses of 960 women

Data for the figure above is reproduced below:

Postnatal care	% 0-3 Days	%4-10 Days	%11-30 Days
Care	15	8	16
Information/advice	16	11	18
Emotional support	26	19	26

during the birth and visited for 10 days after. Consistency of care was important – I was able to build up a relationship which helped a lot in labour and after.' (First baby, London)

Those who did not have good continuity of carer said this was an area in need of improvement.

'Staff tried hard but didn't have enough time to give everybody the individual attention they needed. I would have preferred just one midwife to visit me at home.' (First baby, Bradford)

'My home-visit midwife came one day, then said 'oh you're fine' and didn't come back for 3 days, then a different person turned up and the same thing happened again.' (First baby, Edinburgh)

Staffing levels

In line with previous national findings,[9] women saw midwifery staffing levels as a problem. One third of the women said there were 'never' or only 'sometimes' 'enough' midwives to provide postnatal care in the first days after birth.

'The first 24 hours on the ward, no one checked me at all healthwise. One midwife was appalling to another lady and threw drugs at me. I received hurried and differing advice about feeding. I left hospital with bleeding nipples because no one showed me how to remove the baby properly. The main problem appeared to be a shortage of midwives and no breastfeeding dedicated staff.' (First baby, London)

Care during different periods

In the period 4-10 days after giving birth, two thirds of the women were happy with the level of care they received from midwives. During this period most women receive postnatal care from community midwives.

'My one-to-one midwife continued to visit after the birth for 10 days and also took anxious phone calls twice in the night when baby could not feed and wouldn't stop crying. She was very reassuring on these occasions.' (First baby, location not provided)

'The midwives who visited always had time to listen to me and sometimes took extra time to explore how I really felt. They understood my perilous emotional state. They did not make me feel inadequate in any way.' (First baby, born by caesarean, Worcestershire)

But the transition between midwife and health visitor care was difficult for some women. Satisfaction with care was lowest in the period 11-30 days after childbirth, when community midwife care tends to be tailing off.

'After the midwife support finished after 10 days there seemed to be nothing – a huge gap with no one to support me. 10 months later I find the health visitor support very poor, many mums use their GP for what I consider routine health visitor matters.' (First baby, Hampshire)

'The hand over from the midwife to the health visitor was not good. The midwives provided fantastic care and support. The health visitor provided little support, little advice, no kindness!' (First baby, Winchester)

Implications for midwifery practice

Although this survey is limited to the views and experiences of selected women who visited the Baby World website or received the National Childbirth Trust journal during one month in 2000, the findings offer some broader insight into aspects of postnatal care within the United Kingdom, especially midwifery postnatal practice:

- There is a need for clearly defined postnatal service strategies.
- A more holistic model of care which acknowledges emotional support needs is warranted.
- Community midwifery care could be extended, in order to provide the continuity of care that women value.

Postnatal service strategies

In line with other research showing a lack of satisfaction with postnatal services,[32] 8-26% of women in this sample did not feel that they were given the postnatal care they needed. 19-26% felt they got little or none of the necessary emotional support. This is likely to be a result of midwifery staffing shortages and lack of clear postnatal service strategies.

This survey provides further evidence that explicit strategies outlining the aims, procedures and resource implications for postnatal support provision are needed. Maternity services, 'clinicians and managers should clarify the objectives and set standards for postnatal care in hospital and at home.'[9] Such service strategies need to be evidence-based and also need to take the needs of women and their families into consideration, as well as the practicalities of health care structures.

In 1997 the Audit Commission concluded that the objectives of postnatal care were unclear:

There is... some uncertainty about what postnatal care is aiming to achieve – whether it is solely to prevent and treat immediate health problems in mother and baby or whether it is aiming to enhance the overall experience, giving mothers time to recover and get to know their babies, possibly avoiding problems later on.[9]

The development of postnatal service strategies by Primary Care Groups, Health Authorities or individual hospital trusts would ensure that the objectives and mechanisms for postnatal care provision are explicitly addressed.

The needs of women and babies after birth should be worked out in detail, using agreed outcome measures as a guide, following consultation with parents and professionals. Local targets should be set to improve the quality of postnatal care, especially for those most in need. Managers should calculate the midwifery and other time needed to meet delivery targets. This could form an evidence-based case for improved staffing levels. A time-costed plan for providing high-quality postnatal care services could be used to attract additional resources and as part of local bids for Sure Start funding.

In this study women having their first baby, those who had complications, and those who gave birth in a hospital rather than at home or at a birth centre were most likely to feel let down by the care they received. This is important since effective postnatal care may be a critical factor in assisting women recovering from more difficult births, coping with a sick baby and adjusting to a birth experience which was unanticipated or disappointing.[1] Postnatal care strategies need to acknowledge those most in need.

Holistic care model

Maternity services should aim to meet both the health and social needs of women and their families. This is particularly relevant in the early postnatal period when the social and emotional impact of having a baby is intense.

This survey shows that women believe postnatal care currently places more emphasis on their physical wellbeing than their need for information and support,[33,34] yet emotional support is extremely important.[32,35] In order to make informed choices and feel in control after the birth of their baby, women need to know what to expect during the postnatal period and be given reliable information about how to take care of themselves and their baby. The historical focus on physical 'recovery' has excluded social and emotional needs as well as the needs of the baby's father and other family members.

In this survey only 40% of women said that they were always treated with respect and that health professionals were always kind and understanding of their needs. This suggests that midwives need to give much higher priority to spending time with women, treating them with kindness, listening to their feelings and concerns, offering emotional support and helping them adjust to motherhood.

Contact with midwives in the early postnatal period is an ideal time for helpful advice and support to be given but midwives are not always perceived as fulfilling this part of their role.[34]

This is of particular importance for those from less advantaged groups.[36,37] Postnatal care is not just about physical checks. We need to work towards a more holistic care model. Ensuring that women and their families have realistic expectations of what health professionals can achieve is also important.

In order for more holistic care models to work, women and their partners need to be consulted about their needs, preferences and experience of existing services; health professionals' pre-qualification education and continuing development should include modules on the impact of the social and emotional changes experienced when a baby is born; and the particular needs of women in lower socio-economic status groups, minority ethnic groups, first time mothers, disabled women, those who have more than one child and young mothers need to be acknowledged.

Extended community midwifery

In this study, the period 4-10 days after giving birth, when most women receive postnatal care at home from community midwives, was rated more positively than that immediately after the birth when many women are in hospital, or care 11-30 days after birth, when access to a community midwife is reducing or no longer available. This suggests that midwifery care could be extended or better ongoing support is needed after midwifery care ends.

During the transition from midwife to health visitor care some women experience a widening of the gap between their needs and the ability of postnatal services to respond. One in four women said that at this crucial stage when their partner might be returning to full-time work, they got little or no emotional support from health professionals. However ad hoc postnatal services can not easily address the situation.[38,39] Instead particular attention needs to be paid to improving care in the first days after the birth and ensuring that care tailored to women's individual needs is available at least up to the end of the first postnatal month. Midwives and health visitors should be proactive in helping to build community support networks and referring women to local support schemes.

This would also enhance continuity of carer which controlled trials[40,41] and other research[21] have suggested as clinically beneficial and psychologically important to women. However the evidence from this study suggests that current staffing levels do not allow midwives to give women all the support they need. Extensions to midwifery care can not occur without a much closer examination of the staffing and support structures needed in order to further develop quality postnatal care, and without formal postnatal care service strategies.

In the past, some maternity health professionals saw their role as ending soon after childbirth. However it is now recognised that ongoing postnatal care is extremely important.[37] By recognising the importance of the early postnatal period, developing levels of emotional support, improving interactions, and working with service managers to develop practical postnatal care service strategies, midwives can make a real difference to the quality of postnatal care provided to women in the United Kingdom.

REFERENCES

1 Department of Health Expert Maternity Group. Changing childbirth. London: HMSO, 1993.

2 Blumfield W. Life after birth. Every woman's guide to the first year of motherhood. Dorset: Element, 1992.

3 Campbell R, Macfarlane A. Where to be born? The debate and the evidence. 2nd Edition. Oxford: National Perinatal Epidemiology Unit, 1994.

4 Figes K. Life after birth. What even your friends won't tell you about motherhood. London: Viking, 1998.

5 Kitzinger S. The year after childbirth. Surviving the first year of motherhood. Oxford: Oxford University Press, 1994.

6 Taylor J, Glossop C, Hames P. Parents' needs for information and support during pregnancy, labour and the first three years of parenthood. London: National Childbirth Trust, 1997.

7 Williams S. Birth and beyond. What every new mother should know. London: Boxtree, 1994.

8 Anderson T, Podkolinski J. Reflections on midwifery care and the postnatal period. In: Alexander J, Roth C, Levy V. (eds). Midwifery Practice Core Topics 3. London: Macmillan, 2000.

9 Audit Commission. First class delivery: A national survey of women's views of maternity care. London: Audit Commission, 1997.

10 McKim E. The transition home for mothers of healthy and initially ill newborn babies. Midwifery 1995; 11(14): 184-95.

11 Acheson D. Independent inquiry into inequalities in health. London: HMSO, 1998.

12 Alexander J, Levy V, Roch S (eds). Postnatal care. A research based approach. Hampshire: Macmillan, 1990.

13 Chamberlain G, Wraight A, Crowley P. The report of the 1994 confidential enquiry into home births. London: Partheon, 1997.

14 Oakley A. Social support and motherhood. Oxford: Blackwell, 1992.

15 May H et al. Group support for parenting skills: Taking first steps.
Community Practitioner 1999; 72(4): 86-7.

16 Moody G. The needs of mothers in Hackney: Action research. Maternity Action 1996; 71: 6-7.

17 Reid M. A RCT of two interventions to provide social support. British Journal of Midwifery 1997; 5(10): 610-12.

18 Sanderson E & Curry J. How postnatal support groups can benefit new parents. Nursing Times 1996; 92(3): 34-5.

19 Moran C et al. What do women want to know after childbirth? Birth 1997; 24(1): 27-34.

20 Benbow A, Wray J. Midwifery practice in the postnatal period. Recommendations for practice. London: Royal College of Midwives, 2000.

21 Farquhar M, Camilleri-Ferrante C, Todd C. Continuity of care in maternity services: Women's views of one team midwifery scheme. Midwifery 2000; 16(1): 35-47.

22 Lawrence JM, Ershoff D, Mendez C, Petitti DB. Satisfaction with pregnancy and newborn care: Development and results of a survey in a health maintenance organization. American Journal of Managed Care 1999; 5(11): 1407-13.

23 Murray D, Ryan F, Keane E. Who's holding the baby? Women's experience of their postnatal care. Irish Medical Journal 2000; 93(5): 148-50.

24 Proctor S, Wright G. Consumer responses to health care: Women and maternity services. International Journal of Health Care and Quality Assurance 1998; 11(4-5): 147-55.

25 Baby World and the National Childbirth Trust provided sponsorship for the study as well as access to their clients for the sample.

26 Formal written informed consent was not sought given the self selection strategy used. The questionnaire was completely anonymous. No demographic or identifying information was

recorded and as such formal ethical approval was not required.

27 Government Statistical Service. The UK in figures, 2000. http://www.statistics.gov.uk/stats/ukinfigs/

28 Office for National Statistics. Living in Britain. Results from the 1996 general household survey. London: HMSO, 1996.

29 Office for National Statistics. Birth statistics. Review of the Registrar General on births and patterns of family building in England and Wales, 1998. Series FM1. Number 27. London: HMSO, 1998.

30 Office for National Statistics. Annual abstract of statistics. 1999 Edition. London: HMSO, 1999.

31 The sample was not selected using probability methods therefore standard statistical indicators can not be readily applied. However given the large sample size, the data approaches a normal distribution, allowing significance testing to be undertaken. In all instances where relationships are discussed in the text Chi-square tests have been conducted and the probability of trends occurring by chance is less than 5% (ie $p < 0.05$)

32 Butchart WA, Tancred BL, Wildman N. Listening to women: Focus group discussions of what women want from postnatal care. Curationis 1999; 22(4): 3-8.

33 Hannula L, Leino-Kilpi H. Good nursing care in the postnatal wards – mothers' views on the aspect of nursing care. Hoitotiede 1998; 10(1): 33-43.

34 Stamp GE, Crowther CA. Women's views of their postnatal care by midwives at an Adelaide Women's Hospital. Midwifery 1994; 10(3):

148-56. Quote from abstract.

35 Singh D, Newburn M. Access to maternity information and support. Women's needs and experiences before and after giving birth. London: National Childbirth Trust, 2000.

36 Kabakian-Khasholian T, Campbell O, Shediac-Rizkallah M, Ghorayeb F. Women's experiences of maternity care: Satisfaction or passivity? Social Science and Medicine 2000; 51(1): 103-13.

37 Zadoroznyj M. Women's satisfaction with antenatal and postnatal care: An analysis of individual and organisational factors. Australian and New Zealand Journal of Public Health 1996; 20(6): 594-602.

38 Kitzman H, Olds DL, Henderson CR Jr et al. Effect of prenatal and infancy home visitation by nurses on pregnancy outcomes, childhood injuries, and repeated childbearing. A randomized controlled trial. Journal of the American Medical Association 1997; 278: 644-52.

39 Morrell CJ, Spiby H, Stewart P et al. Costs and effectiveness of community postnatal support workers: Randomised controlled trial. British Medical Journal 2000; 321(7261): 593-8.

40 Hodnett ED. Continuity of caregivers for care during pregnancy and childbirth. Cochrane Database Systematic Reviews 2000; 2: CD000062.

41 Waldenstrom U & Turnbull D. A systematic review comparing continuity of midwifery care with standard maternity services. British Journal of Obstetrics and Gynaecology 1998; 105(11): 1160-70.

Is breast always best?

Nicky Bean

'There is nothing wrong with breastfeeding; breastfeeding is good. What is worse is the message that, if you bottle feed, you are monstrous and unnatural.' (Knight, 1995)

Having recently had a baby and breast fed her till she was 12 months old, I am obviously not against breastfeeding. Yet as a new mother, I have become increasingly concerned after my discussions with other mothers and midwives about the climate in which women are making their choices about how they feed their babies.

Most of the information and support given to women on infant feeding focuses on breastfeeding, and women who bottle-feed from the start or at sometime in the child's first year seem to be finding it increasingly difficult to get the information or support they need. Many also appear to suffer from incredible anxiety and guilt, often feeling as if they have failed as a mother if they bottle-feed. In this article I want to question whether current practices are helping to transform a practical childcare issue into a moral crusade which makes it almost impossible for women to make an informed choice about whether to breast or bottle-feed. The term bottle-feeding will be used throughout to refer to feeding a baby with formula milk.

Much of the current practice in both the hospital and community setting can be traced back to the UK Baby Friendly Initiative (BFI) which is part of a World Health Organization and UNICEF campaign to improve breastfeeding rates worldwide. The campaign aims to 'support every mother's right to choose', 'ensure that breastfeeding is a positive experience for everyone' and to 'ensure that parents then feel supported in their chosen method.' (UNICEF). The initiative sets out standards that services need to adhere to. Some of these standards, however, either in themselves or in their over-enthusiastic implementation create an atmosphere in which women sometimes feel coerced by an unhealthy climate of guilt and ignorance instead of feeling encouraged and supported.

Lack of bottle feeding information and support

Some women report that they have received little or no information about bottle feeding and studies indicate that whilst women who bottle-feed either initially or at a later stage do have some knowledge of bottle-feeding, their knowledge is incomplete (Hughes & Rees, 1997; Cairney & Alder, 2001). It has been suggested that the BFI may have contributed to this lack of information being given to potential and active bottle feeders (Cairney & Alder, 2001).

One of the aspects of the BFI is the prohibiting of the display or distribution of materials which promote breast milk substitutes, feeding bottles, teats or dummies. Whilst the initiative does not stop maternity facilities from providing their own information about bottle-feeding, very few do, and all of the women I talked to who had decided to bottle-feed had received or been offered little information in either the antenatal or postnatal period. Typical comments included: 'In hospital when I said I had decided to bottle-feed, I was pretty much left to get on with it' and 'There was so little information that when I finally did give my baby a bottle I was so frightened of the whole process!' (The Pregnancy Book and Birth to Five books are given to new mothers but information on bottle-feeding is frequently not pointed out or discussed.)

Women are often confused by all the different milks on the market and the differences between them. One told me that when she asked her midwife for information she was told: 'They are all as crap as each other'. In the absence of health professionals providing the information they need, many women try to approach formula milk manufacturers. These organisations are limited in what they can provide by the International Code of Marketing of Breastmilk Substitutes. If you surf the Internet, usually a rich source of information on any topic, all you will find is information on the dangers of formula milk, produced by a number of breastfeeding lobbies.

Antenatal group discussions about infant feeding, as well as one-to-one discussions with the midwife, focus on the importance of exclusive breastfeeding for the first 4-6 months, the benefits of breastfeeding and basic breastfeeding management. If bottle-feeding is discussed at all, it is around the potential hazards of this method. The demonstration of formula preparation as part of routine antenatal group instruction is prohibited because this is perceived as 'normalising bottle-feeding'. One mother spoke about her experience when her antenatal classes covered 'infant feeding'. She said she particularly enjoyed the session on breastfeeding when a mother came in and demonstrated feeding. When she asked the midwife when the session on bottle-feeding would be held she was told there would not be one because 'midwives did not do that' (Hughes & Rees, 1997). Most women would however appreciate being shown how to make up a feed, advice and anticipatory guidance (Hughes & Rees, 1997).

One of the arguments used by midwives for not giving women information about bottle-feeding in the antenatal period is that it would encourage women either not to try breastfeeding or encourage them to give this up at an earlier stage by 'normalising' bottle-feeding. However, women seem to make their feeding decisions prior to pregnancy or in the early weeks, with only a tiny minority altering their decisions during late pregnancy. Therefore it seems unlikely that giving women information about bottle-feeding during pregnancy would affect their decisions (Cairney & Alder, 2001).

It is suggested that much of the information about bottle-feeding can be given to women in the postnatal period if they decide they wish to bottle feed, but in practice this does not often happen (Hughes & Rees, 1997; Cairney & Alder, 2001). One midwife commented: 'I am very concerned that women who bottle-feed are not given the information they need. People assume that all mothers need to do is read the instructions on the tin. My experience is that if a mother asks for a bottle, that is usually all she gets. No information on how to hold a baby, how much to give, how often to give it, how to store it, dental advice, how to make up a feed, or that it is recommended to introduce a cup by six months and stop the bottle by one year...'

Women do not complain only about a lack of information in relation to bottle-feeding, they also comment on a lack of support from health professionals. A young woman with twins experienced many problems with bottle-feeding but was offered little support. She commented bitterly that had she decided to breastfeed, 'the midwives would have been here all the time'

(Hughes & Rees, 1997). Another woman told me that the leaflet given her by her health visitor listed a number of reasons about which she could contact her. Breastfeeding was listed, bottle-feeding was not.

Pressure to breastfeed

Today, the benefits of breastfeeding are well established and accepted by the general public. In this climate, a woman who bottle-feeds her baby exposes herself to the potential charge that she is a 'poor mother' who places her own selfish needs, preferences or convenience above the welfare of her baby (Murphy, 1999). Many women who bottle-feed feel this pressure from the outset and others who breastfeed for a short while can feel that they have failed if they give up.

Some women report that many midwives respond to women who say they intend to bottle-feed with a mixture of apparent indifference, disapproval and coercion. When women in one study were asked how they were going to feed their babies, their responses met with comments such as 'Don't you know you should be breastfeeding?' One woman said her midwife continually asked her if she was sure about her decision to bottle-feed. Another was told by her GP it was positively dangerous not to breastfeed (Murphy, 2000).

Other women feel that they were coerced to breastfeed either by the antenatal discussions or by their experience postnatally. Because of the BFI, all women are encouraged to breastfeed straight after the birth though they may have declared their intention to bottle-feed. Some women find this experience pressurising and embarrassing. Several women told me they would not be allowed to leave the hospital until their baby had fed from the breast. Kate from Nottingham said 'I was told "you won't be leaving this hospital until you have breast fed", so I discharged myself'. Another mother I spoke to said 'I don't feel as though I was given a choice as they (health visitors and midwives) didn't talk to me about anything apart from breastfeeding, and made me think that anything else would have been unthinkable'. Others just say they are going to breastfeed knowing they will stop when they get home, simply to avoid confrontations with the midwives (Davidson, 2001).

A number of studies have highlighted the inseparable association in women's minds between 'breastfeeding and being a good mother' (Murphy, 1999; Schmied, Sheehan & Barclay, 2001). This belief means that some women maintain a strong commitment to breastfeeding despite enormous difficulties. Often women think that if they cease breastfeeding their relationship with their baby will be shattered. Those that discontinued often struggled with enormous guilt and felt that they had failed as mothers. One commented, 'I was too embarrassed to admit that I no longer breastfed, I felt guilty about not "doing the best for the baby".' Another said: 'I just needed someone to reassure me that I wasn't a loser for not continuing to breastfeed – it can be quite soul destroying when you are not successful' (Schmied, Sheehan & Barclay, 2001).

Not all women find breastfeeding a positive or rewarding experience, despite having a supportive environment. One study indicated that for some women, breastfeeding could be distressing and disruptive to their sense of self. Some women in this study described breastfeeding using metaphors such as 'being a feeding machine', 'a walking talking cow',' the milk bar', 'a battle ground' and 'a fight' (Schmied, Sheehan & Barclay, 2001).

These women found their experience of breastfeeding interfered with their relationship with their baby and created a feeling that they were working in opposition to each other. In describing their babies they used comments such as 'an uncivilised creature', 'the rotten sucking little leech' and the 'child from hell'. Despite an enormous amount of physiological and emotional problems with breastfeeding, the women struggled to maintain their commitment to breastfeeding in an attempt to maintain their goal as breastfeeding mothers (Schmied, Sheehan & Barclay, 2001).

Some midwives are concerned that the current professional practice around infant feeding does encourage women to focus their identities as mothers around the experience of infant feeding, with breastfeeding being associated with 'good' or 'successful' mothering. They highlight the amount of distress some women suffer if they do not continue to breastfeed for whatever reason. They are also concerned that some midwives and other health workers may unwittingly contribute to this distress by conveying that it is necessary to preserve with breastfeeding despite excruciating pain. One example is highlighted in an article which describes the intensive support one midwife gave to a woman who had been sexually abused. She encouraged her to continue with breastfeeding despite the feelings of revulsion the new mother experienced during her six long months of breastfeeding (Minchin, 1999).

Bottle feeding as a rational choice

Many breastfeeding lobbyists are very keen to publicise problems, no matter how remote, that can be associated with bottle-feeding babies, and clearly see it as an unsafe choice. A remark from Catherine McCormick at the RCM illustrates this point. 'We are up against a society in Britain which believes that bottle-feeding is safe...' (Waters, 1997). Other comments to me by midwives on this issue have included: 'I'm not surprised they feel guilty – after all it's got to be quite brave, to face the possible risks and still to take the chance', and 'If women feel guilty at not breastfeeding... we should not be taking it away from them. It is their guilt, not ours.'

The underlying message of the current approach around infant feeding seems to be that women are thought not to have sufficient intelligence to take on board information about breast and formula feeding, to weigh up the consequences and to make an informed decision. Furthermore, if a woman chooses to bottle-feed either from the outset, combine it with breastfeeding or introduce bottle feeds following a period of breastfeeding, she must have had inadequate information and/or support from the health service, from family and from society in general. But bottle-feeding a baby with formula milk can be a rational, sensible and safe choice. It is also a choice which many mothers make without adversely affecting the health of their babies.

Several studies have indicated that women who bottle-feed were well aware that breastfeeding was best but this was overridden by other factors, which meant that breastfeeding was considered 'not right for me'. As one woman put it: 'You have to be happy with what you are doing' (Hughes & Rees, 1997; Earle, 2000). Factors influencing women's decision to bottle feed included being employed and wishing to keep financial security, the need for the childminder and mother to feel confident about infant feeding methods before she returned to work and the need to be able to share the responsibility of feeding including paternal involvement (Hughes & Rees, 1997; Earle, 2000). The advantages centred very much on the mother and the social aspects of motherhood.

There are lots of health benefits for a baby who is breastfed and there is nothing wrong with women being informed of them and supported to breastfeed when they make that choice. But the current campaign to promote breastfeeding has become a kind of moral crusade, in which advice is turned into a form of moral blackmail (Furedi, 2001). I think that health professionals today need to consider how they can improve on the information given and support offered to women who either bottle-feed from birth or introduce bottle feeding during or after a period of breastfeeding. The decision to bottle feed, rather than being seen as a problem, should be understood as a rational response to a practical childcare issue in particular circumstances (Hughes & Rees, 1997).

REFERENCES

Cairney PA, Alder EM. 2001. A survey of information given by health professionals, about bottle-feeding, to first-time mothers in a Scottish population. Health Bulletin, 59(2), 97-101

Davidson M. 2001. When to recognize that breastfeeding is not an option. Pediatric Nursing, 27(1), 49

Earle S. 2000. Why some women do not breast feed: Bottle-feeding and father's role. Midwifery, 16(4), 323-30

Furedi F. 2001. Paranoid Parenting. Abandon your anxieties and be a good parent. London: The Penguin Press

Hughes P, Rees C. 1997. Artificial feeding: Choosing to bottle-feed. BJM, 5(3), 137-42

Knight I. 1995. The Formula for Mother's Happiness. The Guardian, June 4

Minchin M. 1999. Good enough breastfeeding or good enough definitions: A contrary view. MIDIRS Midwifery Digest, 9, 94-6

Murphy EA. 1999. 'Breast is best': Infant feeding decisions and maternal deviance. Sociology of Health and Illness, 21(2), 187-208

Murphy EA. 2000. Risk, responsibility and rhetoric in infant feeding. Journal of Contemporary Ethnography, 29(3), 291-325

Schmied V, Sheehan A, Barclay L. 2001. Contemporary breastfeeding policy and practice: Implications for midwives. Midwifery, 17, 44-54

UNICEF. The UNICEF UK Baby Friendly Initiative. London: UK Baby Friendly Initiative

Waters J. 1997. Investing in breastfeeding. Nursing Times, 42(93), 56

Sock it to me

Using a breast model to enable women to establish lactation

Alison Blenkinsop

I am the proud owner of a prize-winning breast. I display it frequently and encourage people to handle it. In fact, it's been touched so often that it needs to go into the washing machine. My breast is made from a sock stuffed with old tights and a shoulder pad. I use it to show women the importance of a good latch in breastfeeding, and to demonstrate hand expression.

I am a midwife at Kingston Hospital in Surrey, and a member of the Breastfeeding Working Group. In 1999 I qualified as an International Board Certified Lactation Consultant. As part of my training, I attended a month-long Breastfeeding Practice and Policy Course at the Institute of Child Health in London. One of the leaders was Dr Felicity Savage-King, a senior lecturer at the Institute, who has taught breastfeeding support in Africa. As several participants came from developing countries, she showed us how to make a breast and a doll from simple materials, and offered prizes for the best. I added a plastic bottle-neck and a balloon to represent the baby's mouth and tongue, and won the first prize of a video about breastfeeding in Kingston Hospital... Jamaica.

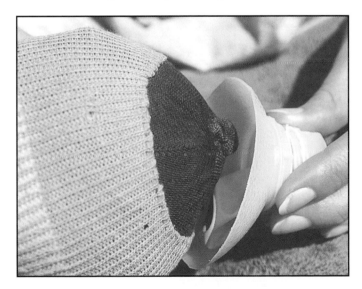

Figure 7.4.1 The breast is made from a patterned sock; the toe has been stuffed, twisted into the heel and the leg part has been twisted and reversed onto the heel part. The heel represents the areola, with a nipple made by pulling out the centre with a purse-string stitch. The leg represents the rest of the breast.

When the baby's mouth comes up to the breast from below, the tongue reaches the lower edge of the areola. The nipple is then level with the oral cavity, and can be drawn to the back of the mouth.

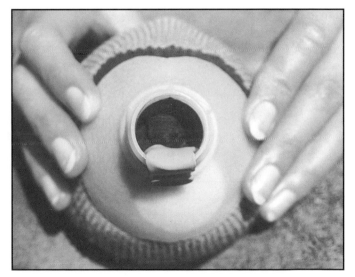

Figure 7.4.2 The mouth is made from the top of a wide-shouldered juice bottle, cut asymmetrically to show that the lower jaw is larger. The screw top and shoulders represent the posterior oral cavity and the anterior oral cavity/lips respectively. The balloon represents the tongue.

The tip of the nipple is level with the screw top opening, to indicate that the baby can draw it to the back of the mouth. There is more areola above the mouth than below. The tongue is applied along the whole nipple and reaches the lower edge of the areola.

A POOR LATCH

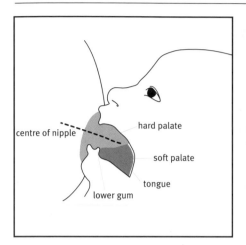

Figure 7.4.3 The baby's tongue is behind the lower gum. The tip of the nipple is pressed against the hard palate, off-centre. The nipple will look wedge-shaped after the feed.

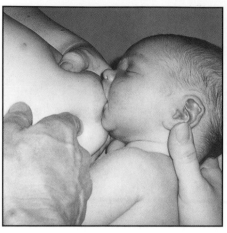

Figure 7.4.4 In this photograph, the latch seems to be good, but note the amount of the mother's areola that is still visible underneath the baby's lower lip.

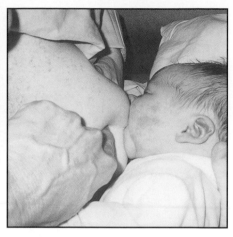

Figure 7.4.5 The mother here is experiencing pain during the feed from a damaged nipple. The baby's mouth is not wide open – compare this with Figure 8.

A GOOD LATCH

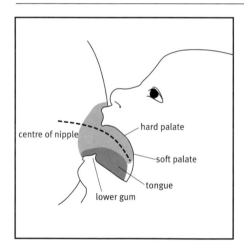

Figure 7.4.6 The tongue covers the lower gum, pushing the lower lip out. The tip of the nipple is drawn back to the soft palate, and is centred. The nipple will look rounded after the feed.

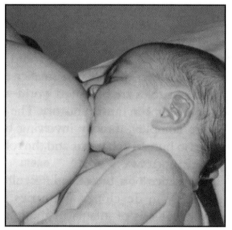

Figure 7.4.7 Compare this photograph to Figure 4 above. The latch is now much better and the baby's lower lip is at the edge of the areola. The mother now feels more comfortable.

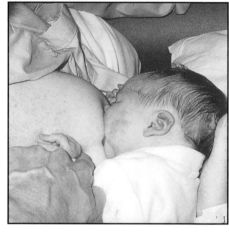

Figure 7.4.8 Compare this photograph to Figure 3 above. It is clear that the latch is now much improved, and the mother is no longer in so much pain.

The problem

I spend a lot of time helping women to establish lactation. Many are distressed by the pain of sore nipples and being unable to settle a hungry baby. Tears turn to laughter as I bring out my breast with a flourish and say, 'Here's one I made earlier'. Most of the mothers I observe feeding – including those who have not complained of a problem – have attached their babies too high, so the tongue cannot reach under the areola and the nipple is at the front of the mouth (see Figures 7.4.3-5). This causes pain, as the nipple is grated against the hard palate, and the resulting trauma may also become infected with thrush. Poor breast drainage, the major cause of inadequate milk supply, blocked ducts and mastitis, is very likely. The babies may feed constantly, but have poor weight gain as they cannot obtain a good flow of milk; some will develop colic from swallowing excessive amounts of foremilk.[1] Unfortunately, many health professionals caring for these mothers and babies do not recognise a poor latch. Is it surprising that many women stop nursing in the first few weeks?

In 1995 two-thirds of British women breastfed their newborns, but by 4 months 73% had stopped. Over 80% of these mothers would have liked to continue, but the majority experienced some of the preventable problems mentioned above.[2] Based on my own experience, I do not expect the next official survey to show much improvement.

A useful solution

In order to help improve these statistics, I explain how important it is for the baby's tongue to reach well under the nipple, with its tip at or near the edge of the areola. I use diagrams and photographs of a baby well and poorly attached to the breast (similar to those in Figures 7.4.3-8), and the sock breast and 'mouth' (Figures 7.4.1 & 7.4.2) to show how to position the baby low enough to achieve this.

I have cut the bottle top asymmetrically, to represent the smaller upper jaw and larger lower jaw. If it is correctly applied to the sock breast, the nipple can be seen through the hole, the tongue reaches the edge of the lower areola, and the upper areola may be visible (Figure 7.4.2). If the baby is positioned in this way, he can easily draw the nipple to the back of his mouth, where it will not be damaged. I also explain that the lower jaw needs to be pressed against the breast so that the tongue can reach the edge of the areola (Figure 7.4.6). To demonstrate, I hold the sock breast in one hand and the bottle-top mouth in the other, showing where to position the baby, and how to keep the hand supporting the breast (if necessary) out of the baby's way. I make the following suggestions, adapted from Jamieson[3] and Fisher and Inch.[4]

- Support the baby with the arm opposite the breast (unless using 'football' hold)
- Support the baby's shoulders and neck or lower side of the head with that hand, so he can tilt his head back
- Support the breast, if necessary, with the 'V' of the hand where the side of the mouth will be and the fingers parallel with the lips, but well away from the areola; this can help the baby to get his tongue further underneath
- Aim to get the baby's chin meeting the breast first, so the tongue can be placed as far from the nipple tip as possible.

Using the models, I can show a mother, without touching her, how to attach the baby herself – a vital step towards successful breastfeeding.[5]

I also use the model to demonstrate hand expression. The Baby Friendly Initiative recommends that all lactating women be taught this skill,[6] in order to prevent or treat engorgement, blocked ducts and mastitis. I imagine that women would prefer me not to handle their breasts unnecessarily, so I use the sock breast to show them where to place their fingers. I also use it to show my colleagues how to teach hand expression and perform it themselves if necessary.

Conclusion

In an ideal world, women learn how to breastfeed by watching other women. In our society, many have to rely on a midwife. The use of a breast model can minimise the need for the midwife to touch a woman's breasts, and increase everyone's understanding of how lactation works. Women who are empowered to breastfeed successfully are more likely to continue, improving their own and their babies' health.[5]

For instructions on making a 'sock breast', send an sae plus 6 2nd class stamps to Mrs AS Blenkinsop, c/o 12 Oakdene, Woodcote, Reading RG8 0RQ.

REFERENCES

1 Mohrbacher N & Stock J. The breastfeeding answer book. Schaumburg, Illinois: La Leche League International, 1997.
2 Foster K, Lader D, Cheesbrough S. Infant Feeding 1995. London: HMSO, 1997.
3 Jamieson L. Getting it together. Nursing Times 1994; 90(17): 68-9.
4 Inch S & Fisher C. Breastfeeding: Getting the basics right. Practising Midwife 1999; 2(4): 35-8.
5 Renfrew M, Woolridge M, McGill H. Enabling women to breastfeed. London: HMSO, 2000.
6 UNICEF UK Baby Friendly Initiative. Baby Friendly News 2000; 5: 3.

Skin-to-skin contact
Benefits and difficulties

Helen Wallace and David Marshall

Skin-to-skin contact facilitates the initiation of breastfeeding, neonatal thermoregulation and the promotion of maternal–infant attachment. However, there are cultural influences in society and in the labour ward that may make implementation of skin-to-skin contact difficult.

Initiation of breastfeeding

All mothers, regardless of how they may intend to feed their infant, should have the opportunity to have skin-to-skin contact with their babies for as long as they wish within the immediate postnatal period. Such contact has been shown to stimulate breastfeeding. Removing healthy babies for gastric suction has no clear advantage,[1] but disrupts pre-feeding behaviour. Babies who have skin-to-skin contact with their mothers, however, show a consistent behavioural pattern resulting in spontaneous rooting and sucking within one hour.

A sample of 72 mothers were allocated to a contact group or a separation group.[2] Of 38 infants in the contact group, 24 were sucking correctly within 50 minutes and four were making attempts to feed. Ten infants affected by Pethidine did not suck. This compared favourably to the separation group where 34 infants were removed for weighing and bathing following 15-20 minutes of skin contact. Seven infants sucked correctly with open mouth and tongue under the areola. Eleven sucked incorrectly and 16 made no attempt to breastfeed. There is the possibility that because the mothers chose which group to join, those in the contact group were more highly motivated. However, this is unlikely to have influenced the results as observations were made solely on the actions of the infant and in neither group was the infant encouraged to breastfeed.

Skin-to-skin contact between mother and baby and early feeding promotes successful breastfeeding in the long term.[3] A randomised controlled trial[4] examined skin-to-skin contact between mothers and their preterm infants. Mothers in the skin contact group lactated for four weeks longer than those mothers who were encouraged to hold their babies, but not skin-to-skin.

Neonatal thermoregulation

Another important benefit of skin-to-skin contact is the maintenance of a newborn's body temperature,[5] which is important for all babies, whether the mother chooses to breastfeed or bottle-feed. Potentially, hypothermia is a risk for all newborn babies delivered wet from liquor into a cooler environment. A standard care of newborns under radiators was compared to skin-to-skin contact.[6] Three groups were identified and babies were randomly assigned to each. The control group subjects were nursed under radiant heat alone. Subjects in the comparison groups were either nursed initially under the radiator, then returned to mother for skin-to-skin contact, or had continuous skin-to-skin contact with their mother. All babies were dried and had sensors applied to monitor temperature. The three groups were similar in all other ways. The results bore out the hypothesis that body temperatures in babies receiving earliest skin-to-skin were warmest. Not only were babies in the control group cooler but a significant number had rectal and skin temperatures below thermoneutral range at 21 and 45 minutes.

A randomised control trial compared skin-to-skin contact and nursing babies, well wrapped, in a cot at the bedside for the first ninety minutes of life.[7] Higher temperatures were again identified in the skin-to-skin contact experimental group. This provided further evidence that the maternal body is both an efficient and reliable heat source for the baby. A small yet valuable trial involving six babies indicated that low risk preterm infants could be safely nursed skin-to-skin and benefit from a rapid rise in temperature to thermoneutral range.[8]

This was confirmed by a larger study[9] where hypothermic neonates as small as 1500 grams warmed to normal temperature with skin-to-skin care much quicker than infants in an incubator. It is suggested that close body contact for healthy newborns might be of minor importance in the west where the delivery environment is generally warm.[7] There is, however, disagreement[5] in that metabolic acidosis and hypoglycaemia can result in babies making the effort to maintain body temperature in the wrong environment. Skin-to-skin contact on the other hand appears to be a safe and cost-effective way of giving optimum care to healthy term babies and to low risk preterm neonates.[9]

Maternal–infant attachment

Not only can skin-to-skin contact be promoted as a safe physiologic method of warming newborns and initiating breastfeeding, but many writers acknowledge that it enhances maternal–infant attachment.[10-12] Initial mother–baby contact, as soon as possible following delivery, is vital in developing the mother–baby relationship.[13] If skin-to-skin contact is accompanied by a feed within the first hour the relationship between them may be enhanced by both a sense of achievement and fulfilment. The time of close physical and emotional contact immediately after delivery has been named as the fourth stage of labour.[14] This idea of a crucial period to achieve attachment between mother and baby appears to be extreme. It would be true to say that sometimes separation is unavoidable owing to the poor health of the mother or baby yet they go on to form a very close relationship. It may be that maternal–infant attachment grows as mother and baby get to know each other and recognise each other's signals. Nevertheless mothers with extra skin-to-skin contact during the first hour showed different behaviour to mothers who had restricted skin contact.[3] After three months the extra contact group spent more time kissing and face-to-face gazing with their infants. Their babies smiled more and cried less frequently.

A randomised controlled study was unable to support the view that extra early physical contact between mother and baby enhanced the relationship.[15] Their evidence suggested there was no difference between the regular contact and extra contact groups. All mothers had contact in the delivery room with their babies but it is not clear whether this was skin-to-skin, and it appears to have been approximately twenty-five minutes after delivery. The contact was interrupted again in the recovery room and the extra contact group were handed their naked babies about ten minutes later. The babies were not placed skin-to-skin and the mothers were given no instruction as to what they might do. There is no indication whether any mothers practised skin-to-skin or wrapped their babies in a blanket. It is not clear whether this work[3] refutes the possibility that extra uninterrupted skin-to-skin contact within the first hour would have produced different results.

Cultural aspects of society

Despite the advantages of skin-to-skin contact, implementation within labour wards is patchy. It has been shown that as well as social class, age and parity, cultural attitudes prevail when women are making a decision about whether or not to breastfeed.[20]

Societal factors are very influential on attitudes toward female breasts.[16] Many men view breasts as sexual symbols and while they may be happy to see naked breasts on television or in newspapers, often regard breastfeeding as 'embarrassing' or even 'disgusting'.[17] Breast exposure is seen as erotogenic, sensual and titillating and, for western women, there appears to be a conflict between the sexual and maternal aspects of female breasts. Indeed, the emphasis appears to have shifted from a functional nurturing organ to a sexual object.[18,19] Some women, influenced by the sexual aspect, may regard skin-to-skin contact as slightly immoral or sleazy and experience feelings of guilt which may be inexplicable and confusing to them, making it unacceptable.

An extensive literature search[20] compared Jewish and Celtic attitudes. Positive Jewish attitudes to breastfeeding were heavily influenced by their own culture, rather than western culture, and were underpinned by scriptural references. The desirability of breastfeeding is consistently emphasised and breasts are seen as necessary for nurturing and not regarded in a sexual way. Celtic populations, however, such as that in Northern Ireland, tended to reflect an attitude of prudishness and embarrassment. While topless images of black women breastfeeding in developing countries are acceptable, images of western women doing the same are often regarded as inappropriate.[21] Within western society some people may regard skin-to-skin contact as savage or uncivilised, thus causing those feelings of embarrassment and a desire not to do it.

Despite this, many women feel immensely womanly and feminine after becoming a mother and gain a sense of completeness. However, partners may well be aware of these feelings and in turn have their own feelings of rejection and jealousy.[19] Men often feel jealous when their partners breastfeed and it could be argued that they may also feel jealous and excluded while a mother and her baby have uninterrupted skin-to-skin contact for as long as the mother wishes.[22] Under these circumstances a woman may feel pressurised to decline skin-to-skin contact completely or stop it prematurely in deference to her partner's feelings.

Cultural aspects of the labour ward

Culture within the labour ward itself may be such that skin-to-skin contact may be hindered rather than encouraged. There is often a contradiction between hospital policy and actual practice.[23] Some professionals may, themselves, dislike breastfeeding and therefore may also have negative feelings about skin-to-skin contact. It should be remembered that midwives are also probably influenced by their culture and while policy may seek to enforce a particular practice, the lack of a support system means they may be unable to deal with their own feelings and prejudices. There may also be a misconception among midwives that mothers must be exposed for skin-to-skin contact, which makes them feel uncomfortable. This attitude can be conveyed to mothers, reinforcing the sexual notion of breasts, and feelings of embarrassment may result.[5]

Implications for midwives' practice

Midwives can help to restore a culture where breastfeeding is more valued.[16] By educating women about the benefits of breastfeeding they may begin to appreciate their nurturing side more and become more open to practices such as skin-to-skin contact in the process. Midwives should, perhaps, consider forming links with schools, as attitudes may well be set in teenage years and therefore be more difficult to address when women present at the antenatal clinic expecting their first baby.[20] More controversially, midwives may want to consider including boys in these education programmes, as prospective fathers' attitudes have been shown to strongly influence their partners.[16]

However, midwives should also be seeking to educate the public about skin-to-skin contact in its own right and not just in association with breastfeeding. There will always be women who choose not to breastfeed and they should not be denied the opportunity to enjoy the close physical and emotional contact with their baby. Not only that, within Northern Ireland 11% of women, in a recent survey, stated that they decided to breastfeed after childbirth.[24] Encouraging skin-to-skin contact for all

women may persuade more of them to at least attempt breastfeeding. Fathers need not feel excluded and midwives can help by encouraging the father to sit close and stroke his baby's head, then leaving the family in private.

Effective communication is vital and mothers need to discuss the issue of skin-to-skin contact before delivery. Misconceptions about nakedness need to be addressed and the reassurance given that the practice is discreet under a nightdress or blanket and that the baby is dried to ensure warmth.[1,9] The ability to provide accurate and consistent information and effective support is underpinned by one's own knowledge and attitudes.[25] While ongoing training with regular updates would seem essential to keep midwives informed, they also need to be reflective practitioners both in listening to women and in examining their own attitudes and prejudices. In this way skin-to-skin contact may be presented in a more sensitive and flexible way, accommodating individual needs without compromising on the evidence.[25]

Conclusion

There are three main benefits of encouraging skin-to-skin contact between mother and baby following delivery. The initiation of breastfeeding is facilitated as babies left in uninterrupted skin contact with their mothers show a consistent behavioural pattern of rooting and sucking. This can result in active breastfeeding within one hour.[1,2] It has been shown that even premature neonates warm quicker and maintain their temperature better when nursed in skin contact with mother.[9] The maternal-infant relationship may also be enhanced, and even at this early stage they can begin to recognise cues and develop responses which help to foster trust.[12,26]

On the other hand, cultural barriers to skin-to-skin contact exist within society. Some women may be confused between the sexual and nurturing function of the breasts, making them view skin-to-skin contact with distaste. This may be exacerbated by the attitude of their partner or even the midwife. Good lines of communication allow the issue to be discussed. Midwives should be reflective in their practice, continually re-examining and informing their own attitudes to maximise their ability to be receptive to the concerns of woman.

REFERENCES

1 Widstrom AM, Ransjo-Arvidson K, Christensson AS et al. Gastric suction in healthy newborn infants. Acta Paediatr Scand 1987; 76: 566-72.
2 Righard L, Alade MO. Effect of delivery room routines on success of first breastfeed. Lancet 1990; 336: 1105-7.

3 DeChateau P, Wibert B. Longterm effect on mother-infant behaviour of extra contact during the first hour postpartum II. A follow-up at three months. Acta Paediatr Scand 1997; 66: 145-51.
4 Whitelaw A, Heisterkamp G, Sleath K et al. Skin-to-skin contact for very low birthweight infants and their mothers. Archives of Disease

In Childhood 1998; 63: 1377-81.

5 Sheridan V. Skin-to-skin contact immediately after birth. Practising Midwife 1999; 2(9): 23-8.

6 Fardig JA. A comparison of skin-to-skin contact and radiant heaters in promoting neonatal thermoregulation. Journal of Nurse-Midwifery 1980; 25(1): 19-28.

7 Christensson K, Siles C, Moreno L et al. Temperature, metabolic adaption and crying in healthy full-term newborns cared for skin-to-skin or in a cot. Acta Paediatr 1992; 91: 488-93.

8 Ludington-Hoe SM, Anderson GC, Simpson S et al. Skin-to-skin contact beginning in the delivery room for Colombian mothers and their pre-term infants. Journal of Human Lactation 1993; 9(4): 241-2.

9 Christensson K, Bhat GJ, Amadi BC et al. Randomised study of skin-to-skin versus incubator care for rewarming low-risk hypothermic neonates. Lancet 1998; 352: 1115.

10 Widstrom AM, Wahlberg V, Matthieson AS et al. Short term effects of early suckling and touch of the nipple on maternal behaviour. Early Human Development 1990; 21(3): 153-63.

11 Mercer RT. Becoming a Mother. New York: Springer Publishing Company, 1990.

12 Maier MJ. Promoting parenting by keeping new families together from birth through dismissal. Kansas Nurse 1996; 71(5): 9-10. Available from: http://biomed. Niss.ac.wk.ovidweb/ accessed 20 Apr 2000.

13 McKay S. Communication and motherhood. Midwives 1997; 110(1312): 122-4.

14 Ball J. Reactions to Motherhood: The Role of Postnatal Care (2nd Edition). Cheshire: Books for Midwives Press, 1994.

15 Taylor PM, Taylor FH, Campbell SB et al. Extra early physical contact and aspects of the early mother-infant relationship. Acta Paediatr Scand Supplement 1985; 316: 3-14.

16 Dykes F, Griffiths H. Societal influences upon initiation and continuation of breastfeeding. British Journal of Midwifery 1998; 6(2): 76-80.

17 Royal College of Midwives. Men's attitudes to breastfeeding. Midwives Chronicle 1993; 106(1271): 473.

18 Hall J. Breastfeeding and sexuality: Societal conflicts and expectations. British Journal of Midwifery 1997; 5(6): 350-4.

19 Jackson KB. Women, men, breastfeeding and sexuality. British Journal of Midwifery 2000; 8(2): 83-6.

20 Ineichen B, Peirce M, Lawrenson R. Jewish and Celtic attitudes to breastfeeding compared. Midwifery 1997; 13: 40-3.

21 Palmer G. The Politics of Breastfeeding. (2nd edition) London: Pandora, 1993.

22 Read L. The sexuality of breastfeeding. British Journal of Midwifery 1996; 4(8): 424-6.

23 Frossell S. If breast is best then what is the problem? British Journal of Midwifery 1998; 6(5): 316-9.

24 Research and Evaluation Services. Breastfeeding, knowledge, attitudes and behaviour in Northern Ireland. Belfast: RES, 1999.

25 Stein J, Dykes F, Bramwell R. Breastfeeding: Midwives meeting mothers in the middle. British Journal of Midwifery 2000; 8(4): 239-45.

26 Christensson K, Cabrera T, Christensson E et al. Separation distress call in the human neonate in the absence of maternal body contact. Acta Paediatr 1995; 84: 468-73.

The instruction in pelvic floor exercises provided to women during pregnancy or following delivery

Linda Mason, Sheila Glenn, Irene Walton and Carol Hughes

Objectives: to examine the instruction in pelvic floor exercises given to women during pregnancy or following delivery, to assess the quality of any instruction provided, and to consider these in light of the women's views about the service.

Design: a postal questionnaire was sent to a sample of women when they reached 34 weeks of pregnancy and a second at 8 weeks postpartum. A sub-sample of women who reported symptoms of stress incontinence at 8 weeks postpartum were interviewed about the instruction in pelvic floor exercises that they received during their pregnancy, or in the puerperium.

Participants: of the 918 women who were sent the first questionnaire, 717 returned it completed (78%). Five-hundred-and-seventy-two of 894 women (64%) completed the second questionnaire. Forty-two of 179 symptomatic women (23%) took part in an interview.

Findings: 55% of women received some form of instruction in pelvic floor exercises by 34 weeks of pregnancy. Eighty-six per cent received instruction following birth. The way the information was given varied, ranging from a brief reminder, to exercising in a class with an instructor. The information was provided by a range of health professionals, and no single profession appeared to undertake responsibility for the service. As a result, the views of the service varied. A few women reported that they had received good quality instruction, others were critical of it, and a small number reported that they had received no instruction at all. The widespread practice of leaving a leaflet by the women's beds during their stay in hospital, was criticised by a large proportion of the women.

Key conclusion: the instruction in pelvic floor exercises by health service professionals was provided on an ad hoc basis. In many instances, the programme of instruction did not meet recommendations made in the literature. It is likely that the success of randomised controlled trials reported in the literature would not be repeated in the 'real world'.

Implications for practice: there is a need for the service to be re-organised so that all women receive high-quality instruction during pregnancy, with a reminder to exercise following birth. This could help to prevent, or relieve, the symptoms of stress incontinence that frequently occur at these times.

Between 6 and 31% of women are reported to experience stress incontinence following childbirth (Dimpfl et al. 1992, Mason et al. 1999a). The main method of treatment for this condition is pelvic floor exercises, first introduced by Kegel in 1948. He described how the muscles of the perineal body are put under strain during delivery, resulting in injury and loss of function. A series of exercises were devised for 'reinnervation, regeneration and re-education (p. 241) of the muscles.' The exercises increase the tone and power of the pelvic floor muscles thereby improving continence in either or both of two possible ways. First, by restoring the tone of the urethral striated muscle, urethral pressure may be increased, and its occlusive action strengthened. Secondly, strengthening of the levator ani muscles will increase support to the urethra and bladder neck, lifting them within the intra-abdominal cavity and thereby improving pressure transmission during periods of stress. Support of the bladder neck may help to restore the urethrovesical angle and decrease the level of funneling of the upper urethra (Norton 1994).

Numerous studies have explored the effectiveness of pelvic floor exercises, with differing success rates reported. For example, Shepherd et al. (1983) found that 27% of study participants achieved continence, whilst a further 27% reported an improvement in their condition. Burgio et al. (1986) reported continence in 15% of their sample, whilst the remaining 85% showed a significant improvement. Burns et al. (1993) reported 3% continent and a 54% reduction in incontinence in the group receiving exercise therapy. The variation may result from differences in the way the instruction is provided and the exercise regime. Variations in the instruction that have a bearing on outcome include the methods of instruction (including whether a check is made to ensure the exercises were undertaken correctly), and the level of supervision.

Research has shown that pelvic floor exercises are difficult to teach correctly. Bump et al. (1991) found that 40% of participants were unable to contract their pelvic floor following brief verbal instruction. One in four women were using a technique that could promote incontinence. The authors concluded that 'simple or written instruction does not represent adequate preparation for a patient who is about to pursue a Kegel exercise programme' (p. 326). Similarly, after being taught on an individual basis, 69% of stress incontinent women reported that they had previously been exercising incorrectly (Bo et al. 1987). One of the difficulties is that many women are unaware of their ability to contract their pelvic floor muscles. In addition to rendering the exercises ineffective, incorrect pelvic floor contractions may, in some cases, also compound the problem. Bearing down could stretch the pelvic floor muscles (Laycock 1997). For this reason, Sampselle et al. (1998) taught their participants muscle identification exercises prior to strength-building ones.

A randomised controlled trial by Wilson et al. (1987) compared a group of women treated with pelvic floor exercises in hospital, to those treated at home. Women who took part in twelve exercise sessions, supervised by a physiotherapist at the hospital, had a significantly better outcome compared to those exercising at home, who had received just one supervised session of exercise. A second study also found a greater improvement in women who exercised with an 'instructor' once per week for 6 months, compared to the group who exercised on their own at home (Bo et al. 1990). The instructor ensured that the women exercised in different positions, with contractions held for six to eight seconds. However, as the women who trained with the instructor also undertook more exercise in comparison to the home exercise group, it is likely that this had a bearing on outcome.

Another factor that may affect the success of a programme of exercise relates to the exercise regime itself. Because of the differences in the study parameters reported in the literature, it is difficult to assess the

Table 7.6.1 Information received

	During pregnancy		Postpartum	
	No.	%	No.	%
Yes	397	55.3	490	85.6
No	320	44.6	80	13.9
Missing	-	-	2	0.3
Total	717	100	572	99.8

Table 7.6.2 The percentage of women receiving information from different health professionals*

	During pregnancy		Postpartum	
	No.	%	No.	%
Hospital midwife	110	15.4	319	55.7
Community midwife	202	28.3	230	40.1
GP	11	1.5	40	7.0
Practice nurse	27	3.8	22	3.8
Physiotherapist	87	12.2	89	15.5
Health Visitor	-	-	110	19.2

(*This may be from more than one source.)

Table 7.6.3 The percentage of women receiving information via different methods

	Method of instruction*		Sole method of instruction	
	No.	%	No.	%
During pregnancy				
Mention/reminder	111	15.6	53	7.4
Leaflet	214	30.0	118	16.5
Verbal instruction	167	23.4	46	6.4
Physical instruction	111	15.6	30	4.2
Postpartum				
Mention/reminder	203	35.4	52	9.2
Leaflet	394	68.8	184	32.1
Verbal instruction	144	25.1	17	2.9
Physical instruction	48	8.4	5	0.8

(*This may be from more than one source.)

nature of an 'optimal' exercise programme. Variations have included the number of contractions stipulated per session/per day, and the length of time the contractions should be held, although most studies have incorporated daily sessions of frequent or sustained exercise. Kegel (1948) himself recommended a daily target of 300 contractions, although more recently Dougherty et al. (1993) found that a reduction in urine loss occurred when pelvic floor exercises were carried out just three times per week. Lagro-Jannsen et al. (1991) recommended building up from five to ten sessions of ten contractions per day. Henalla et al. (1988) recommended that the contractions were held for three to four seconds, with equal numbers of fast and slow for up to ten minutes, and repeated every hour. Dougherty (1998), however, argued that recommending too many repetitions does not result in improved outcome as it reduces motivation and adherence to the regimen. Indeed, Sampselle et al. (1997) found that just 30-40 repetitions were sufficient to produce a significant improvement in symptoms. A review by Wells (1990) found that the recommended duration for a contraction to be held varied from two to thirty seconds. However, Dougherty (1998) discussed the rationale for undertaking ten second contractions, that is, they are thought to recruit both type II muscle fibres and activate type I fibres. A meta-analysis concluded that exercise programmes should include both short- and long-duration exercises, with daily or twice daily regimens of increasing repetitions until fatigue sets in (Berghmans et al. 1998). According to Miller et al. (1994), because the ability to contract the pelvic floor muscles varies from woman to woman, any exercise programme should begin at the appropriate level for each woman. Once pelvic floor muscle strength has built up, the exercises should be continued, albeit at a lower intensity, in order to maintain the effects.

The evidence suggests that the exercises need to be carried out over a substantial period of time for most women to obtain relief (Benvenuti et al. 1987, Henalla et al. 1988, Tapp et al. 1988, Bishop et al. 1992). Participants in one study (Bo et al. 1990) demonstrated some increase in muscle strength after one month, although those undertaking intensive exercise continued to improve over a six-month period. Participants in another study (Hahn et al. 1993) showed improvements with increased duration of training. Only after 3-4 months were more than half of the participants cured or improved. Some women reported improvements in stress incontinence soon after starting pelvic floor exercises. However, it is likely that the improvement occurred as a result of the women learning to contract their muscles during times of stress (Miller et al. 1996). It appears that, whilst pelvic floor exercises are an effective treatment for stress incontinence (Berghmans et al. 1998), the success is partly dependent upon the instruction provided. As no recent studies were found which describe the routine teaching of pelvic floor exercises to women at around the time of childbirth, the present study was set up to investigate: (a) the instruction provided routinely to women during the antenatal and postpartum periods; (b) whether the service met the recommendations made in the literature; and (c) the needs of the women themselves.

Methods

Permission to undertake the study was obtained from the two Local Research Ethics Committees responsible for the health authorities where the study was to be carried out. Each woman attending the antenatal clinic during a five-month recruitment period was presented with an information sheet outlining the research and invited to take part. If she agreed, she was then asked to sign a consent form. A decision was taken to exclude anyone under the age of 16 from the study. This was due to the issue of having to get parental consent as well as that of the participant. Women were also excluded from the study if there was any doubt over whether they were still pregnant at 34 weeks gestation. Checks were made either via the computer or her records. Further exclusions were made at stage two if a stillbirth or neonatal death was recorded.

The data were collected using both questionnaires and interviews. The questionnaires were used to gather quantitative data from a large sample of women. This was in order to explore the prevalence of any incontinence, the coverage of instruction in pelvic floor exercises, the ways in which it was provided, and also which health professionals were responsible for providing the information. The qualitative interviews were used to gather more detailed information on the above from a smaller number of women. This provided a cross check against the information collected by the quantitative methods and enabled the women's views of the instruction and the ways in which it could be improved, to be collected.

Whilst the methods used to gather data are outlined briefly below, for more detailed information on the quantitative methods see Mason et al. (1999a), and for the qualitative methods see Mason et al. (1999b).

The Questionnaire Survey

The questionnaires were administered at 34 weeks of pregnancy to women recruited at the antenatal booking clinic from two hospitals in the north-west of England. A reminder was sent two weeks later. Nine hundred and eighteen questionnaires were posted and 717 returned, giving a response rate of 78%. A second questionnaire was administered at 8 weeks postpartum and a reminder posted two weeks later. Eight hundred and ninety four questionnaires were sent out and 572 returned, giving a response rate of 64%.

The following questions were used to elicit details on the presence of symptoms of stress incontinence, and any instruction received on pelvic floor exercises:

Do you leak any urine during physical activity or exertion, for example, whilst coughing, laughing, lifting heavy objects, climbing stairs, during sex, etc.?
Yes   No

Since becoming pregnant (since giving birth), have you been given any information or instruction on pelvic floor exercises?
Yes   No

Who gave you this information or instruction? (please tick as many as apply)
Midwife
GP
Health Visitor
Physiotherapist/Nurse (at the health centre/GP practice)
Nurse (at the hospital)

How was the information or instruction given to you? (Please tick as many as apply)
Brief mention or reminder to do them
Leaflet/written instruction or drawn diagram
Verbal instruction
Physical instruction/demonstration

The data were analysed using the Statistical Package for the Social Sciences (SPSS for Windows Release 7.0.1)

The qualitative interviews

All of the women who reported symptoms of stress incontinence at 8 weeks postpartum were invited, by letter, to participate in an interview. Of the 179 symptomatic women, 42 gave consent (23%).

Procedure The interviews took place in the women's homes and all were conducted by one of the authors (LM). The interviews followed an unstructured but focused format, gathering information on the instruction the women had received, their views on the way it was imparted, and their suggestions for any improvements needed. Each reply received an appropriate response from the interviewer so that the interview took the form of a conversation. This allowed the women to concentrate on those issues that they felt were pertinent, rather than having a strict agenda set by the interviewer. Not all women wished to be recorded on cassette tape so the answers were written down on paper in shorthand, and transcribed in full on return to the office.

Data analysis The transcripts were read through several times until the data became familiar to the investigator, and they were coded as topics, themes, and patterns. Some data were listed under more than one heading. Each of the coded items was then considered in turn. The transcripts were reread and recoded until no new items were found. The narratives were further explored using both content and inductive analysis (Patton 1990), which allowed data to be sought in response to specific questions or ideas, whilst other phenomena emerged naturally from the data. Descriptions, recurring themes and patterns, contrasts and negative and deviant cases were found. Each transcript was re-examined to consider the data as individual cases rather than looking at items across cases. Contradictions and repetitions became evident at this stage. To assure credibility (Appleton 1995), the raw data were returned to repeatedly to check that the issues described had not been taken out of context, over represented, or exaggerated. As the findings emerged, each transcript was checked to verify whether an issue was evident. The number of interviewees for whom the issue was relevant was then counted. It was thought that showing the numbers of women involved in each item would provide some indication of the importance of the issue.

Findings

The questionnaires

Questionnaire 1 The instruction in pelvic floor exercises during pregnancy appeared to be provided on an ad hoc basis. Just over half of the women (55.3%) received some information (Table 1). This was provided by a range of staff from different professions (Table 2) and the method also varied from a reminder only, to practising the exercises in a class (Table 3).

Questionnaire 2 The majority of women (85.6%) received instruction following birth (Table 3). Whilst again the source varied, a large proportion of women received it from a midwife (either a hospital-based or community midwife). Although again the method varied, most women received the information via a leaflet.

The qualitative interviews

Characteristics of the interviewees Forty-two women were interviewed. Their ages ranged from 21 to 45 with a mean of 31 years. Two of the women were Asian, one was black, the remainder were white. Fourteen of the women were para 1, 18 were para 2, 4 were para 3 and one each were para 4, 5 and 7 (information on 3 of the women was missing). The severity of the women's condition ranged from 'less than one episode of incontinence per week' to 'daily incontinence'.

Information provided during the pregnancy The major source of information during this period came from the various voluntary classes, with the antenatal class providing information to the greatest number of women – 12 in total. In some classes, the physiotherapist provided much of the information, whilst in others it was provided by a midwife. The following quote illustrates a case where a woman felt that the instruction provided had been very good:

The physio, apart from saying what's what, we did them in class. She said you can feel the muscles contracting if you go to the loo and stop. She also gave out leaflets as well. She had diagrams she'd photocopied from the manual or book. Explained what was what, how to do them and how often. She got us to do some there and then and asked if we could feel the muscle, tried to explain what muscle it was ... She made sure your partner can feel it. She said to do them every time you remember – in the bus queue, when you're having dinner, short ones hold for ten, even whilst making love and occasionally when you're on the toilet. (09)

The other classes where information was provided were parentcraft classes (three women), National Childbirth Trust classes (two women), aquanatal classes (four women) and relaxation classes (three women). Some women attended more than one of these and consequently received information from a number of sources.

Twenty-two out of the forty-two women interviewed mentioned that they were not provided with any information on pelvic floor exercises during their pregnancy. Few women received information during their routine health checks, although seven women reported that a midwife, either at the antenatal clinic, or on a home visit, had provided some information on pelvic floor exercises. In two instances, the women reported that they had to ask for it themselves. The information ranged from:

...at the first midwife visit when I first became pregnant she gave me a leaflet which was in the pack with other leaflets. Just told to read them. That has been the only time. (13)

to

... the midwife told me verbally what to do, was very easy to understand. Very good at just getting it across just verbally. May also have been given a leaflet. She motivated me into doing them. (27)

Information provided during the postnatal period All of the women were asked whether they had received any information following the birth of their baby. Thirty-two reported having received a leaflet during their stay in hospital following birth. One had been given three copies of the same leaflet within three days. Six women said that they had not received a copy whilst four were not sure whether they had received one or not.

Seventeen women said that the leaflet was the only source of information on pelvic floor exercises that they had received. Generally they thought this to be unsatisfactory. Many commented upon the fact that the leaflet was just left by their bed and felt it was not the best means of communicating the information:

I was left a stack of leaflets straight after the birth. Anonymous leaflets, down to me to sort the information out. It was just put at the end of the bed, nothing was said. It wasn't satisfactory. It would be helpful if somebody went through the

leaflets, it's like junk mail – just given a stack of mail, very easy to dump them. If that's common practice then something should be done. (07)

Altogether, 20 women made a negative comment during their interview about receiving the information in this way. The following criticisms were made:

The timing was poor.

The leaflet was left without any introduction, and it didn't appear to be associated with stress incontinence.

The description of how to do the exercises was inadequate, which meant that some women could not follow the instructions. The leaflet needed explaining in person; it did not stress the importance of doing pelvic floor exercises.

Providing the information with many other leaflets was not an effective way of making sure the information was seen and read, particularly when it was left with other leaflets, including one on cot death: After the birth some leaflets were left by the bed for when I came back from theatre. No one actually said 'here's some leaflets'. I just happened to notice it. It needed pointing out really. It was strange (03).

The leaflet's given with other things, nobody went through it. You need somebody to go through and check you can do the exercises (33).

...but the handouts don't detail what to tighten, just said pelvic floor but didn't say what the pelvic floor is. Need to explain what the muscles are. (04)

One woman made an additional point that '*nobody checked to see that I could read*'. (19)

Following discharge from hospital, some women were asked if they were doing pelvic floor exercises, or they were reminded to do them, by either a midwife or health visitor. A few had reminders from more than one health professional. One woman mentioned that her GP had asked her whether she was doing her pelvic floor exercises at the six-week postnatal examination. Four women were annoyed that nobody had reminded them or checked to see if they were doing them correctly.

Seven women suggested that they received little information because they were not first-time mothers. They felt that whilst the health professionals assumed they knew what to do from previous experience, they themselves did not feel this to be the case:

They possibly assumed that someone with seven children should know what they're doing but it shouldn't be assumed. . . it's always assumed because I've got a lot of children and I'm educated that I'm going to pick up on things but there's always a new situation to crop up and I'm likely to panic as the last person. (34)

Suggestions on how to improve the services Five women stated that the service they had could not be improved:

The care I got before and after was good. It was sufficient, I understood it, thought the physio was brilliant, she couldn't stress it enough. (09)

All of these women had attended antenatal or aquanatal classes (both, in some cases). During these classes an explanation was given as to why they needed to do pelvic floor exercises. They were also instructed on how to do them and some time was spent practising the exercises. The women also received leaflets during their stay in hospital, and had a midwife, health visitor or both, remind them of the need to practise the exercises.

The others felt that the services had scope for improvement. Five main topics emerged. These were: the importance of doing pelvic floor exercises, the way information was given, the timing of the information, whether the exercises were being performed correctly and the content of the instruction.

The importance of doing pelvic floor exercises

This was the most important issue to emerge from the interviews, with 18 women mentioning this during the course of their interview. Two ways of stressing the information were suggested. Fourteen women thought that the consequences of having stress incontinence should be stressed, along with the importance of doing pelvic floor exercises to prevent or alleviate the problem.

They (health professionals) don't stress the incontinent side – just to get everything back in place. Don't know if everyone's aware of it . . .the fact that you're going to wet yourself every five minutes is not mentioned. . . .They should stress more on the problems that you can have. When you're young you think 'it won't happen to me'. (17)

Six women suggested that health professionals should frequently remind women to practise the exercises.

The way the information was given

Half of the women requested that the information be given verbally, for a number of reasons: the information was understood more easily when explained in person; it added more emphasis and stressed the importance of doing the exercises; it also provided the opportunity to ask questions. Five women asked for a handout to reinforce the information, and which could be perused at a later date.

The timing of the information

Most women received a leaflet whilst they were in hospital at the time of birth, yet many felt the timing was inappropriate. Eleven requested that the information was given during pregnancy for the following reasons: a number of women experience problems at this stage, practising the exercises antenatally could help get women into the routine of doing them, and women are more receptive to the information at this time because:

'all hell breaks loose after delivery'. (09)

Whether the exercises were being performed correctly

Seven women suggested that someone – usually the midwife – should check to see that the women were doing the exercises correctly. For some, a check seemed to consist of having someone on hand to provide instruction whilst the exercises were being performed. Others described a physical check

. . . thought it would have been better if someone was there when you're doing the first exercises to see that you are doing them properly. Somebody just feeling you to see that you're pulling in the right muscles. (40)

Six more women, whilst not specifically requesting that someone should check they were doing them correctly, stated that they weren't sure if they were doing them properly.

The content of instruction

Whilst few chose to mention the contents of the instruction, three issues were raised: the instruction should be more in-depth or explicit; more detail is needed on which muscles are involved; and information should be provided on the frequency with which the exercises should be performed.

Discussion

A limitation of the study was that only a small proportion i.e. 23%, of the symptomatic women responded to the request to be interviewed. It is thought that this reflected the method used to recruit the interviewees. Women who reported on the questionnaire that they had symptoms of stress incontinence were sent a letter asking if they would like to take part in an interview. A reply slip was enclosed for their convenience, which necessitated some action on their behalf. This may have resulted in some element of self-selection bias and possibly a lower response rate than if the women had been invited to participate in person, or over the telephone. It is possible that those women who responded felt more at ease talking about their condition. However, the final sample included 42 women who represented all ages, parity, ethnicity and degree of severity with respect to their condition, and they also appeared to have been in receipt of very different levels of service. In addition, as the themes were repeated throughout the course of these interviews, it was felt that saturation had occurred, and increasing the sample size would not enrich the findings of the study.

With hindsight, it would also have been useful to obtain data on the information the women received through informal sources such as their family and friends. As the original aim of the study was to look at the provision of services by healthcare professionals, questions regarding other sources of information were not included in the questionnaire.

A further limitation of the study was that detailed information was not collected on the nature of the exercise regimes, and the recommended time period. Few women mentioned the length of time they were instructed to practise or the number of contractions to be performed. However, a couple of women did request that information should be given on frequency. This suggests that women were not provided with all of the necessary information. The literature itself is unclear as to how many contractions should be performed and over what time-period. Many studies have not provided information on the nature of the exercise regime, and where this is reported, it appears to vary between studies. Whilst Bo et al. (1990) found a better outcome amongst women who were enrolled in an intensive exercise group compared to those in a home exercise group, other factors such as the degree of supervision may have influenced the findings.

In their review, Berghmans et al. (1998) concluded that pelvic floor exercises are an effective form of conservative treatment for stress incontinence. Because of the numerous mechanisms involved in promoting continence, pelvic floor exercises would not be expected to help all women. However, approximately two-thirds to three-quarters of women, embarking on a course of exercise, may be expected to be 'cured' or show improvement in their symptoms, provided that the exercises are carried out correctly over a substantial period of time (Henalla et al. 1988, Lagro-Jannsen et al. 1991, Hahn et al. 1993). The way the instruction is given and the exercise regime itself can affect the efficacy of the exercises. The randomised controlled trials which have found pelvic floor exercises to be effective included the following components:

- detailed instruction on how to perform pelvic floor exercises, usually comprising one or more practice sessions with a physiotherapist. (Henalla et al. 1988, 1989, Bo et al. 1990, Lagro-Janssen et al. 1991);
- a test to ensure that each participant can perform an effective pelvic floor contraction (Henalla et al. 1988, Henalla et al. 1989, Bo et al. 1990, Lagro-Janssen et al. 1991);

- a three-month, or longer period over which the exercises are carried out (Henalla et al. 1988, Henalla et al. 1989, Bo et al. 1990, Lagro- Janssen et al. 1991);
- a series of fast and slow contractions performed on a daily basis, or at least three times per week (Henella et al. 1989, Bo et al. 1990).

The instruction provided to the women in the present study did not meet these criteria in many cases. The instruction was provided on an ad hoc basis which meant that, whilst some women received very detailed instruction, 5% received none at all. Frequently the information was provided in the form of a leaflet. Of the 572 women who responded to both questionnaires, 314 women received the information, if at all, by means of a reminder and/or leaflet only. In many cases, they received no other form of instruction. Bump et al. (1991) reported that brief verbal instruction was ineffective, and the women in the present study agreed with this finding.

Much criticism was made of the practice of leaving a leaflet by the bedside at the time of birth. As well as the method, it was thought to be an inappropriate time. Although easy to understand, the leaflet did not stress the importance of the exercises, particularly as it was frequently left with no introduction. The practice of leaving it amongst a pile of other leaflets attracted much criticism as there was too much information at one time. Consequently, priority was given to those such as one on cot death, which was deemed to be more important, although much rarer.

Few women had the opportunity to practise alongside a supervisor, although research suggests that a better outcome is obtained when this is the case. Where this had happened the women agreed this was good practice. It was felt that the information provided during antenatal or aquanatal class was the best source of information for the following reasons: it was provided during the last trimester, the instruction was usually detailed and the women were usually given the opportunity to practise the exercises alongside an instructor who could answer any questions if necessary. However, although the quality and timing of the information at these classes appeared to be good, they were not accessible or accessed by all women. According to Hancock (1994) less than half of the women who present for antenatal care also attend classes in childbirth preparation and those who do, appear to be unrepresentative of the population as a whole. Nolan (1994) found that irrespective of whether the class was provided by the voluntary sector, or the hospital, the women attending tended to be older than the national average for childbearing women, and predominantly middle-class. Cliff and Deery (1997) found that young unmarried working-class women were particularly poorly represented at antenatal classes.

These findings were in agreement with previous studies (O'Brien & Smith 1981, Lumley & Brown 1993). It can, therefore, be assumed that a large proportion of women, particularly those who are younger and less advantaged, would not receive detailed instruction in pelvic floor exercises.

Although common practice in the randomised controlled trials, few women in the present study received a check to ensure that they were exercising the correct muscles. A number reported that they were not sure if they were doing the exercises correctly, whilst others specifically requested that a health professional check that they were doing them properly. This would appear to confirm the difficulty in teaching pelvic floor exercises (Bo et al. 1987, Bump et al. 1991), and the need to make sure that the women could perform an effective pelvic muscle contraction before embarking on a regime of exercise. A number of ways of assessing the strength of pelvic floor contractions are described in the literature. These include: digital assessment, whereby the pelvic floor muscles are squeezed around the examiner's finger/s (Laycock 1994), the perineometer (Kegel 1948), the urine stream interruption test (Sampselle 1993) and palpation of the perineal body. Laycock (1987) recommended that the latter technique is adopted during pregnancy, although experience is needed to assess this accurately. If women are to be taught pelvic floor exercises during pregnancy as suggested, this non-invasive technique may be the most appropriate method of verifying a correct muscle contraction.

In summary, it would appear that the routine instruction of pelvic floor exercises during pregnancy or following childbirth was provided on an ad hoc basis. Whilst some women received good-quality instruction, many others received information which did not meet standards set in the literature. Indeed, the women themselves often criticised it, and gave suggestions for improvement. Consequently, it is doubtful whether the success rate reported in previous research studies would be achieved by women receiving routine antenatal or postpartum instruction in the 'real world'. The following suggestions to improve current service provision and the programme of exercise are drawn from the findings of the study.

The organisation of the service provision

- Instruction in pelvic floor exercises could be made explicit in the policies and protocols governing practices, not left to the discretion of the individual carer. Providing instruction to women in pelvic floor exercises could be made the sole responsibility of one of the healthcare professions.
- Responsibility for the task may be best held by the midwives, as they provide care for women during pregnancy when the women suggest information should be given.
- The instruction could be provided routinely as part of antenatal care, rather than during antenatal or other voluntary classes, which are only attended by a proportion of the women.
- It could be useful to adopt a multidisciplinary approach with respect to reminding women to exercise their pelvic floor.
- The 'optimal' exercise programme could be defined and adopted by all instructors.
- The practice of leaving leaflets for women during their stay in hospital, without introducing the subject, could be discontinued in favour of a more appropriate means of instruction (see below).

The programme of exercise

- The instruction could be given both verbally and visually, providing women with the opportunity to ask questions.
- A good handout could be devised and provided – not for instruction purposes but to serve as a permanent record or reminder. A video would provide an alternative source of record for those women who are unable to read.
- The instructor could be made aware of the difficulty women have isolating the correct muscle group.
- The need to avoid contracting the abdominal, gluteal or thigh muscles, could be emphasised, as well as the need to avoid 'bearing down'.

The instruction could incorporate a check to ensure that each woman can perform an effective pelvic floor contraction. Although vaginal palpation is a method used by many experts, if the exercises are being taught during pregnancy, a less invasive check such as self palpation, may be more appropriate and acceptable to the women. The 'optimal' exercise programme provided to the women would appear to include both sustained and maximal contractions, and regular sessions of exercise per day, or several times per week. A gradual schedule, in which women can build up their muscle strength and endurance according to their differing abilities, may be the most effective means of exercising the pelvic floor.

Acknowledgements

The authors would like to thank the women who participated in the study and also staff at the two hospitals in which the study was undertaken.

REFERENCES

Appleton JV 1995 Analysing qualitative interview data: addressing issues of validity and reliability. Journal of Advanced Nursing 22: 993-997

Benvenuti F, Caputo GM, Bandinelli S et al. 1987 Re-educative treatment of female genuine stress incontinence. American Journal of Physical Medicine 66 (4): 155-169

Berghmans LCM, Hendriks HJM, Bo K et al. 1998 Conservative treatment of stress urinary incontinence in women: a systematic review of randomised clinical trials. British Journal of Urology 82: 181-191

Bishop KR, Dougherty M, Mooney R et al. 1992 Effects of age, parity, and adherence on pelvic muscle response to exercise. Journal of Obstetric, Gynecologic and Neonatal Nursing 21 (5): 401-405

Bo K, Larsen S, Oseid S et al. 1987 Knowledge about and ability to correct pelvic floor muscle exercises in women with urinary stress incontinence. Neurourology and Urodynamics 7: 261-262

Bo K, Hagen R, Kvarstein B et al. 1990 Pelvic floor muscle exercise for the treatment of female stress urinary incontinence: effects of two different degrees of pelvic floor muscle exercise. Neurourology and Urodynamics 9: 489-502

Bump RC, Hurt WG, Fantl MD et al. 1991 Assessment of Kegel pelvic muscle exercise performance after brief verbal instruction. American Journal of Obstetrics and Gynecology 165 (2): 322-329

Burgio KL, Robinson JC, Engel BT 1986 The role of biofeedback in Kegel exercise training for stress urinary incontinence. American Journal of Obstetrics and Gynecology 154: 58-64

Burns BA, Pranikoff K, Nochajski TH et al. 1993 A comparison of effectiveness of biofeedback and pelvic muscle exercise treatment of stress incontinence in older community dwelling women. Journal of Gerontology 48: M167-174

Cliff D, Deery R 1997 Too much like school: social class, marital status and attendance at antenatal classes. Midwifery 13: 1339-1145

Dimpfl TH, Hesse U, Schussler B 1992 Incidence and cause of postpartum urinary stress incontinence. European Journal of Obstetrics, Gynaecology and Reproductive Biology 43: 29-33

Dougherty M 1998 Current status of research on pelvic muscle strengthening techniques. Journal of Wound, Ostomy and Continence Nursing 25 (2): 75- 83 Dougherty M, Bishop KR, Mooney RA et al. 1993 Graded pelvic muscle exercise: effect on stress urinary incontinence. Journal of Reproductive Medicine 38: 684-691

Hahn I, Milsom I, Fall M et al. 1993 Long-term results of pelvic floor training in female stress urinary incon- tinence. British Journal of Urology 72: 421-427

Hancock A 1994 How effective is antenatal education? Modern Midwife 4 (5): 13-15

Henalla SM, Kirwan P, Castleden CM et al. 1988 The effect of pelvic floor exercises in the treatment of genuine urinary stress incontinence in women at two hospitals. British Journal of Obstetrics and Gynaecology 95: 602-605

Henalla SM, Hutchins CJ, Robinson P et al. 1989 Non- operative methods in the treatment of female genuine stress incontinence of urine. Journal of Obstetrics and Gynaecology 9: 222-225

Kegel AH 1948 Progressive resistance exercise in the functional restoration of the perineal muscles. American Journal of Obstetrics and Gynecology 56 (2): 238-248

Lagro-Janssen ALM, Debruyne FMJ, Smits AJA et al. 1991 Controlled trial of pelvic floor exercises in the treatment of urinary stress incontinence in general practice. British Journal of General Practice 41: 445-449

Laycock J 1987 Graded exercises for the pelvic floor muscles in the treatment of urinary incontinence. Physiotherapy 73 (7): 371-373

Laycock J 1994 Pelvic muscle exercises: physiotherapy for the pelvic floor. Urologic Nursing 14: 136-140

Laycock J 1997 Physiotherapy assessment of the pelvic floor. Proceedings of the 4th Biennial Pelvic Floor Conference. Harrogate December 1-2. Copies avail- able from J Laycock, The Culgaith Clinic, Culgaith, Penrith, Cumbria, UK

Lumley J, Brown S 1993 Attenders and non-attenders at childbirth education classes in Australia: How do they and their births differ: Birth: Issues in Perinatal Care 20 (3): 123-130

Mason L, Glenn S, Walton I et al. 1999a The prevalence of stress incontinence during pregnancy and following delivery. Midwifery 15: 120-128

Mason L, Glenn S, Walton I et al. 1999b The experience of stress incontinence after childbirth. Birth: Issues in Perinatal Care 26 (3): 164-171

Miller J, Kasper C, Sampselle C 1994 Review of muscle physiology with application to pelvic muscle exercise. Urologic Nursing 14 (3): 92-97

Miller J, Ashton-Miller J, DeLaney JOL 1996 The knack: use of precisely timed pelvic muscle contraction can reduce leakage in stress urinary incontinence. Neurourology and Urodynamics 15: 392-393

Nolan M 1994 A comparison of attenders at antenatal classes in the voluntary and statutory sectors: education and organisational implications. Midwifery 11: 138-145

Norton P 1994 Aims of pelvic floor re-education. In: Schussler B, Laycock J, Norton et al (eds) Pelvic floor re-education: principles and practice. Springer, London

O'Brien M, Smith C 1981 Women's views and experience of antenatal care. The Practitioner 224: 123-125

Patton MQ 1990 Qualitative Evaluation And Research Methods. Sage, Newbury Park

Sampselle CM 1993 Using a stopwatch to assess pelvic muscle strength in the urine stream interruption test. American Journal of Primary Health Care 18: 14-20

Sampselle CM, Burns PA, Dougherty MC et al. 1997 Urinary incontinence: ambulatory management. Journal of Obstetric, Gynecologic and Neonatal Nursing 26: 375-385

Sampselle CM, Miller JM, Mims B et al. 1998 Effect of pelvic muscle exercise on transient incontinence during pregnancy and after birth. Obstetrics and Gynecology 91 (3): 406-412

Shepherd AM, Montgomery E, Anderson RS 1983 Treatment of genuine stress incontinence with a new perineometer. Physiotherapy 69: 113

Tapp AJS, Cardozo L, Hills B et al. 1988 Who benefits from physiotherapy? Neurourology and Urodynamics 7: 259-261

Wells TJ 1990 Pelvic floor muscle exercise. Journal of the American Geriatric Society 38: 333-337

Wilson PD, Sammarrai TA, Deakin M et al. 1987. An objective assessment of physiotherapy for female genuine stress incontinence. British Journal of Obstetrics and Gynaecology 94: 757-582 64

Reflecting on the postnatal experience

- Do you talk with women about issues of relativity between beliefs in different cultures and societies, and how the concepts of 'right' and 'wrong' can be culturally relative? Is this an important topic to put on the agenda, for instance during 'preparing for parenting' sessions?

- In your opinion, is it better to promote breast milk, artificial milk, or choice? What do you honestly feel about this? Is there a difference between what you 'objectively think' you should promote, and what you feel? To what extent are your feelings coloured by your own experiences? How can we work to remain true to who we are, and the things that we think are important, while also offering the best care we can to women?

- Do you discuss the issues around co-sleeping with women and, if so, at what point? Are you aware whether the women you work with are practising this kind of parenting, and for what reasons? Do they have positive, negative or neutral feelings around this? What can we do to inform women about this option and reduce the possibility of negative feelings or worries in the women who are doing this instinctively?

- How can we ensure that women are receiving the information they need within a busy postnatal service? What information do you offer women, and what do they think about it? Are we effectively linking with lay or professional colleagues who can sometimes offer women more time on areas such as breastfeeding support or postnatal exercises than we can?

Reflecting on the postnatal experience

Focus on:
Parenting

SECTION CONTENTS

Putting parents at the heart of classes

Mary Nolan

As an NCT Antenatal Tutor, I spend a lot of my time observing classes run by student and qualified teachers and giving feedback afterwards. One of the questions I ask teachers is 'What percentage of this class was made up of you talking, and parents listening?' Nearly always, it's a high percentage. The desire to share with our clients all the information we have can over-ride what we know about adult learners – namely, that they retain only a little of the information given to them, and reject information that they do not perceive to be relevant.

How then do you get parents talking, and identifying for themselves the information they need? This article looks at how to involve parents attending antenatal classes in agenda setting, the decision about when to come into hospital in labour, and nappy changing. All the activities aim to:

- model a relationship in which parents' knowledge is valued alongside that of healthcare professionals
- boost parents' confidence in their innate understanding of birth and parenting.

Agenda setting

It can be very dispiriting to make a determined effort to ask parents what they want to cover during their antenatal classes, and be met with an embarrassed silence, or a few ideas that quickly peter out.

Try to reflect parents' ideas back to them in order to encourage them to explore their ideas further.

The start of the first class should be hard work for the educator – you have to think of lots of questions to get parents talking, give plenty of positive verbal and non-verbal feedback, and ensure that, as far as possible, everyone participates.

Flow chart for agenda setting

(Educator's questions are printed in italic, and parents' possible responses in bold.)

What would you like to cover during these classes? Give me some ideas. What are the things that are worrying you that you need to find out about?

WAIT for a reply!

Pain!
OK. What is it about 'pain' that you want to talk about?
  - **What you can do to help yourself**
  - **Drugs – pethidine, gas and air, epidurals**
  - **TENS**

What happens?
Do you mean what happens in a normal labour?
  - **Yes. What's the normal sequence of events?**
  - **What happens when something goes wrong?**
  - **What procedures do you have in hospital during labour?**

Control.
Can you explain what you mean by 'control'?
  - **How to make sure we don't have anything done to us we don't want doing.**
  - **Can we make choices? Or are the choices made for us?**
  - **Who's who in the hospital? How do you know who you're talking to?**

Eating in labour.
Why do you ask about that?
  - **I've heard that some hospitals let you eat in labour and others don't**

Is there anything that the fathers and the people who are going to be labour companions want to cover?

Partner's role.
Do all the partners want to have a role in labour?
  – **Not sure – depends on what partners might have to do.**
  – **Definitely – want to be as involved as possible.**
  – **Is it OK to leave the room for certain procedures?**

What about after the birth? Is there anything you want to know about?

Caring for the baby.
What are you particularly interested in?
  – **Feeding**
  – **Bathing**
  – **Nappies**
  – **Sleeping arrangements**
  – **Coping with crying**
  – **How you know if the baby's ill.**

Postnatal depression.
Is that something you're worried about?
  – **It seems to be very prevalent**
  – **What are the symptoms?**
  – **What treatments are there?**

Greet every suggestion with a smile and a nod, and write it down on the flipchart. Make sure that everyone's contribution is valued. Reassure the group that they can add to the agenda as they think of other items, but that you'll start with their immediate concerns.

Discussion on when to go to hospital in labour

This is a key issue for parents, and especially for labour companions! After spending some time making sure that parents understand the signs of labour, try the following exercise. Prepare slips of card describing events of early labour.

- Four contractions in the last hour
- Contractions lasting 10 seconds
- A show
- Low back-ache
- Wet underwear
- Seven minutes since the last contraction
- Can still chat and watch TV during contractions
- Contractions lasting 30 seconds
- No change in contractions
- Ouch! With a contraction
- A contraction every 10 minutes
- Contractions getting stronger

- Definite gush of water down the woman's leg
- Contractions lasting 45 seconds
- Diarrhoea

Shuffle the cards and hand them to a parent. Ask the parent to read out the first card. Ask: *Would anyone want to go to hospital if this was happening?*

Ask the parent to continue reading the cards and placing them one underneath the other. Prompt the rest of the group to share their thoughts about when they would go to hospital. *Does anyone feel that they'd be ready to go now?*

The point of this exercise is that there are no right or wrong answers. The decision about when to go to hospital will depend on when each woman or couple feel that they would be more relaxed in the hospital environment than at home. Some couples will want to rush into hospital at the first twinge; some will want to stay at home as long as possible. You will want to remind parents that they must ring the hospital if they think that the woman's waters have broken, but your role is to reassure parents that their decision about when to come in will be the right one for them.

Nappy changing

You need two dolls with plastic bodies. Smear nappies with mustard (representing the motion of a breastfed baby); put them on the dolls and dress the dolls in baby clothes.

Divide the group into men and women (if teaching couples).

Give each group a doll, cotton wool balls, a bowl of water and a clean nappy. Ask them to change the 'baby's' nappy. Insist that the doll should be treated as a BABY at all times. Supervise at a distance, answering questions only when there is no one in the group who knows the answer. Or make a list of things which parents seemed doubtful about, and cover them at the end of the exercise.

The point of this exercise is that any group of reasonably intelligent parents will be able to work out for themselves how to change the baby's nappy! Working with the doll will prompt many questions such as:

- Are disposables better than terries?
- Is there a local nappy-laundering service? How much does it cost?
- What about talc?
- When do you use nappy creams?
- Is water best for cleaning? Does it have to be boiled first?

The group members will have plenty of ideas on these subjects. Your job is simply to correct any incorrect or dangerous information that the parents hold, and, otherwise, to let them make their own decisions.

Finally...

As you gain confidence as an educator, you will find that you do less and less talking, and the parents come increasingly to the fore of your classes. Now you are educating them for independence, empowering them to make their own decisions and trust their instincts. You are weaning them off the kind of dependence on health professionals that is limiting for them, their children and for you.

Our children's safety

Jenny Fraser

Parents have a crucial responsibility for the safety of their children and they must consider how to prepare their children for the hazards of life. (Fraser, 1997)

How difficult is it for parents to get the right balance between protecting their children from harm but feeling relaxed enough to allow the natural curiosity of the child which enables their personal growth? Without a child being inquisitive about the world around them, how can they gain knowledge which develops from this interest?

An A&E statistic

According to statistics, one million children aged 14 and under attend an accident and emergency department every year following an injury in the home (www.childalert.co.uk/stats).

Such a child was brought to our A & E department earlier this year, aged only five weeks old, having been attacked by the family Alsatian. The baby was sleeping in its cot unattended with the dog roaming freely. The baby sustained horrific injuries including fractured ribs and punctured lungs, necessitating the removal of one lung immediately and further surgery is needed. The baby has been left with substantial physical scarring on its face and body from the mauling, which will remain for life. The long term physical and emotional sequelae of this scenario are difficult to imagine.

Whilst this story is horrific, it falls within our role as midwives to recognise which parents may need extra help and tuition in order to keep their babies safe. At the end of the day, the baby's safety is part of the remit of the parents and not the midwife; however, to have been instrumental in pointing out the danger, providing the said advice was acted upon, could have saved that baby.

In most instances it should not be a problem to leave a sleeping child unattended; however, the parents have a duty to make sure that their baby is safe, as the baby cannot obviously undertake this task for itself. Dogs, cats and other children need to be thought of as well as the temperature of the room and the place of the cot; such a lot of parental responsibility.

Oblivious

I remember many years ago working with parents needing enhanced parenting classes. They were mainly sent to the class by social workers and had to attend. It was amazing how the parents would often be oblivious to the safety of their babies. I clearly remember one mother placing her baby on a high surface with no barriers whilst she wandered off to light a cigarette, heedless of her baby's safety. It took many, many sessions to try and instil the basic principles of child safety into these parents. It is a long arduous road with such parents. If they cannot see the issues when their child is a baby how much worse it will be, regarding safety, when they need to transfer their limited ability to a mobile baby/toddler.

The most serious accidents are caused each year in the kitchen. Fifty thousand children each year suffer from burns or scalds. Thirty thousand children suffer poisoning, usually having swallowed domestic cleaning substances.

This risk of accidents has become a billion-dollar industry in the United States and Canada where over twenty thousand qualified professionals will set about teaching parents how to childproof their home. This 'childproofing' is said to provide protection for not only your child but also your property.

This industry is set to become more commonplace over here. Ann-Marie Ciccini trained in the US and is a member of the International Association of Child Safety. She says:

'In America the first thing you do when you know you are having a baby is call in the BabyProofers. They go around to your house and point out all the potential problems. Over here

there is nothing like that, a lot of parents have no idea how many hidden hazards are lurking in their homes.'

On the other hand, what long-term problems arise from over anxious parents who do not allow their child any freedom to explore thus restricting the baby's innate potential to learn? It appears that the issue of children's safety has acquired obsessive proportions. The International Association of Child Safety is not just concerned with safety in the home but safety outside the home, nannies, strangers, nurseries, equipment, cars, shopping, holidays, cot death and so on. Frightening stuff, really, knowing that such an abundance of dangers are lurking in every nook and cranny. How can a parent feel relaxed with such a battery of worries?

Additionally, if they rely on professionals to make their homes safe, parents may not acquire the common sense and judgement that they are going to need for many years of childrearing. What next, professionals in your home to deal with teenage outbursts? Furedi (2001) has this to say:

'This obsessive fear about the safety of children has led to a fundamental redefinition of parenting. Traditionally, good parenting has been associated with nurturing, stimulating and the socialization of children. Today, it is associated with monitoring their activities. Today, allowing a child to play outside on its own is seen as an act of neglect.'

Overanxiety

Of course, it did not need a professional in child safety to have alerted the family with the Alsatian dog to the dangers, any thinking adult could have responded just as well. Thankfully such families are rare and in Paranoid Parenting, Frank Furedi (2001) tries to redress this obsession with parenting as an anxious profession. He recalls a teacher friend of his who has recently given up working as a teacher. Whilst he felt prepared for dealing with rowdy children, he could not cope with the relentless stream of anxious parents! He tells of the mother who insisted on driving behind her son's coach to France to make sure that he arrived safely, and the trip to the seaside that had to be cancelled because parents were concerned about whether the cars would be roadworthy, who would accompany their child to the lavatory, and whether their children would become victims of passive smoking...

The Tesco club appears on the surface to offer more balanced information (http://www.tesco.com/youand yourchild). The information on the introduction pages looks positive: 'baby stays safe whilst she has fun'. At last information giving a balance between keeping babies safe and letting the baby have some fun along the way. Entering into the site revealed a different story. The information on safety aspects is excellent and well laid out. It discusses the safety issues of different age bands in many different scenarios. Parents following the good advice on this site would stave off the need for BabyProofers. However, even searching very closely, the promised information on the baby having some fun was not found. Tesco quite rightly point out that the kitchen is the most dangerous room in the house for the baby. How nice it would have been to have added how the baby could have fun in the kitchen, for instance, not having locks on all the doors but having a low cupboard with plastic containers and wooden spoons in, so that the baby could be curious and explore this cupboard safely.

So where is our middle ground? What do babies need in order to thrive and grow safely in our world and for parents not to be over anxious and therefore free to enjoy their children thoroughly? Of course parents have to accept responsibility for their children but they must also be free to accept the fun and challenges on the way. Life with a baby can be enjoyable without all the untoward daily anxiety that danger is hiding around the corner and the child will be harmed without a doubt.

Babies have an innate ability to develop and in order to foster this process they need a quality interaction, without undue stress, between themselves and their parents. A natural awareness of safety issues is obviously paramount in order to keep baby safe but a balance has to be maintained between looking out for the baby and becoming apprehensive about these aspects.

Whilst other factors such as personality are obviously highly relevant, ironically the paranoid obsession to keep a baby safe and free from danger may result in over anxious adults with long term difficulties in coping with life. As Furedi concludes 'Is there not a danger that if we so desperately try to protect children from every possible risk we may end up causing more harm than good?'

REFERENCES

Fraser J. 1997. Child Protection: A guide for midwives. Oxford: Books for Midwives.

Furedi F. 2001. Paranoid Parenting. London: Penguin Books Ltd.

Motherhood

Unrealistic expectations?

Jacqui Gibson

The birth of a baby is a major life event and, at the same time, an important life-changing experience. Becoming a parent is a long-term commitment with irreversible side effects! Parental responsibility can last a lifetime, and yet many people who become parents have little understanding of the realities of parenting and the effect that the birth of a child will have on their lives. Price[1] states that 'motherhood can be the best or worse emotional experience of a woman's life'. For most, motherhood is a combination of these extremes.

Many girls grow up with the belief that they will become mothers one day. Women can face a lot of pressure: it is anticipated that a woman will have children and, somehow, being a mother gives them credibility as a woman.[2]

Many women have children before they themselves have reached emotional maturity. Psychologically, they are not ready for motherhood.[1] Whilst one could easily relate this to teenage mothers, of which there are a growing number, the author's personal experience of caring for new mothers has involved many encounters with women of all ages, who are not ready for the realities of motherhood.

Parenting has become a hot political topic. Perhaps that is due in part to increased media attention on the pregnancies and lives of famous celebrities and politicians' wives. Perhaps it is related to reports that blame lack of parental support for children who lead a life of crime. Perhaps the influence of organisations such as Childline and the NSPCC also has a part to play. Whatever the reason, anything that helps people understand more fully the realities of parenting, and can aid in the development of the important and unique child/parent relationship, has to be beneficial.

In our society, there has been a great deal of change to the family structure. Single parent families, and people who (through work or relationships) have moved away from their relatives, often lack the support systems and confiding relationships which have been shown to be vital in the prevention of depression following childbirth. Postpartum depression can lead to a breakdown of the mother-child relationship and has possible long-term effects on the emotional, behavioural and cognitive development of the infant.[3,4]

Paradice[5] suggests that early onset of postnatal depression may not necessarily be an abnormal response to childbirth, but a rational response to the changes and adaptations that are required when a woman becomes a mother. Therefore, if a woman embarks on a pregnancy with unrealistic expectations of motherhood, lack of support and no one to confide in, this would seem to place her in a high risk category for suffering from depression and all its possible consequences.

Young women today are seldom exposed to babies and their needs before embarking on a pregnancy and consequently their expectations of how a baby behaves and what motherhood entails are unrealistic. They do not perceive how much their lives will change and the adaptations that they will have to make. The responsibilities of motherhood are always there, even when the woman is not the full time carer of the baby. Arrangements have to be made for childcare; the time the child has to be delivered to and collected from a nursery can be quite specific. If the nursery closes at 6.00pm that is the time the child has to leave! What happens if the child is ill? And of course, if you ever want to go out without the child, arrangements have to be made for someone else to take care of the child. The mother is constantly juggling her life to accommodate the child and not many women realise before becoming mothers the extent to which this happens.

The myth of motherhood

Unrealistic expectations of motherhood are often influenced by what has been called the 'myth of motherhood',[6] or the 'Madonna and child' effect.[7] Motherhood is idealised and portrayed by the media with images of young beautiful women, with perfect hair and makeup, immaculate clothes, a beautiful serene baby and a loving, attentive, understanding partner. The parents always seem to know what to do and the right words to say in any situation. In reality this is often far from the truth. The mother has not had the time or money to go to the hairdresser, or put on her makeup, and the baby has been sick down her blouse. Her skirt does not fit and her partner is at work or down at the pub to get out of the house where the baby never stops crying.

The new mother is often uncertain about what to do. Elliot[7] and McKay[8] both suggest that if a mother feels that she is not fulfilling her perceived idealistic role, whatever that may be, guilt, depression and despair can set in. In 1988, Price[1] stated that young mothers often asked why no one had told them what motherhood was really like. It would seem that little has changed over the past twelve years.

A confiding relationship

One of the reasons why the reality of motherhood is not portrayed is the extent to which our culture is dominated by male mythology.[1] If a woman is brave enough to speak out, she runs the risk of being labelled a 'bad mother', a fate which most women would avoid at all costs. The woman prefers to believe she is at fault, rather than blame society.[1] It has been shown that unless the mother has a previously established confiding relationship with another mother, she will not discuss any difficulties that she may be having with parenting with other pregnant women or mothers.[7] It is unlikely that, over coffee at the Thursday morning mother and toddler group, a mother will admit that she reached a point last night where she wanted to throw her baby out of the window when he/she would not stop crying, or that she does not know what to do about her two-year-old child's temper tantrums.

The majority of housework and mothering is done in the privacy of one's own home, behind closed doors. This provides women with little opportunity for comparison or feedback with other women on their performance. The stresses of motherhood are not discussed for fear of being labelled incompetent. Unrealistically high standards of housework and mothering skills can be set up. The myth of motherhood is so widespread, women maintain the view that other women are performing the tasks more efficiently and more easily than they do. This can confirm feelings of inadequacy and lead to feelings of guilt.[7]

Elliot[7] suggests that as women do not wish to be the bearers of bad news to other pregnant women, the myths of motherhood persist. There is a lack of recognition that motherhood can at times be one of the most stressful occupations there is. A new mother is unlikely to consider that any feelings of tiredness, irritability, difficulties in coping or low mood she may be experiencing are just part and parcel of being a mother, her introduction into motherhood.

As midwives we have a unique role in caring for women and their families, but many of us are also mothers and those who are not have seen the realities of parenting firsthand. It is time we put a stop to this 'myth of motherhood' and started to portray to our clients the realities of parenting.

Can those midwives who are mothers admit to women that they have at times been a 'good', even 'wonderful', mother but at other times their skills as a mother left a lot to be desired and most of the time their abilities are 'satisfactory'? Can we admit that while we always love our children, there are days when we do not like them very much? Discuss the realities of parenting with your colleagues, get it out in the open, you may be surprised to find that 'supermum' has problems too!

Being a parent can be the most frustrating, stressful, unrewarding job in the world, but it is also the most enjoyable and rewarding job you could ever want. Those of us who are fortunate enough to take on this role (and there are many who cannot), should equip themselves with some of the skills necessary to carry it out. We don't have to apply for the post, or be interviewed before we are accepted as parents, yet parenthood is a great responsibility that lasts a lifetime. It is not a role that you can easily resign from if you find you do not like it!

Only by having realistic expectations of what they are letting themselves in for, can women empower themselves to carry out the role to the best of their ability, and avoid unnecessary heartache and worry. Mothers cannot and do not have to be 'perfect' all the time.

REFERENCES

1 Price J. Motherhood: What it does to your mind. London: Pandora Press, 1988.
2 Di Matteo MR, Khan KL, Barry SH. Narratives of birth and the postpartum analysis of the focus group responses of new mothers. Birth, 1993; 20(4): 204-11.
3 Clement S. Listening visits in pregnancy: A strategy for preventing postnatal depression. Midwifery, 1995; 11: 75-80.
4 Holden JM. Counselling in a general practice setting: Controlled study of health visitor intervention in treatment of postnatal depression. British Medical Journal, 1989; 298: 223-6.

5 Paradice K, Postnatal depression. A normal response to motherhood. British Journal of Midwifery, 1995; 3(12): 632-5.

6 Prince J, Adam ME. Minds, Mothers and Midwives. London: Churchill Livingstone, 1978.

7 Elliot SA. Commentary on 'Childbirth as a Life Event'. Journal of Reproductive and Infant Psychology, 1990; 8: 147-59.

8 McKay S. Communication and Motherhood. Midwives, 1997; 110(1,312): 122-4.

Nine women, nine months, nine lives

Delivering psychology into our preparation for parenthood

Sandra L Wheatley

Over the last six years I have worked on a variety of research projects exploring the emotions it is both usual and unusual to feel when becoming a mother for the first time. Over the years our multi-disciplinary team has included obstetricians, occupational therapists, community mental health nurses, psychiatrists and epidemiologists amongst many others. This somewhat diverse mixture of clinicians, nurse practitioners and academics has stood us in good stead. The most well-known part of our work in the area is the ongoing 'Preparing for Parenthood' research project.

Preparing for Parenthood attempted to reduce the likelihood of postnatal depression occurring by encouraging first-time mothers-to-be to come along to an antenatal course of classes. During these classes – which were held six weeks earlier than the standard antenatal parentcraft classes so that the women did not feel they had to choose between the two – various life skills were addressed. For example, these included assessing and developing:

- The physical and emotional support they had available to them now and how they expected that would change over time when the baby arrived – preparing themselves for the best and worst case scenarios in advance so that they did not feel let down because their expectations of others were unrealistic and could not be met
- How they currently dealt with problems (relationships, housing, money) and just how good they were at helping themselves to overcome difficulties – learning new coping skills and not always to attempt to cope alone, or alternatively, not always to rely on others (most often partners and parents) to solve problems
- What they knew about emotional changes around the time of having a first baby and whether they would know if what they felt was unusual – if that did arise, informing them about where to go, who to see and what would happen to them if they went for some extra help.

The essential aim of the Preparing for Parenthood course was to help the women to empower themselves – not to do it for them. The research I describe below, and the focus of this article, was initiated due primarily to my own embarrassment at discovering that women's real-life experiences of pregnancy and motherhood are rarely reported. When I was asked by the pregnant women attending the course to recommend an honest, balanced book to read I had very little to offer them!

Fact finding

In order to attempt to rectify this apparent oversight, I recently spoke to nine women from Leicestershire about their experiences of having their first child; qualitative interviews with the nine randomly chosen individuals were completed shortly after their first child was one year old.

Basically, the qualitative interviews consisted of me going to see them at home, having a cup of tea or two (or three) and a chat with the tape recorder running. Rocket science this is not.

To ensure some common ground between the women I had a set of questions I asked of everyone, but the direction that our conversation took us was very much determined by their individual experiences. These recorded conversations were then transcribed by myself and analysed using the grounded theory technique.

From the moment they saw the blue line on the pregnancy test up until their child's first birthday I asked them what they had expected to happen and how they had expected to feel. I also asked them what had actually happened and how they had actually felt. The two did not always match up – for better or for worse.

A varied sample

Just to give you a feel for the nine women who participated in this research, they were from nine very varied backgrounds, besides culture. They ranged from 17 to 31 years old when discovering they were pregnant. One was undergoing fertility treatment, six had not planned to get pregnant at the time. Some were married, one was single, most worked, several wanted to return to work after the baby was born, and many changed their minds when the time came. Some were terrified of the birth, others couldn't wait to have as many children as possible. Several of them felt let down by their partner, a few couldn't speak of him highly enough.

None of them encountered postnatal depression but all of them had very real ups and downs and all of their experiences came under the umbrella of 'normal' – although I personally prefer to think of them as more or less 'not unusual'.

Unrealistic expectations

One of the most concerning findings was that the nine women felt, with the benefit of hindsight, that far too little information was given to them about what to expect to feel when they had their first child. Little wonder that their ideas of motherhood and their actual experiences of motherhood did not always match up!

Many of them were amazed to find that the first few months of motherhood were a time of mixed emotions. The joy of having the baby they had been carrying for nine months in their arms at last, was often combined with the everyday worries of meeting the needs of this little, but very loud stranger, who hadn't had the courtesy to arrive with a set of instructions!

Quite simply, they had not expected this extreme combination of intense happiness and desperate frustration, nor the disproportionate ratio of (too) little up to largely down. They recounted how relatives, friends and, most shockingly, health professionals, including midwives and health visitors, often continued to perpetuate the image of the mother as a woman who is truly fulfilled. They all had times when they did not feel fulfilled. At those times they felt exhausted and betrayed.

Feeding back to the professionals

A couple of months ago these findings were presented to a group of health professionals and academics from the local area. Unsurprisingly there was quite a heated debate about the roles and the difficulties that those at the coalface – the midwives, GPs, and health visitors in the main – have in treading the tightrope of informing and empowering pregnant women without propelling unnecessary panic and fear through the veins of the public at large. A very tricky balancing act if ever there was one. And yet many of those present felt they had not been trained to walk this line, nor had they any great confidence in what they practised on a day-to-day basis. For those that had had children, having their own experiences (and having made their own mistakes) was felt to not necessarily be enough of a base to draw upon.

Several wailed 'We do tell them – we do really!' – but 'they just don't listen – they don't want to know about the difficult bits!' We all unanimously agreed that this is, quite simply, human nature. After all, it's much easier (not to mention nicer) to talk about the wonderful things that happen when you have had your first child and how great you feel – for both the talker and the listener.

However, we could not distance ourselves from the fact that part of the health professional's role is portraying a balanced picture of how day-to-day life is likely to change so that an individual does not feel shocked or out of their depth when the baby arrives. This means the health professionals involved in a woman's care feeling comfortable and confident when talking about the range of emotions it is usual to feel when going through the transition to motherhood.

So what to do?

How to help the expectant woman hear that 'forewarned is forearmed' became quite a focus of our discussion and has continued to do so since. To try and inject some psychology into the non-perpetuation of the 'Myth of Motherhood', meetings were subsequently arranged, open to all health professionals including health visitors, community midwives, community mental health nurses and social workers. Our exchanges of ideas have resulted in some very positive actions already!

One thing we came up with was that a small change in the way that information is presented to a pregnant woman and her partner can make a huge difference in helping them to be realistic about life as a parent. Instead of not mentioning the fact that many people have selective hearing when it comes to the realities of parenting, go out of your way to mention it!

In general, somebody telling us 'the majority of people tend not to take in or remember what I am about to say...' makes us feel like we want to be different from the crowd. We sit up and listen to prove the other person wrong – 'other people may not remember but I will!' Try it, and watch the flicker in the other person's eyes!

In addition, the book I have written presenting the findings of the research into these nine women's expectations and their actual experiences of pregnancy, birth and early motherhood entitled *Nine women, nine months, nine lives*, is now being utilised in a variety of settings.

Midwives are using it as a teaching tool in parentcraft classes, to illustrate the many different emotions (both positive and negative) women feel as mothers.

Health visitors are using it as a catalyst to begin relaxed and honest discussions within new mum groups, and social workers involved with pregnant women and families with infant(s) currently experiencing social difficulties have also reported that the book is useful.

Not to mention its recommendation as a useful wider reading text for student nurses, midwives and doctors – incredibly this has also extended to mainland Europe!

One local health visitor has attempted to stimulate discussion about expectations of motherhood at her new mums group by getting mums to write a job description for the post of 'Full-time Mother – no experience necessary'. She asks participants to reflect back on what they would have written before having their baby and compare it with what they now know. This encourages the individuals themselves to realise that their expectations were unrealistic – a similar use of psychology to the way that the women who attended the Preparing for Parenthood course were empowered. The facilitator reminds the mothers of the changes they have weathered in the last twelve months, and points out that it is likely that there will be just as many challenges in the coming twelve months – some of which they will cope well with and some of which they won't.

Realisation is always best followed up with reassurance. Each new mum realises that she is not alone in having had unrealistic expectations, and this often acts as a catalyst to discussion – the health visitor may have to risk unpopularity when the meeting and discussion has to come to an end!

Stories and reflection

SECTION CONTENTS

This final section needs little introduction; it is primarily a compilation of the kinds of anecdotes, stories and reflection, which midwives have always used to share their experience and wisdom. I think it is sad that the term 'anecdotal evidence' is often used in a negative way, to differentiate women's and midwives' subjective, experiential knowledge from the more scientific kind (although whether medical research can be termed scientific, and whether science is the best way of gathering knowledge are both highly debatable points). I have probably learned more from midwives' anecdotes than from any textbook which lays out 'the rules' of how birth and midwifery should be – which, of course, are there to be broken, disproved and generally mown over by the incredible mysteries of nature and women's and baby's bodies.

In here, you will find midwives' and women's stories about how it is to be a woman, a midwife and a student midwife. Pam Connellan reflects on information found in a book her grandmother owned, while Lorna Davies, having experienced both, considers whether being in labour and running a marathon really are similar experiences. Nessa McHugh has written an original article to complement this section, exploring the different ways in which we 'know', and looking in depth at narratives, and Susan Battersby and Ruth Deery consider some of the issues surrounding the use of listening, communication and research skills in hearing the voices of women in research and practice. In this volume the last word belongs to Jane Bowler, who has recently moved on from her post as Managing Editor of *The Practising Midwife*, where she helped many midwives to get their voices 'heard' in print.

Telling the tales and stirring the tea

Nessa McHugh

'She laughed a midwife's laugh,
Thick with birth jokes, coated with the dirt of centuries.'[1]
(From *Labour Day*, by Angela Cooke)

What makes a midwife a midwife? Of course it is undertaking and passing a recognised programme and being admitted to the relevant part of the NMC register; but that only tells you about part of the mechanism of professional regulation and control. It says nothing about the culture, passions, beliefs and struggles of modern midwifery. More importantly, it says nothing about how midwives perceive themselves and how as a social subgroup we have evolved a unique knowledge base and identity, both of which are constantly under threat in terms of changing professional role and the identification of what is real knowledge.

Concepts of authoritative and legitimate knowledge are pivotal in understanding how we identify ourselves as midwives and knowledgeable practitioners.

Key point: How do we grade evidence and whose evidence do we choose to consider?

The acknowledgement that these concepts have not remained fixed throughout the history of the midwifery profession is central in understanding the contemporary challenges faced by modern midwifery.

The changing dynamics of valued knowledge, of who are the knowers and who are the doers, places midwifery and childbirth in a unique position which reflects the politicisation and gendering of knowledge. The control of birth knowledge both in terms of those women who give birth, and those women who support them, offers crucial insights into the places occupied by women within social structures. For a woman, giving birth is a form of interconnection both with herself, her child and with the experiences of generations of women before her. As midwives we also navigate those connections, both in cultural, spiritual, emotional and knowledge-based terms. Where it is perceived as negative we talk about work-based gossip and subliminal reinforcement of stereotypes.

'For many women being a mother as well as having a woman as a mother provides a profound experience of human connection. That adult experiences as well as childhood experiences contribute to the evolution of a sense of connection is consistent with our observations that connectedness with others is one of the most complicated human achievements, requiring a high level of development.'[2]

Until the emergence of the last wave of feminism in the late twentieth century it would have been impossible to consider that there are many ways of knowing something and that there are just as many ways of learning about something. It would also have been inconceivable that there may be a gender bias in the ways in which knowledge is ranked and acquired.

As a midwife I believe that there have always been differing ways in which midwives have expressed and passed on their knowledge. We might have called it 'sitting with Nellie', recognising that we learnt by observation and action. Now we have adopted the mentorship system. It all means the same thing – that a crucial part of receiving knowledge is to work with someone who is skilled and experienced. However, when we think about learning the job, what exactly are we learning? The anecdotes or stories that are shared between a midwife and her student or between colleagues also ensures that a belief system is passed on and a shared way of being comes into existence. Where this is recognised as having a huge impact on the growth and development of the profession we talk about apprenticeship and the embracing of interactive, situational learning.

'When I hear a midwife say to someone "I'll make a midwife of you yet" there is an ever present pride in the accomplishment of teaching someone an acceptable standard of practice but also

the underlying idea of a distinctive way of being, behaving and knowing.' (Personal Communication 2003)

It has been proposed amongst some feminist theorists that the acquisition of knowledge is a gendered activity and that historically women shared and passed on knowledge in ways that were fundamentally different to those ways used by the dominant masculinist traditions. Cheek and Rudge[3] have highlighted how the failure to acknowledge personal and subjective knowledge has acted as a way of devaluing a rich source of experience and skills.

When I decided to become a midwife, my mother told me that my Gran would have been so proud, if only she was alive to see me. I never knew my grandmother was a midwife, let alone that she moved from house to house around Ireland delivering babies. What tales she could have told me, I never knew until it was too late, and her stories remain untold because no one else was interested. Perhaps we might have disagreed about aspects of practice but I would have delighted in listening to her experiences and comparing them with my own.

Stories and narratives can give us a connection to both our personal and collective pasts. A story grows in the telling and can take on an identity of its own. Oral history traditions rely on the transmission of knowledge through the retelling of stories because they pass on a sense of continuity through shared knowledge and shared beliefs. In the end the minute factual accuracy of the story becomes less important than the shared perspectives and ways of viewing the world.

Key point: How do you determine fact and fiction? What do we learn from fictional sources of information such as poems, folk stories and novels?

Narratives can give us a different kind of knowledge. A narrative is in effect a story told in the first person. To listen to someone tell their own story is to gain a window into their world. To take the time to listen to someone and understand that what he or she has to say is valid and authoritative, and is to recognise his or her importance as an individual. It is recognising the difference between a life event and a set of signs and symptoms. In listening to someone narrate their experiences we take part in an age old tradition of storytelling which has implications far beyond a sentimental connection with the past. We move beyond the objective reporting of events and partake of the deeper emotional, social and spiritual significance those events have for the person who experienced them. In applying narrative knowledge to clinical practice we have the experiences/narrative of the woman leading the care she receives. So in an equilineal approach her experiences are part of the history that is recorded, lead

the treatment decisions that may need to be made and consequently inform the knowledge base of those who enter into a caring/supportive or healing dialogue with her. The woman is not the passive recipient of controlled received knowledge.

Key point: What do you see written about clients in their hand held notes? What does this tell you about the woman's experience of pregnancy as opposed to the health professionals' perspective on her pregnancy?

From Table 9.1.1 it is possible to see how western authoritative knowledge has been dominated by a defined perspective. The search for truth and evidence are important both in terms of clinical practice and terms of collective and individual development. Unfortunately when that perspective is confined to a limited philosophical perspective then the impact on participants and recipients can become distorted. There are many well documented accounts of why childbirth has become so medically controlled.

'In the field of midwifery the confiscation of women's knowledge was evident in the ways in which barber surgeons and physicians gained knowledge of childbirth, first through the observation of midwives practices, then confiscated this knowledge for their own.' [4]

Medical care is commonly seen as expert and authoritative, regardless of evidence base or need.[5,6] Women are still seen as needing professional advice to protect them from the scare mongering of other women and mothers (malicious gossips with wagging tongues!). Subliminally, we hold onto the belief that only medical intervention can ensure that a woman has a safe outcome. Kirkham[7] observed that in the earlier editions of the highly influential medical text *The Active Management of Labour* [8] it was stated that the recounted experience of multiparous women was seen as a real threat to their view of labour.

Despite the 1902 Midwifery Act, which ensured the legality of midwifery as a separate profession, historically midwifery education was often run by people who had a nursing or medical orientation; it would be very naive to assume that midwifery education is no longer under such threats. Lose control of your education and you lose control of your profession.

Women's stories are dangerous because they might show another way of knowing, might instil the ability to fight, but what of midwives' stories?

How do midwives learn the difference between midwifery knowledge and medical knowledge? Textbooks often reiterate a medically defined agenda. Until 1902 there was little, if any, education for midwives; historically, midwives as women had been barred from educational institutions and the majority of them were far

Table 9.1.1 Traditional Dominant Western Knowledge Forms versus Narrative Knowledge Forms

Traditional dominant Western Knowledge Forms	Purpose	Narrative Knowledge Forms	Purpose
Hard facts	The need to determine irrefutable truth which is a fixed concept	Interpretative	The recognition that truth is not fixed and subjective
Quantative	Repetition of facts establish reliability	Qualitative	Information is dependent on lived experiences and these are a valid form of insight and knowledge
Reductionist	Reduce an object/concept to its component parts in order to understand it	Contextual	Knowledge needs to be seen as a relative concept and that to reduce lived experience into small units of knowledge misses the experiential wholeness
Positivist	True knowledge is based only on that which can be perceived	Perspective	There are many layers of perception. We can only perceive an aspect of truth at any one time and our perceptions are coloured by our experiences
Controlled	Knowledge is a form of power and as such access is limited by gatekeepers	Connection	We are all experts in our own experiences and the gateway to knowledge is through interconnection and recognition of the validity of others
Patrilineal	Institutions of the state operate under predominantly masculinist traditions, which dictate the gatekeepers. The politics of the system are gendered, so gatekeepers may be female but fail to see the gendered imbalances of control and knowledge	Equilineal	Systems of knowledge are synthesised to allow context and validity to develop into an effective knowledge base. The experiential account is recognised as informing the objective account and both are blended together to enable access and validity

Figure 9.1.1 Qualitative educational gains from narrative-based forms of learning

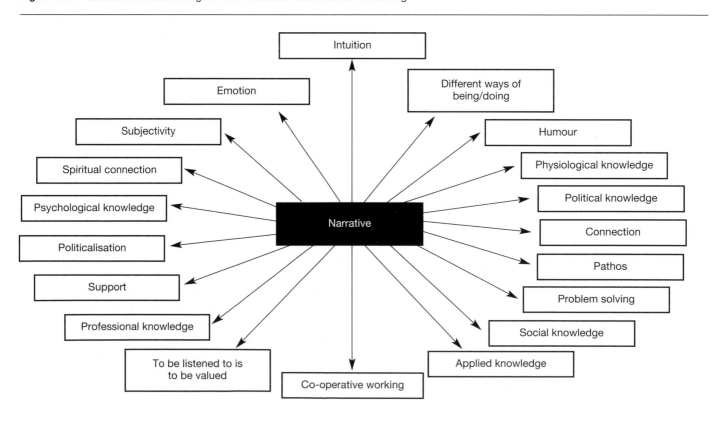

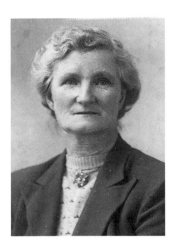

Figure 9.1.2 The author's grandmother, Anne Stacey, was also a midwife

too impoverished, illiterate and isolated to even contemplate accessing whatever formal education was available to them.[9] For the reasons already stated, and for the fact that midwives were women, the propaganda of the ignorant and dangerous midwife began to take hold.

In Europe, the women who were called to attend the birth of women were known as gossips, and when a child was being brought to church for the christening the midwife took her place with the gossips. The gossips are thought to have served a number of purposes. Firstly, they would often be the women who had whatever birth expertise was available, women who had given birth themselves or attended many births. They would also be the women who acted as a support to the labouring woman, talking and distracting, talking and encouraging and sometimes, even terrifying her. The midwives, whoever they were, would have knowledge of many births and also of deaths. It has been suggested that the women who attended birth also knew some methods of abortion.[10] The *Malleus Maleficarum*[11] detailed the tortures of the witch trials and places midwives under particular suspicion: midwives were thought to surpass all others in their wickedness. The only real way to gain knowledge was through attending births, but the association with birth was not valued and at certain times in the history of midwifery, midwives were themselves put under suspicion and in danger.

Midwifery survived in Britain but the price of survival was a large degree of control by the medical profession; midwives internalised the dominant knowledge base whilst seeming to forget their own origins. We are left with a legacy of dismissing old wives' tales and stories as subjective, unscientific and – the new axiom – not evidence-based.

However, as we recognise the struggles to maintain our own practice base and as we metamorphose into an educated rather than a trained profession, the possibilities are opening up to us. Reflectivity and reflexivity are now an established part of our professional identity. When we

work in a truly woman-orientated way we listen to the women who are our clients. If we embrace feminist principles of knowledge and education then we value the prior knowledge and experiences of those people who chose to become midwives. A feminist approach to knowledge is about interconnection and relational knowledge which alters the way we think about ourselves as knowledgeable and how we view the people that we work with and work for. This has moved us away from an imposed reliance upon orthodox models of education and medicine. It would be good to think that we had re-remembered the importance of being amongst the gossips! We are reaching the stage where we recognise that gossip or story telling has a history and as such is a legitimate form of authoritative knowledge.

Lave and Wenger[12] recognise the importance of situational learning and the absorption of culture, it can be argued that a pivotal part of that culture is the sharing of information. The stories that I hear as a midwife from other midwives and women have informed me more fully than the content of text books, because they represent a way of looking at birth that is not disembodied and that is embodied in a way of being.

'Participation in the cultural practice in which any knowledge exists is an epistemological principle of learning. The social structure of this practice, its power relations, and its conditions for legitimacy define possibilities for learning.... Conflict is worked out through a shared everyday practice in which differing viewpoints and common stakes are in play.'[11]

Curtis[13] observes that through the use of storytelling midwives are able to reconstruct our perception of midwifery and remove the bogeyman (woman) image foisted onto us by other groups. James[14] debates the issue of confidentiality in practice and the dilemma of working to a feminist ethic or a biomedical ethic. Which approach supports the woman and the midwife? James argues that the feminist approach to stories and friendship absorbs and reclaims the image of gossip and recognises the value of eliminating the autonomy – paternalistic dichotomy and claims the importance of creating community and identity.

'If I do not facilitate ... connections to others, both in actual connections and in the telling ... of stories am I cutting off a valuable source of information and positioning myself in the seat of power in terms of this information.'[14]

Using stories to pass on knowledge is a valuable way of passing on fading skills and reclaiming them. It is also crucial in focusing on who is the centre of that story, not the midwife but the woman and re-learning that a gossip was a support and a midwife was with woman. If we are to be woman-centred then we must look to our stories and value them and the women in them.

'So I'm letting out one a' my secrets. I don't want to bury 'em. There's so much that I don't want to die with. Not sharing it with somebody.'[15]

REFERENCES

1. Cooke A. Labour Day. In: Palmeira R (Ed). In the Gold of Flesh. London: Women's Press; 1990 p86
2. Field Belenky M, McVicker Clinchy B, Rule Goldberger N, Mattuck Turule J. Women's Ways of Knowing: The development of self, voice and mind. New York: Basic Books; 1997
3. Cheek J, Rudge T. Been there, done that? Consciuos Raising, Critical Theory and Nurses. Contemporary Nurse, 1994; 3: 58-63
4. Davies D. Embracing the Past, Understanding the Present, Creating the Future. NZ College of Midwives Journal 1999; 20: 5- 10
5. Donnison J. Midwives and Medical Men. London: Historical Publications; 1988
6. Oakley A. The Captured Womb: Towards sociology of childbirth. Oxford: Martin Robertson;1984
7. Kirkham M. Stories and Birth. In: Kirkham M and Perkins E. (Eds) Reflections on Midwifery. London: Bailliere Tindall; 1997.
8. O'Driscoll K, Meager D. Active Management of Labour. London: WB Saunders; 1980
9. Acterberg J. Woman as Healer. Dorset: Shambhala; 1990
10. Chamberlain M. Old Wives Tales: Their history, remedies and spells. London: Virago Press; 1981
11. Sprenger and Kramer (1486). Cited in: Acterberg J. Woman as Healer. Dorset: Shambhala; 1990
12. Lave J, Wenger E. Situated Learning. Cambridge: Cambridge University Press; 1991
13. Curtis P. Supervision in clinical practice. In: Butterworth T, Faugier J. (Eds) Clinical supervision and mentorship in nursing. London: Chapman and Hall; 1992
14. James S. Gossip, Stories and Friendship: Confidentiality in midwifery practice. Nursing Ethics 1995; 2:295-302.
15. Onnie Lee Logan. Cited in: Clark K. Motherwit: An Alabama Midwife's Story. New York: EP Dutton; 1989

Midwifery and research

Comparable skills in listening and the use of language

Susan Battersby, Ruth Deery

The importance of research in midwifery is widely recognised with the move towards a profession that is evidence-based. (Sandall, 1998). The foundations for policies, procedures and guidelines have mainly arisen from quantitative research, especially in the form of randomised controlled trials (RCTs) (NHS, 1996). The NHS Executive in 1996 stated that only recommendations based on RCTs should be used in contract setting (NHS, 1996).

With these recommendations there is a risk of elevating the importance of quantitative research to the detriment of qualitative research. It is important to recognise that practice can be enlightened by giving equal recognition to qualitative research methods.

Communication is an area that is amenable to qualitative research methodology and is an area that has been increasingly highlighted in Changing Childbirth (DoH, 1993), Making a Difference (DoH, 1999) and The NHS Plan (DoH, 2000) as an important aspect of midwifery care. This reinforces the significance of the midwife-mother relationship as fundamental to midwifery practice where the midwife constantly works within a cycle of interactions with women and their families, doctors, colleagues and researchers. This paper will therefore focus on communications within midwifery and on the qualitative aspects of research that can assist, build on and develop good communication skills as a necessary part of midwifery care.

The art of communication

The art of communication is based on a reciprocal process of sharing information and knowledge between two people (Kirkham, 2000) and is complex and multifaceted. The NHS Plan not only highlighted the importance of good communications but also recommended inter-professional collaboration (DoH, 2000). As two researchers who have encountered barriers to communication when conducting qualitative interviews we recognised the parallels between communications in the interviewing process and midwifery practice, and believe that sharing midwifery knowledge with other professions and vice versa can help to enhance and develop professional practice.

Interview or inter view?

The initial antenatal interview has been criticised for its task oriented approach which has been adopted by many midwives in order to complete what would appear to have become nothing more than a checklist within restricted time parameters (Methven, 1989). This may have resulted in midwives bombarding questions at women and expecting, and getting nothing more than, monosyllabic responses. The woman may then feel that she has not been listened to. When discussing interviewing within qualitative research Kvale (1996) states that 'an interview is literally an inter view, an interchange of views between two persons conversing about a common theme' (pp 44). Further to this Oakley (1981) emphasises the conversational nature of research interviews and that they should not be sterile, one way communication processes. Richens (1999) argues that in our quest for evidence-based practice we now turn to policies and protocols to inform our care, often forgetting that the woman herself is a valuable source of evidence.

Risk management

Our listening skills as midwives have been further undermined by the advent of risk management. Pregnancy and childbirth will always carry the possibility of unexpected and unwanted outcomes. This has led to high litigation rates in maternity units with management seeking ways to reduce this cost. The introduction of risk management as a systematic process to identify, analyse, evaluate and correct both potential and actual risk (DoH, 1994) has been utilised to this end. However, Aslam (1999) argues that enhancement of client care should be the principal driving force of risk management not the reduction of litigation.

Unfortunately risk management has led to an increase in documentation which has reduced the time that the midwife can spend with women. It has also regimented midwifery practice with an increase of policies and protocols that can reduce the value of the woman's contribution to her individual plan of care.

Learning to listen

Both the midwife and the researcher need to acknowledge the importance of facilitating women to 'tell their own stories' when probing for information in order to plan care or collect data. Listening is a crucial element within the research interview and is also fundamental to the midwife-mother relationship (Kirkham, 1994). Midwives might like to consider the fact that when listening to the women they care for skills are utilised that are similar to those of the researcher. Developing an understanding of these skills can enhance the development of the midwife-mother relationship.

Again the initial antenatal interview provides a good example. The purpose of this interview is to gain knowledge of the mother's medical, social and psychological needs and to try and ensure that the foundation for a partnership in care is initiated. However, the midwife undertaking the interview may feel that it was the risk assessment component of the interview that was the dominating factor rather than the woman's individualised needs and anxieties. Likewise a researcher may have had a situation where they thought they were 'leading' the interview. This may result from an interviewee or interviewer feeling muted or silenced because of a perceived unequal partnership. These situations arise even though the researcher or midwife may not intend their voice to override that of the woman or interviewee; rather the purpose in both these scenarios is to facilitate the woman or interviewee to tell their story.

Hitchcock and Hughes (1995) state that when undertaking interviews the researcher must recognise the influence of a variety of social, cultural, institutional and linguistic factors. The same principles apply to midwives who are striving to provide woman-centred care that takes into account the woman's social, psychological and cultural needs. This emphasises the fact that childbirth extends beyond medical considerations.

This is very pertinent at the present time when there is a growing body of knowledge and increasing awareness of issues surrounding domestic violence and sexual abuse (Price & Baird, 2001). It is only by developing ways that enable women to disclose and inform midwives of these issues that information can be gained to facilitate the women to share their experiences and difficulties. Perhaps by listening and tuning in to women and enabling them to tell their stories midwives can develop intuitive knowledge of the women they care for. This would help midwives to perceive the woman individually rather than 'just another pregnancy.'

Overbearing attitudes

Other barriers can arise to prevent women telling their stories, such as the midwife being seen by women as the holder of an authoritative knowledge base on childbirth. Battersby (2000) highlights this dilemma within the field of breastfeeding where women feel they are being coerced by midwives and health professionals into a feeding method contrary to their wishes. Within midwifery practice today the midwife no longer needs to be viewed as holding superior, authoritative knowledge but rather a partner in care provision whose knowledge base runs parallel with the woman's own knowledge base.

On reflection this devaluing and non acceptance of each others' knowledge base might well stem from past styles of education, which has exposed midwives and women to didactic and authoritarian styles of teaching where the teacher was always right.

To enable partnerships to develop between women and midwives, and interviewers and interviewees the language used must be acceptable to both parties. If this is not undertaken then again barriers to communication can arise. Hitchcock and Hughes (1995) state that if the interviewer concentrates on the 'words, phrases and idioms,' (p169) within an interview then the interview becomes more meaningful. It enables the researcher to concentrate on the conversational aspects of interviewing and not on the technical issues which can so often mask the linguistic style of the interview (Mishler, 1991). We need to make sure that the terminology used within midwife mother interactions facilitates the woman to take control of her own health by making her own choices about her health care.

Medicalisation of language

Miller (1973) states that language is '... by all odds the most subtle and powerful technique we have for controlling other people.' The language used by midwives is intrinsically linked with the use of medical definitions applied to midwifery care and this again is linked with the authoritative knowledge base of the profession. It can be argued that obstetricians have created a power base that has subsequently allowed them to control childbirth. Midwives have accepted and utilised the obstetricians' knowledge and language, and have therefore been granted power over childbearing women (Shirley & Mander, 1996) through the obstetricians.

Within research, a different vocabulary has emerged that can enable the researcher to hold power over the interviewee. It would seem sensible to all concerned to value each other's knowledge whilst at the same time developing a shared vocabulary that is comprehensible to all concerned. Within midwifery this will be even more important in the future when any letters written between health professionals regarding clients will be copied to them (DoH, 2000). Clearly midwives need to develop an awareness of the way in which they interact with their clients (Deery, 1999), as doing this inappropriately can leave long lasting impressions on the mothers and their family which can impinge on future childbearing and the wider health agenda (RCM, 2000).

In conclusion it can be seen that there are clear parallels between how the midwife and the researcher need to listen and use appropriate language within their respective fields. Communication is identified throughout the literature as being of paramount importance to the midwife/mother relationship.

Listening is an important skill that needs to be used effectively by midwives to facilitate women telling their stories; likewise the researcher needs to use the same skills to enable the interviewee to tell their story.

Language has been identified as a barrier to communications. Having a mutually acceptable language base for communications can help to reduce the power differentials between midwives, researchers and woman. Sharing knowledge from different disciplines has highlighted within this paper is just one of many ways in which communication awareness can be developed.

REFERENCES

Aslam R. 1999. Risk management in midwifery practice. Br J Midwifery, 7(1), 41-4

Battersby S. 2000. Breastfeeding and Bullying: Who's putting the pressure on? The Practising Midwife, 3(8), 36-8

Deery R. 1999. Improving Relationships through Clinical Supervision: Part 1. Br J Midwifery, 7(3), 160-3

Department of Health. 1993. Changing Childbirth, Part 1. Report of the Expert Maternity Group. London: HMSO

Department of Health. 1994. Risk Management in the NHS. Leeds: NHS Executive

Department of Health. 1999. Making a Difference: Strengthening the nursing, midwifery and health visiting contribution to health and healthcare. London: HMSO

Department of Health. 2000. The NHS Plan: A plan for investment, a plan for reform. London: HMSO

Hitchcock G, Hughes D. 1995. Research and the Teacher: A qualitative introduction to school-based research. 2nd Edition. London: Routledge

Kirkham M. 1994. Research skills as midwifery practice skills. Br J Midwifery, 2(8), 390-2

Kirkham M. 2000. The Midwife Mother Relationship. Basingstoke: Macmillan

Kvale S. 1996. InterViews. An Introduction to Qualitative Research Interviewing. London: Sage Publications

Methven RC. 1989. Recording an obstetric history or relating to pregnant women? A study of the antenatal booking interview. In Midwives, Research and Childbirth. Vol 1, eds S Robinson & AM Thomson. London: Chapman and Hall

Miller GA. 1973. Communication, Language and Meaning. London: Basic Books. Cited in Shirley KE, Mander R. 1996. The Power of Language. Br J Midwifery, 4(6), 298-300 & 317-18

Mishler EG. 1991. Research Interviewing: Context and narrative. London: Harvard University Press

NHS Executive. 1996. Clinical Guidelines. London: HMSO

Oakley A. Interviewing women: A contradiction in terms. 1981. In: Doing Feminist Research, Ed H Roberts. London: Routledge & Kegan Paul

Price S, Baird K. 2001. Domestic Violence in Pregnancy. The Practising Midwife, 1(7), 12-14

Richens Y. 1999 Listening to mothers: Improving evidence-based practice. Br J Midwifery, 7(11), 670

Royal College of Midwives. 2000. Midwifery Practice in the Postnatal Period: Recommendations for Practice. London: RCM

Sandall J. 1998. Bridging the gap between evidence and practice. Br J Midwifery, 6(10), 624-6

Shirley KE, Mander R. 1996. The Power of Language. Br J Midwifery, 4(6), 298-300 & 317-18

For midwifery care, choose a midwife!

Virginia Howes

A pregnant woman does not have to see her GP. When a woman becomes my client, I always write a polite, professional letter to her GP introducing myself, and inviting them to be supportive in the client's choices. I have yet to receive a polite reply! One GP stated that his patient is foolhardy in her choice of home birth and that maybe if she wants support she should look elsewhere for a GP! Another refused a client any antenatal blood tests unless she booked with 'his' midwives. Eventually I had to ask the local Supervisor of Midwives to intervene.

Libby

Libby booked my care at 16 weeks. She had had an early bleed at 10 weeks. I was appalled that her GP had vaginally examined her during the bleed, but it was done, and having discussed the issue with the NHS community midwife based at the surgery, we felt that we could move on with Libby's care. At 30 weeks, Libby had the tiniest spot of pale blood. After establishing the wellbeing of both baby and Libby we both felt that there was no need to investigate further as long as there was no more bleeding. Libby wanted a rest from work and visited her doctor for a sick certificate. Libby told the doctor that her midwife had no concerns about the pregnancy. The doctor palpated Libby and told her that her baby's head was low, that the baby was 'stressed' and wanted to be born! He refused to give Libby a sick certificate unless she went the next day to the hospital for a scan. Libby telephoned me, upset and worried for her baby, certain that labour was imminent. But no one can put their hands on a soft, normal abdomen and claim to feel a stressed baby or imminent birth. Given her early, threatened miscarriage, Libby had had quite a few scans. I told her that repeated scans should be kept to a minimum. But Libby needed a reassuring scan now. When she went back to her GP, proudly showing off her normal scan, the goal posts shifted. Now he was only willing to give the

certificate if he performed a vaginal examination to confirm a closed cervix. Libby later told me that although she did not want this examination and instinctively felt it was not appropriate, she felt powerless to refuse it. I told her I would support her if she made a complaint. Surely if the GP believed there was a problem, he should not have been carrying out vaginal examinations in the community with no back-up on hand? He had two professional opinions, as well as that of the pregnant woman herself, that this was a normal pregnancy. He made a little problem into a big one and put his patient at risk both physically and emotionally.

Maxine

Maxine suffered from herpes and wanted a home birth. She knew that, should she have an outbreak of blisters at the time of the birth, it was advisable to have a Caesarean section, and she wanted to avoid that. We reviewed the literature together and found that according to Enkin, a short course of Acyclovir at term reduces the incidence of an outbreak. She discussed this with her doctor who later informed her that he had taken advice and was not prepared to give her the prescription. She had a photocopy of the article and references but he was still not prepared to give the drug until she mentioned that, should she get an outbreak and need to go to hospital for a Caesarean, she just may want to sue him!

Following a lovely primip water birth, the GP phoned to tell me that the baby had physiological jaundice. When I got there, I found a pink, warm, healthy, breastfeeding newborn, but distressed parents, upset by the GP's cold, off-hand manner. Didn't she know that jaundice at less than 24 hours is not physiological – and if the baby did have it, what was she doing walking away from a sick baby? This couple's complaint was not acknowledged.

I was overjoyed when a client reported that her female GP supported her choice of a home birth, having had one herself. It was a lovely birth and Janine went on to breastfeed Robert wonderfully. At her six-week check she proudly showed off her fully breastfed baby to the GP. The GP raised the topic of bottle feeding, but Janine said: 'I couldn't give him formula, my midwife worked so hard in helping me to breastfeed well and after all it is made from cow's milk with all those added risks'. The GP replied: 'Oh, no, formula milk has many constituents but it is not cow's milk'. Please! I rest my case.

Transition

Reflections on becoming a student midwife

Anna Fielder

'No situation can become favourable until one is able to adapt to it and does not wear ...[oneself] out with mistaken resistance.' [1]

During my initial weeks and months as a student midwife I have reflected a number of times upon these words from the ancient Chinese text, the *I Ching*, for it seems to me that they express much about the nature of transition. Certainly my own transition to becoming a student midwife has been a gradual process of adaptation in which I have, and continue to, let go of certain fears and apprehensions that I have about my new role. Each time I overcome an element of resistance, I am one step closer to understanding why I have chosen midwifery and to feeling fully comfortable with that choice. The purpose of this piece of writing is not to provide a definitive account of the events that have brought me to my current place in that transitional process, but to reflect upon some aspects of my journey so far.

To start the pre-registration midwifery diploma at the University of Salford, I left my research job at a university in the north of England, where I had been working for nearly five years. Although I greatly enjoyed my time there, I needed more creativity and compassion in my 'number-crunching', 'report-writing' reality. As I spoke with friends who are midwives and delved into some classic texts on holistic, woman-centred midwifery[2,3,4] I became increasingly aware of something that I had sensed for a long time; that perhaps midwifery offered scope for a combination of art, compassion and science that escaped me in the world of academic research.

At the birth of my sister's first child my thoughts were confirmed: I watched with admiration at the calmness, warmth, clinical expertise and obvious job satisfaction of the midwives – one of whom was my mother. The birth of my niece was the most life-affirming event that I have ever had the privilege to share, and as if to demonstrate that birth and death are part of the continuous cycles of life, our grandfather passed away within days of my sister's labour. I am sure that the low-tech homebirth of my niece helped me to deal more fully with the death of my grandfather in hospital. Both played a role in encouraging me to fill in the application form for midwifery.

I feel incredibly privileged that I was offered a place on the course, that I am part of a group of what I consider to be very special student midwives, and that I am entering the profession of my dreams. Whilst observing my first normal birth as a student, not only was I filled with admiration at the mother for achieving a spontaneous birth in a comparatively medicalised environment, I was also proud of myself for having eventually taken the necessary steps to be with her for that event.

However, leaving behind my previous job has not been easy. I often find myself longing for the world of university research, where interaction is with computers or 'research subjects' and where there are ideas, concepts and numbers to work with rather than bodies, mucus, emotions and tears. It was a world that I knew, and one in which I was skilled and valued. Suddenly I am utterly unskilled again, and even the simplest tasks, like taking a blood pressure, are a challenge. Also, childbearing women do not respond in the same way as computer databases (thank goodness)! That is what I love about midwifery: working with human life on such a basic and fundamental level. Yet that is also what is so daunting for me about the job. Human life is so precious, and through midwifery it is possible to add great joy and value to that life, or on the other hand to destroy it. I am just beginning to get a sense of the responsibility that my new role will entail.

As the daughter of a midwife, I am also aware that although I have chosen her own beloved trade I must grow and develop into a midwife in my own right. How do I become a midwife who does not stand in the shade of the woman who gave birth to her; who is privileged enough to learn from that person but to also develop her own independence and confidence as an autonomous practitioner?

My partner recently suggested to me, in his ever supportive and insightful way, that perhaps I have experienced a little 'resistance' (to recall the words of the *I Ching*) to becoming a student midwife, because I am afraid of subsuming my own identity to that of my mother. Maybe he is right: as well as learning to be fully 'with woman', as a midwife I also have to learn to be fully with, and of, myself.

Ten weeks into my training, I am now closer than ever to 'feeling like', as well as actually being, a student midwife. However, becoming a student midwife has been, and still is, a process of personal as well as professional development. It is as if I am learning a whole new way of being, as well as how to become a midwife. Perhaps that is why the birth analogy seems so appropriate: after transition and great effort a baby is pushed into a new and exciting world. I am now emerging from what I feel has been an important transitional period, and I sense the anticipation as new life is waiting to be born.

REFERENCES

1 I Ching or Book of Changes. [The Richard Wilhelm translation, rendered into English by Baynes CF] London: Arkana, 1989.
2 Gaskin IM. Spiritual midwifery. Summertown, TN: The Book Publishing Company, 1977.
3 Davis E. A guide to midwifery: Heart and hands. New York: Bantam Books, 1983.
4 Flint C. Sensitive midwifery. London: Heinemann, 1986.

Having a baby is like running a marathon because...

Lorna Davies

I was introduced to this analogy by Andrea Robinson in her book *Empowering Women – Active Birth in the 1990s*, where she advocated using parallels between events in people's lives and childbirth/parenting experiences, as an activity in preparation for childbirth sessions. I later heard Michel Odent denounce the notion of comparing marathon preparation to preparing for the day of labour, reviling the idea of 'coaching' pregnant women for an event that in reality requires the relinquishing of conscious control.

In April this year, I ran the London Marathon and now, having completed both of these events, I feel that I am in a position of authority to pass comment and opinion on the similarities and differences of these two momentous occasions in life. It could be suggested that the memory of the marathon still looms larger than that of childbirth, the former completed only weeks ago, and the latter seven years ago. But as many who have given birth will agree, the years may pass but the experience retains an exceptional clarity.

In my particular case, the decision to undertake a marathon was given notably more deliberation than that of having a baby, and was made with a greater degree of informed choice. Nonetheless, I did have the full support of my partner on both occasions. It seemed however, that he, as a 'been there, run it, got the T-shirt' marathon competitor, was able to support me to a greater extent in my marathon endeavour. There was a sense of empathy which had been less obvious in labour. I always suspected that during my pregnancies he harboured a degree of uterus envy! He certainly appeared to be more sympathetic of my needs after the marathon, and informed everyone how proud he was of my achievement. After the birth of my first child, he told everyone that it was 'a piece of cake', the proverbial 'pea from a pod'.

The role of supporter would appear to me to be of equal importance in each event. The focus on the encouragement of those around you becomes increasingly significant as the toil continues, and the complete trust and belief in that support is invaluable. I remember clearly my third birth, a VBAC following a section for the second. Although my belief in my own body to achieve a normal spontaneous birth was resolute, the knowledge that those who were with me felt the same, spurred me on through labour.

Likewise, after 'hitting the wall' at eighteen or so miles during the marathon, the momentum of the crowd calling my name (emblazoned across my chest as advocated by seasoned marathon vets) and willing me to complete, became my raison d'etre.

Transition

The point at which the support of the crowd became so significant can be compared to transition in labour. The enormity of the task in hand was almost too much to bear. If my partner had deigned to run with me, I probably would have been blaming him for the ills of the world at this point, from my aching thighs, to the cultural destruction of global capitalism.

A friend of mine has suggested that offering a woman an epidural at this stage in her labour is akin to offering a marathon runner a lift in a car when they hit the wall. Such temptation, I have to say, would have been great for me at that time in the event.

However, early recognition of 'the wall' brought with it the acknowledgment that my endocrine system would soon kick in and help me out. I was positively relishing the thought of the forthcoming endorphin rush, and embraced its pain-nullifying effect when it arrived. My euphoric expression, complete with extremely dilated pupils in the post-event photographs bear witness to this phenomenon.

I feel that this is a status sometimes witnessed during the early post-partum period, when the mother has been blessed with an active birth, where those around her believed in her ability to birth her baby, and didn't interfere with the process. It is the look that proclaims 'We did it ourselves'.

Nutrition

There are some interesting similarities in the nutritional requirements for marathon running and labouring women. The 'carbo loading' encouraged in the weeks running up to the marathon prepares the runner to store quantities of carbohydrate to utilise when the glycogen stores deplete at around the 17-20 mile stage of the event.

The average marathon runner will have used somewhere between 2000 and 3500 calories during the race by this stage. It is believed that the average woman may use up to 700-1000 calories per hour whilst labouring. I spent the early part of labour feeling ravenous and wanting to eat for England, and then having to ask the midwife to kindly 'pass the sick bag, Alice' in the latter part of first stage. I could no more have eaten once in established labour than I could have abseiled down the wall of the maternity unit.

Likewise, I had made arrangements for a 'chocolate stop' at fourteen miles during the marathon, but on arrival at the rendezvous, found I really didn't really want it. However, the offer of 'Liquid Power' (a high calorie, isotonic drink) at 3-4 mile intervals was essential, and I felt made the difference between completing and not completing.

There may be a lesson to be learnt here. The solution prevented me from becoming too ketotic and provided me with essential minerals, which ensured adequate hydration. Sounds familiar as a preferred state for a labouring woman, doesn't it?

Euphoria

Crossing the finishing line and pushing my babies out also brings to mind a range of parallel encounters. The tears, the triumph, the sense of relief, the exhaustion, the pain!

I was able to share this glory with partner and friends after my babies had been born. Sadly, because of the organisational arrangements, I was unable to share the immediate post-marathon experience with anyone other than the official photographer. As I staggered along The Mall clutching my medal, I became aware that if I sat down I would never get up again. I needed my supporters, and finding them and being greeted with warmth and admiration made me feel very special in a way that I have rarely experienced since birth.

My friend who was looking after my children during the event stated that I took on the semblance of a new mother to such an extent that she felt the need to midwife me there and then. She helped me out of my sweaty apparel, into clean fresh clothes, simultaneously providing me with nourishment, though in the form of sandwiches and mineral water, not tea and toast.

Conclusion

Having associated with female runners over the course of the past few years, I am aware of their extensive knowledge of the physiological effects of running on their bodies and systems. By being so attuned they are able to utilise coping strategies to deal with the hurdles along the way. They recognise the value of preparing for running events by ensuring that their bodies are in an optimally nourished state. They recognise the value of preparing physically for the task of long gruelling runs, thus minimising the risk of injury.

How many of our labouring women really understand the physiology of birth? Do we really offer them the opportunity to discuss the physiological peaks and troughs in labour and how to adopt coping strategies that enable them to carry on? They frequently appear to have an awesome knowledge of the choices on the 'pain relief menu', yet have little faith in their own body's resources to cope.

How often do we remind the mother that nature rarely deals more than we can bear, and of the powerful effect of our own hormonal systems? Do we inform them that pain in labour has purposes, about the benefits of experiencing the power and strength of contractions?

How much value do we place on nutrition during pregnancy? Most antenatal education sessions begin at 30+ weeks when the opportunity to discuss the benefits of good nutrition have been lost.

The experience of running the marathon has given me the opportunity to reflect on what made it achievable for me, a woman with a very full life, and as described, I feel that many of those factors can be applied to the needs of a woman in labour.

Would I do it again? My midwife friend reminded me recently that my first comment on greeting her at the end of the race was 'Never again, no one told me it was going to be so hard.' Yet now, several weeks down the line, I am seriously contemplating my entry for next year, because I'm sure I could be quicker next time round!

In conclusion, I think the maxim which sums up both experiences for me, when I look at my children, and of course my marathon medal, was extolled on the T-shirt of a runner at about the 22 mile point: 'The pain will subside – but the pride lasts forever!'

Carly is sixteen

Jenny Fraser

Carly is sixteen. Last year she gave birth to a baby boy. Carly is learning disabled and spent her school years away from home during term time, at a school especially chosen for her needs. Whilst in her last year at school Carly became pregnant; the father, Gary, attended the same school.

Carly is the eldest of five girls. Her mother was very emotionally needy, having had several disastrous relationships and four different fathers for the five girls, all the relationships breaking down in bitter fashion. As Carly was the eldest she had to undertake care of the smaller children, when home, in place of her mother. Her childhood years were spent either at school or looking after her sisters and the home; she did not feel that she was ever allowed to be a child.

Carly liked Gary; she liked the care and affection he gave her. He appeared strong, capable and convincing. He made decisions. Carly felt safe in his presence, he looked out for her and at last she was not in the caring role.

Living at home

Carly had to leave school when she became pregnant and started living full-time at home again with her mother and sisters. This broke down when her mother became more and more needy of her and Carly had to spend all her time shopping, cooking, washing clothes, cleaning and getting the younger children to school; and all this whilst pregnant.

Meanwhile Gary, after Carly had left school, committed burglary in the local village, inflicting actual bodily harm on the owner of the property. He was arrested; court proceedings duly followed and he received a custodial sentence.

Carly decided to move in with her father to escape the life she was leading with her mother and sisters. Her father had lived on his own for many years and was an alcoholic. Carly was in a no-win situation within her life scenario.

The booking visit

Carly presented for her first antenatal appointment when she was 24 weeks pregnant. She looked unkempt and distracted. It was a difficult antenatal as obviously many issues needed to be addressed, the most vital being to gain her trust in order to be able to help and support her. Carly had no eye contact; she was lost in such an encounter.

Following this antenatal many parenting issues were obviously at stake:

- The assessment of Carly's mothering skills
- Her housing – living with an alcoholic father was not the best place to bring up a baby
- How would Gary respond to a new baby?
- How could some appropriate antenatal education be organised for Carly?

Initially some support for her learning disabilities was necessary as Carly could not read or write which put her at an immediate disadvantage. A phone call revealed the availability of a learning disabilities support worker.

Maggie, a qualified learning disabilities nurse, at Carly's request accompanied her to most of her antenatal consultations. Carly was particularly happy about this, as at last she had accessed some care for herself. Maggie was then able to have individual learning sessions with Carly to make sure she understood what was happening. She could also explain the many leaflets that Carly had, and undertook practical sessions such as making up feeds and changing nappies safely. This was all very important information in order for Carly to have some chance of caring for her own baby. This was obviously a wonderful support because someone knowledgeable about Carly's specific special needs was undertaking this time-consuming task.

Aggression

On one occasion Carly came to an antenatal with her

father. Her father could not read or write and could not read a message left on the door of the surgery which was informing the women of a different venue for the antenatal clinic. Carly and her father waited in the usual place and unfortunately a receptionist asked why they were waiting there and why they had not read the message. At this, Carly's father, who had been drinking prior to arrival, erupted and became very aggressive and abusive, so much so that the police had to be called to restrain him.

Carly naturally was very upset by this scenario during the antenatal. However, this untoward event led to some revelations from Carly. She confided that her father was regularly drunk and regularly hit her and she herself felt concerned about the welfare of this baby under her father's roof. Carly's vulnerability was profound. Worse still, she confessed that Gary was out of prison and visiting her. He also was showing signs of violence towards her and had also hit her.

Poor Carly, what a life, what an awful dilemma. Meanwhile Carly at 36 weeks pregnant had a small-for-dates baby, she smoked 20 cigarettes a day. An antenatal appointment was made at the hospital. An ultrasound confirmed a small baby but all else was normal. Carly found this visit daunting and confusing; she was 'told off' by midwives and doctors for her smoking habits, which distressed her. Whilst we all know the dangers of smoking on an unborn baby, in this instance it appeared that there were worse dangers in store for the baby than smoking. Carly would not go back for any further growth scans but regularly attended her antenatal appointments in the community. It is obviously difficult in a busy clinic when a woman is not known to the professional as the maternity records do not give a full and accurate picture of what life may really be like for the woman.

Physical violence

At 39 weeks of pregnancy Carly was admitted to the labour suite having been kicked and punched in her stomach. The CTG was satisfactory but Carly had bruises over her abdomen and arms. The midwives caring for Carly this day voiced their concerns and from this occasion help from Social Services was speedily mobilised because of the threat of violence towards Carly and her baby by both the baby's father and grandfather.

The domestic violence unit at the local police headquarters were involved. This specialist unit visited Carly and an alarm was fitted into the house for her to receive immediate attention if necessary.

It became evident that if she stayed living with her father then child protection concerns would be raised for the fear of physical abuse directed towards the baby. Carly's housing problems needed immediate attention; she was living in one room in her father's house.

Within a few days Carly was accommodated into 'umbrella housing'. This scheme gives young women like Carly independence with their own flat but also the security of a warden-controlled block of flats. The warden monitors visitors, and men are not allowed to stay overnight.

A fresh start

This was a wonderful new beginning for Carly; from her early hesitancy of living alone she gradually became independent and started to take pride in her surroundings. This was a vital first step and once Carly had given birth she received lots of support from midwives, Social Services and Maggie.

Carly very quickly became proficient in physically caring for her baby: this was simple compared to caring for four younger sisters, but she did find it hard initially to meet her baby's emotional needs. She would avoid eye contact and was not comfortable talking to her baby. With specialist play therapy sessions organised by Social Services Carly started to relax, began to smile again and enjoy her baby. The enhanced quality of their two-way interaction became evident.

This may or may not end up as a 'happy ever after' story, but it is a true story of positive steps that can be taken to enhance the relationship between a mother and baby and some of the steps that can be taken in order to reduce violence to women in the home.

Carly grew in strength and eventually moved to a council flat having got the measure of living alone and caring for her baby. She talks now of the dark clouds that were there for her every day without any break. Carly made the decision herself to keep her address secret from Gary and she has no contact with him. Her father does visit but only if the domestic violence unit is informed in advance.

Conclusion

This story seeks to address some of the issues of need and violence towards women, the complexities it raises for us as midwives and some of the steps that can be taken to help women in our care. Midwives must access information and mobilise support from other agencies before it is too late. Networking and specialist professionals should be used for their expertise and working together in this way pays off dividends; we cannot deal with all the issues alone. The input of all these professionals can help create a better life for these women.

The alternative scenario would have been the cost, both in money and emotions, of the child protection proceedings, the continuation of violence towards Carly and maybe the removal of her baby. This would have done no one any favours, particularly Carly.

Hospital infection
The scourge of childbirth

Prunella Briance

When I was looking for a safe place to have my first baby, many years ago, I visited a famous gynaecologist and his hospital, where everyone went. His examination couch had dirty blood marks on it – even then I knew this was wrong. In the nursery I was shocked to find about fifty babies lying side by side and a woman sloshing water over each one from a running tap using always the same cloth. The babies I saw had headless boils over their faces or bodies. At that time my ignorance of staphylococcus infection was appalling, but I retreated fast, and common sense sent me to a small maternity clinic. Later, I encountered a sad funeral cortege. A young man had lost his wife in that very hospital through a caesarean section resulting in staphyloccoccus infection. The baby boy, being cared for by his grandmother, also had headless boils all over him and one can only pray that he survived to grow up. No wonder hospital borne infections linger in my mind.

Birth, if kept mainly in the home where it was originally intended to be, would remain free of this scourge. Midwives would be restored to their rightful place in society, mothers would learn and re-learn the art and instinct of good, happy birthing and GP obstetricians would 'stand-by' which is what their name actually means and as Dr Grantly Dick-Read often said 'with their hands in their pockets, preferably'.

Back in 1956, when I founded the then Natural Childbirth Trust and then Sonia Willington founded the Association for the Prevention of Cruelty to Women in Childbirth (now AIMS) women were undoubtedly being pushed around during birth.

Nowadays things are by no means perfect. At some antenatal classes women are frightened with stories of what can go wrong, and are informed about caesarean section and various forms of pain relief. Grantly Dick-Read never found it necessary to talk about pain relief, it was always available if necessary. In his experience over 97% of healthy women given the opportunity were able to give birth without any medical interference whatsoever. His main emphasis was on the Fear-Tension-Pain syndrome and the teaching of simple relaxation and breathing techniques to overcome the anxiety associated with birth.

As regards the spread of infection; recently I noticed dirty floors being left urine-stained and only on a Sunday did a cleaner appear to polish the floor – it was never properly washed or disinfected. I have noticed carpeted wards with awful marks which should certainly be eliminated but how do you disinfect a grubby carpet without renewing it wholly? I have seen overcrowded wards with double-glazing and no fresh air. I have noticed new babies being put next to central heating or air conditioning, both an invitation to cot death through dehydration, to say nothing of the spread of sticky-eye and glue-ear.

There is much to be done and nothing to be complacent about. Obstetric skills are important, and should be available, but we should never interfere routinely with the natural process. If the mother has chosen home birth then a paramedic on a motor bike could be sent for – far better that the medical team goes to the mother than that she should undertake a hazardous journey only to deliver in the hospital carpark. If any difficulty is anticipated then the birth should be planned as if at home but in the birthing room of a maternity clinic, well away from general hospitals and their proved risk of iatrogenic infections.

Grantly Dick-Read's books should be part of the curriculum of all who deal in birth. The 5th edition of *Childbirth Without Fear* would be a good starting point. All midwifery students should know the story of Dr Ignaz Semmelweis, the Hungarian martyr who died in 1890 in proving that childbed fever was due to surgeons going from the morgue to the childbed and unwittingly infecting their patients. No one would pay attention, any more than in Grantly Dick-Read's time. Doctors were not prepared to take the time to try to understand the beauty and simplicity of natural birth, and would interfere. Semmelweis took a drastic step, he infected himself with the dreaded puerperal fever vaccine and died an agonising death. Is his name known today outside Hungary? It is for this reason that I insist that our babies would be better born away from general hospitals and I hope that someone will pay attention.

Grandma's gynaecology

Pam Connellan

Many homes have hidden in a secret place a book which is not meant to be seen by the children. I was always intrigued by a musty-smelling volume which my grandmother kept hidden in her carefully folded night-dresses, far away from curious eyes. Once I had spotted the ancient book and realised she didn't want me to see it, I was determined to investigate.

The Works of Aristotle, in Four Parts, published in 1808, had intriguing chapter headings such as 'The Experienced Midwife', 'The Secrets of Nature Displayed', and 'Of The Secret Parts of Men and Women.' This sounded useful stuff for a curious twelve-year-old, although even I wasn't so ignorant about 'Virginity; what it is; how it may be lost; and how a person may know that it is so.'

When I eventually realised that the old-fashioned letters which I had thought were F were in fact S, the pages began to make more sense. And when the section on women's anatomy taught me that 'The clitoris suffers erection and falling, stirs up lust and gives delight in copulation, for without this the fair sex neither desire nuptial embraces nor have pleasure in them', I realised why Grandma had been briskly evasive when asked to explain what the book was about.

The tone of the author is often wryly humorous: 'Though the parts of the generation in all creatures are not perhaps the most comely, in compensation of that Nature has put upon them a more abundant and far greater honour than on other parts', and he notes bluntly that even if man or woman is 'endowed with angelic countenances and the most exact symmetry and proportion of parts', if their sexual apparatus is defective in some way they will not be appealing to the opposite sex.

The essential similarities between the sex organs of men and women are expressed in rhyme:

For those that have the strictest searchers been,
Find women are but men turned outside in,

And men, if they but cast their eyes about,
May find they're women but inside out.

Having given cheer to any nineteenth-century transsexuals, the author offers full and fascinating descriptions of the sex organs including an account of how the womb functions, its blood vessels, muscles and nerve endings. I hadn't expected such detail in such an early publication.

I felt we were really getting to the nitty-gritty when the question was raised: 'At what age are young men and women capable of copulation?' The author warns that by 14 or 15, girls have spirits 'brisk and inflamed, and by eating sharp salt things and spices, their desire of venereal embraces becomes very great.' It made me wonder if the teenage habit of eating mountains of crisps was more deadly than realised. I read on avidly to find a warning that if these desires weren't satisfied, girls would fall victim to something called the green sickness, so it was wise to be married by 18 or so.

Apparently at the time of writing marriage was regarded by some as 'a most insupportable yoke', yet a good wife 'is the best companion in prosperity and in adversity the surest friend... How much more satisfaction a man received in the embraces of a loving wife than in the wanton dalliances of a deceitful harlot'.

The author notes with disappointment that however valuable virginity is, young people 'care not how soon they are honestly rid of it.' The section on virginity concluded with an interesting story of a courtesan who convinced clients that she was still a virgin with the aid of a bath of comfrey roots. The herb's astringent properties apparently made her most valuable assets as good as new again. Years later I wonder if comfrey roots might also work as a face-lift, but I don't think I'll risk it.

The advice on how to get pregnant is offered 'with that caution, as not to give offence to the chastest ear', and the humour which the reader has now come to expect. We are advised to get into the mood by enjoying looking at each other's bodies, but 'if there is anything like imperfection (for nature is not alike bountiful to all) be covered with a veil of darkness and oblivion.' And men are advised not to waste seed as 'Women are better pleased in having a thing once done well than often ill done.' Well, quite.

Grandma's gynaecology (2)

Pam Connellan

Advice on pregnancy from my grandmother's book, '*The Works of Aristotle*', published in 1808, is a little strange (to say the least!) but absolutely fascinating.

To couples wishing to conceive promptly, Aristotle suggests 'Let care and business be banished from thoughts, and afterwards leave the woman to her repose with all calmness possible. Coughing and sneezing should be avoided.' Those who didn't have any success with this method were advised to eat partridges, quails and sparrows, because apparently these are birds 'addicted to lechery'! Women are advised to avoid having sex too often because 'the grass seldom grows in a path commonly trodden'.

If all has gone well, there are signs of conception to look out for. The veins under a woman's eye might be swollen, she may have stomach cramps and changes in her breasts, or, more alarmingly, 'sour belchings'. A sure-fire test is to store her urine in a glass bottle for three days, then strain it through linen; if she is pregnant there will be 'small living creatures' in it. An alternative approach is to take a nettle, put this in her urine and examine it next day to see if it has red spots on it.

It was believed that for the first ten days there would be no change in the womb, but in the next six days a round lumpy matter would be formed. Two days later, the heart, brain and liver of the fetus would be formed, and in the next seven days the other limbs would develop. How physicians concluded this so precisely is not explained! Forty days after conception it was believed God would give the child the true breath of life and a living soul.

For parents keen to know the sex of their child some guidelines are offered which are similar to today's folklore. If the woman has a higher and more rounded stomach she will be carrying a girl, and if the baby is felt more on the right hand side, it will be a boy. To double check, in late pregnancy a drop of breast milk can be dropped in water: the milk will sink in a drop to the bottom if a girl is to be expected while it will spread out and stay on the top of the water if the baby is a boy.

Once pregnant, a woman should avoid marshy ground so as not to be infected with fogs. I thought the warning to 'avoid as poisonous anything which causes and creates wind' must be sensible in any day and age.

When pregnant, the woman should have infrequent sex in the first four months, none in months five and six in case of miscarriage, and lots of sex in the last six weeks as this will facilitate the birth. To avoid stretch marks, 'take the caul of a kid and a sow, add chicken and goose grease, the marrow of a red deer and rose water' to make an ointment. The author adds helpfully that if these ingredients are not readily available, dog's grease, whale oil and almond oil will do just as well. And, quite sensibly, pregnant women are told to avoid loud ringing of bells and 'the discharging of great guns'.

The role of midwife is seen as one of paramount importance. 'It is indeed the most necessary and honourable office, being indeed a helper of Nature.' Women are advised to 'Choose a midwife of middle age, with a lady's hand, a hawk's eye and a lion's heart. She should be sober and affable, bountiful and compassionate, and her temper cheerful and pleasant that she may better comfort her patient.' She should also have a proper fear of God and have short fingernails.

The author tells would-be midwives that they must have a thorough knowledge of the relevant anatomy but adds loftily: 'I shall avoid all unnecessary and impertinent matters with which books of this nature are for the most part too much clogged, and which are more curious than needful.'

There then follows further information about conception, how the baby grows in the womb and finally detailed, practical advice on midwifery in an era where there were no monitors, no anaesthetics and little understanding of how infection or other calamities could be put right. It makes for fascinating reading and a sense of deep gratitude for all the maternity care available in the developed world.

Grandma's gynaecology (3)

Pam Connellan

Imagine if you had become a trusted local midwife in the mid-nineteenth century, in an age where there was no Milton to sterilise equipment or come to that, hardly any equipment ; 'The Experienced Midwife', part of my grandma's book, '*The Works of Aristotle*', would have been invaluable to any literate woman.

Aristotle's instructions for midwives start with advice to give a strong laxative to women at the start of their labour so there 'is more space for the dilating of the passage', then to offer light but nourishing food such as eggs and broth to keep up their strength. The breaking of the waters is not recommended: 'these waters, if the child comes presently after them, facilitate labour, so let no midwife use unnatural means to break them'. However, the author approves of the practice of anointing with hog grease to soothe and help with delivery. A linen cloth 'in many folds' should be placed under the woman so that blood and waters can be covered up by opening folds, thus making everything fresh and pleasant. The woman's feet should be pressed against a log, and another two women should be enlisted to hold her shoulders. More grease, preferably fresh butter, is recommended to help delivery.

Being upright and moving about as much as possible is suggested for speeding up labour. I had thought these ideas only spread in modern times, but my grandmother, hearing my revolutionary plans for giving birth in a squatting position, had been unimpressed. She had delivered her three at home, standing with her back cosily warmed by the bedroom fire to ease the discomfort. Her midwife had urged her to keep walking up and down and had urged her back onto her feet when she had wanted to give it all up as too much hard work. In my grandmother's day, books like Aristotle's Works had been invaluable and she had found the advice to keep moving had worked well.

When the head has crowned, the author says 'the woman feels herself scratched or pinched with pins and imagines the midwife hurts her'. The advice on how to actually deliver the child is careful and practical ('make sure the midwife keeps her finger ends pared') with instructions to ease the head out not in a straight pull but moving gently side to side so the shoulders can slip into place. Where feet appear to be coming first, the midwife is told to check which foot is the left and which the right, then to make doubly sure the second foot isn't that of a second child before pulling carefully. In the days when there were no scans, the possibility of twins could only be checked late in labour, and midwives are reminded several times to ensure there are no other babies waiting to be delivered. Hands were seen to be safer than crude instruments unless they were absolutely necessary. Nowhere did I find advice on the importance of cleaning these instruments.

When there are concerns that the baby is in great danger, it is suggested that linen dipped in parsley juice is placed on the neck of the womb to speed things up. And 'many children that are born seemingly dead may be brought to life if she squeeze six or seven drops of blood out of the navel string and give it the child inwardly.' If the afterbirth also proves difficult, a sneezing powder is recommended.

When the woman is safely delivered, she should be warmly wrapped in sheepskin or if not 'the skin of a hare or rabbit taken off as soon as it is killed' would do nicely. Later the woman should be bound in linen, apart from her breasts. Strong light was to be avoided for three days as her eyesight as well as that of the baby was felt to be vulnerable. The baby has to be cleaned and oiled, then swaddled with arms and legs bound in straight lines. The midwife is warned not to bind the stomach tightly so the poor mite can actually breathe and suckle. In case we might feel this swaddling is unnecessary, the author tells us 'it is to give its body a straight figure, which is most decent and proper for man'.

Power to the woman

Virginia Howes

Having waited for it for two weeks, when the telephone rang at 3am I knew exactly who it was. Alison told me that her contractions were coming every five minutes. 'Never trust a multip', I heard ringing in my ears, and so with a quick call to my partner Kay, who was to act as second midwife, I was on my way to my first independent homebirth.

Alison had booked me when she was sixteen weeks pregnant. When I visited her she was contemplating an elective caesarean section, as the birth of her first baby, James, six years previously, had been very traumatic. She had felt totally out of control, was not able to facilitate any of her choices regarding place to labour, pain control or position for birth, and had sustained a third degree tear from an extended episiotomy. She had suffered slight incontinence, postnatal depression and a fierce unnatural possessiveness over James that almost destroyed her marriage.

Throughout the pregnancy we discussed what had happened at that time, and read the research evidence pertaining to the events and actions that may have contributed to the previous poor birth experience. Gradually Alison's confidence grew, and she became a blooming, excited, empowered woman! She decided a homebirth was what she wanted and I began to get as excited as she was.

Waiting

When I arrived at her house Alison appeared to be contracting strong and regular. We had discussed vaginal examinations and Alison wanted to avoid them if possible. I saw no reason not to respect her wishes. Baby was in a perfect position for birth, everything was normal, and so we awaited events... and waited...

Alison took a bath, walked about, took her homeopathic remedies. The sun rose, but baby William did not put in an appearance. However, he was a healthy boy with a strong variable heart rate and so we waited some more.

At 9am Alison decided that she now wanted a vaginal examination. I found her to be 8cms dilated with bulging membranes and the baby's head at mid cavity. I could not define the position due to the bulging membranes but on palpation baby was direct OA, deeply engaged and so an excellent finding. We now knew it would not be much longer...

By mid-day I was beginning to wonder if we would ever see this baby. I suggested an examination. Alison was now 9cm dilated with the baby still the same distance away. Kay and I were in agreement that although taking its time, everything was OK.

At 3pm, with an ear-shattering scream, Alison ruptured her membranes. She began to make familiar grunting noises a few minutes later. We expected to see the baby's head very soon, but Alison had not followed any 'averages' so far, so I suppose we were wrong to expect her to start now. Alison was in second stage for three hours. This was the part of her labour that Alison had feared. Kay and I felt that psychologically she was not letting go, due to her fear of tearing. This theory was reinforced at a recent conference (Childbirth at a Turning Point, 11.11.2000) at which Michel Odent explained the inhibiting effects of fear on the production of oxytocin. Alison was using the intellectual part of her brain rather than letting the primitive part take control, which promotes the release of oxytocin. She needed love and reassurance to encourage confidence in her body.

At 06.10 William was finally born, pink, lusty and in perfect condition. His arm and elbow were up around his neck which may have contributed to his slow arrival. Alison did not sustain any perineal damage and to her that was an achievement like reaching the peak of Mount Everest.

Alison and Andrew both feel that William's birth has gone a long way to healing the emotional trauma and strain that their love and marriage only just endured after the awful time surrounding James' birth.

Furthermore Alison is convinced that had she had William in hospital she would have had interventions to speed up the process in the first stage and maybe even an assisted delivery in the second given the unusual amount of time it took.

How sad to think she may be right.

A word about language

Say what you mean – mean what you say!

Jane Bowler

As an Editor, I think my role is to help midwives to share their experiences and to learn from each other. You could call me a 'facilitator'. Sometimes I feel more like an archaeologist, gently brushing away confusing phrases and general muddiness to reveal the stark beauty of a simple point, well made.

Every article that has been published in *The Practising Midwife* since January 1999 has been through my hands, and I've read every word. Recently, I've noticed reports getting wordier, lists of references getting longer, trains of thought and argument becoming more difficult to follow. Simple and brilliant conclusions are getting buried in management-speak.

Management-speak

Management-speak is contagious, and in some offices it really is possible to play 'buzzword bingo' during meetings. Watch out, midwives, it is coming soon to an office near you. The language of industry is seeping into the NHS, and midwives are starting to pick it up. Based on recent articles, I would suggest top contenders to appear on an NHS bingo card would include empowerment, clients, transaction, paradigm, synergies, mission, vision, and quality. If you hear all of these during one meeting, you win the game, but you probably won't feel like celebrating!

The trust and moral commitment between a midwife and a mother are implicit and unique. For some reason this gentle, feminine, intuitive bond is gradually being forced into the rigid and brisk vocabulary of business. The care given by midwives is now a 'transaction' between a healthcare professional and a client. Language like this is self-perpetuating. In a chapter entitled 'Total Quality Management for Physicians: Translating the new paradigm', in an American book called *The Textbook of Total Quality in Healthcare*, Merry[1] suggests that healthcare practitioners who fail to respond positively to the introduction of 'industrial quality processes into healthcare' are exhibiting 'failure' to achieve 'self-actualization' and that such clinicians are 'in denial'.

Sometimes trying to characterise the world of healthcare by using terms which are fashionable in the world of business and coporate management gives rise to buzzwords that are really quite meaningless. A new book, *Ethics, Management and Mythology* by Michael Loughlin,[2] gives as an example the concept of 'health gains', a term which was apparently popular in the NHS in the early 1990s. It was 'heralded as a massive advance in thinking about healthcare management'.

The basic idea was that identifying and comparing the health gains that could be made from two different approaches to a healthcare problem would enable managers to make decisions relating to healthcare funding, prioritising and (indirectly) the rationing of the limited services and equipment available. Yet in the same articles that praised and supported this revolutionary new concept...

'authors admitted that they could not say what 'health gains' were and that no known method existed to define or measure them. 'Research' into the concept typically took the form of highly paid administrators writing to their colleagues in other parts of the country asking them what they felt the term 'meant to them' and collating any responses received.

Unsurprisingly, answers received usually made reference to the idea that 'producing health gains' had something to do with making people healthier, although it also had a lot to do with 'empowering' people, 'developing' them, and so forth... it will come as no great shock to the reader that the activity of translating the language of 'making people healthier' into talk of 'producing health gains' did not, in fact, produce any 'measurable benefits' to the 'consumers' of healthcare.'

What is quality?

Like 'health gains', quality is a concept that has proved

extremely difficult to define. Everybody wants quality of care, and generally we know it when we see it, but try writing down exactly what it is and you'll end up with an over-complicated and over-generalised framework that isn't much use to anybody.

'We live in an age obsessed with the production of regulatory frameworks, sets of guidelines, codes of practice and the like. On the basis of little or no evidence it is declared that spending massive amounts of money on producing such frameworks, and then checking that everyone is following them (requiring the constant monitoring of people's behaviour) is the best way to improve practices in healthcare, education and elsewhere.'[2]

You know that women want the freedom to choose the positions in which they labour and give birth. You know that birthing places should be comfortable and friendly. You know that women need to be given facts so that they can make decisions. How many questionnaires do you need to send out? Do we really need to put our time and effort into devising sets of rules and guidelines that basically tell us to use our common sense?

It is instructive to look at why the concept of 'quality' and by extension, Total Quality Management (TQM) has taken on a life of its own in the world of industry. With greater automation of production processes, formerly highly-regarded skilled workers were relegated to carrying out short repetitive tasks as part of a larger production line – each worker was reduced to being a cog in a machine. Workers had once felt involved with their product, and proud of it. Once the sense of ownership was gone, the inclination to care about producing 'quality' work was next to go. Quality control, quality assurance and eventually Total Quality Management evolved to 'replace the individual's engagement with the work that mass production had destroyed.'[2]

Genuine empowerment

The management-speak that is creeping into midwifery may be a sign of the splitting of the profession. Midwifery management assumes the top level of the heirarchy. It devotes its time to the development of guidelines, the analysis of questionnaires, and the formulation of rules to govern the work of the midwives who are working at the 'coalface'. It is anxious to see midwives taken seriously and regarded as equals by other 'managers'. Meanwhile, perhaps practising midwives, like the skilled workers mentioned above, are in danger of becoming de-skilled and subject to rigid doctrines which are designed to prevent them from making mistakes in their work, but also effectively stop them from thinking twice about their practice.

As the government has suggested that midwives should play a wider role in community health, now may be the ideal moment to become aware of the blinkers that can limit our perceptions of the world. It is sometimes hard to look beyond the daily demands of the work we do and see the bigger picture. Louglin[2] offers an example which should set us all thinking:

'The position is like that of a battlefield doctor who continues to patch up the bodies brought in, but who never questions why the war is going on or whether it should be being fought at all, because that's not his job: such questions are the concern of the generals. How 'responsible' this stance is is surely a matter for debate.'

Reflective practice is in danger of becoming a meaningless buzzword. It deserves to be salvaged. It is vital to lift one's eyes from the work in progress from time to time, and to remember why one chose to take the work on. Midwives can only provide informed care of women if they take the time to develop an understanding of the circumstances in which the women in their care are living. Continuing education is in vogue for midwives, but perhaps our ideas of what constitutes relevant training need to be broadened.

'We should not aim to supply a new set of 'answers' but instead we should strive to enable people to find good answers for themselves... We must abandon the search for formulae to determine what is right or good, in exchange for investigating methods of intellectual and moral training that will equip individuals to think well and live well, despite all the barriers they are likely to encounter in the diverse situations they must face.'[2]

'We do not need sets of principles for doctors, nurses and managers: we need reflective people able to analyse problems, aware of their limitations and able to distinguish sense from nonsense.'[2]

REFERENCES

1 Merry M. Total Quality Management for Physicians: Translating the new paradigm. In: Al-Asaf AF & Schmele JA (Eds). The Textbook of Total Quality in Healthcare. Delray Beach, Florida: St Lucie Press, 1993.

2 Loughlin, M. Ethics, Management and Mythology. Manchester: Hochland & Hochland Ltd. (In Press).

Index

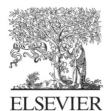

ELSEVIER

 Books *for* **Midwives**

  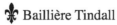

CHURCHILL LIVINGSTONE   Mosby   THE PRACTISING MIDWIFE   Baillière Tindall

MIDWIFERY PUBLISHERS OF CHOICE FOR GENERATIONS

For many years and through several identities we have catered for professional needs in midwifery education and practice. Leading publishers of major textbooks such as *Myles Textbook for Midwives* and *Mayes' Midwifery: a Textbook for Midwives*, our expertise spreads across both books and journals to offer a comprehensive resource for midwives at all stages of their careers.

Find out how we can provide you with the right book at the right time by exploring our website, **www.elsevierhealth.com/midwifery** or requesting a midwifery catalogue from Health Professions Marketing, Elsevier, 32 Jamestown Road, Camden, London, NW1 7BY, UK Tel: 020 7424 4200; Fax: 020 7424 4420.

We are always keen to expand our midwifery list so if you have an idea for a new book please contact Mary Seager, Senior Commissioning Editor at Elsevier, The Boulevard, Langford Lane, Kidlington, Oxford, OX5 1GB, UK (m.seager@elsevier.com).

 Have you joined yet?
Sign up for e-Alert to get the latest news and information.

Register for eAlert at www.elsevierhealth.com/eAlert Information direct to your Inbox

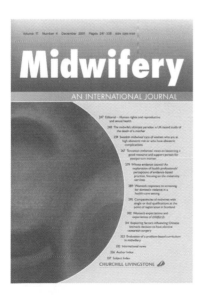

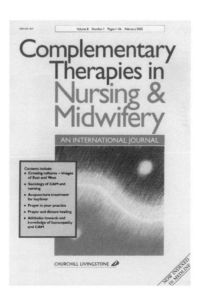

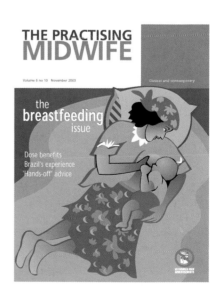